CARDIAC LEFT VENTRICULAR HYPERTROPHY

DEVELOPMENTS IN CARDIOVASCULAR MEDICINE

CARDIAC LEFT VENTRICULAR HYPERTROPHY

edited by

H.E.D.J. TER KEURS
J.J. SCHIPPERHEYN

Department of Cardiology
Leiden University Hospital
Leiden, The Netherlands

1983 **MARTINUS NIJHOFF PUBLISHERS**
a member of the KLUWER ACADEMIC PUBLISHERS GROUP
BOSTON / THE HAGUE / DORDRECHT / LANCASTER
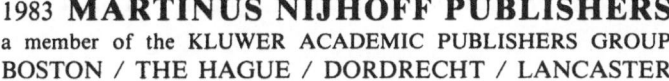

This publication is based upon a Boerhaave course, organized by the Faculty of Medicine, University of Leiden.

Distributors

for the United States and Canada: Kluwer Boston, Inc., 190 Old Derby Street, Hingham, MA 02043, USA
for all other countries: Kluwer Academic Publishers Group, Distribution Center, P.O.Box 322, 3300 AH Dordrecht, The Netherlands

Library of Congress Cataloging in Publication Data

```
Keurs, H. E. D. J. ter.
  Cardiac left ventricular hypertrophy.

  (Developments in cardiovascular medicine ; v. 33)
  Includes index.
  1. Heart--Hypertrophy.  I. Schipperheyn, J. J.
II. Title.  III. Series.  [DNLM: 1. Heart enlargement--
Congresses.  WG 280 C26503 1983]
RC685.H9K48 1983        616.1'2        83-19484
```

ISBN-13:978-94-009-6761-8 e-ISBN-13:978-94-009-6759-5
DOI: 10.1007/978-94-009-6759-5

CONTENTS

INTRODUCTION

Left ventricular hypertrophy (LVH) is usually considered to be a compensatory adjustment of heart muscle to an inreased work load. LVH develops in the course of valvular or congenital heart disease, or when part of the myocardium is damaged by long-standing ischemia or infarction. In the hypertrophied heart the muscle fibers increase in size, not in number. The fibers are found to contain a larger number of myofibrils and the cell organelles are larger.

From epidemiologic studies it is known that even mild LVH is associated with myocardial ischemia, ventricular arrhythmias, and sudden cardiac death. Most cases of LVH show focal degenerative tissue changes including cellular atrophy, myofibrillar disorganization, interstitial fibrosis, and loss of intracellular connections. Myocardial dysfunction develops and, unlike the functional adaptive changes found in pure hypertrophy, is not reversible by surgical treatment of the valvular heart disease or medical correction of hypertension. Interstitial fibrosis, intracellular changes of muscle cells, and loss of contractile tissue lead to poor mechanical function and undoubtedly increase the risk of ischemia, arrhythmias, or sudden death, a well-recognized problem in patients with a variety of heart diseases. Even when successfully treated, the patients may remain at risk if the compensatory hypertrophy is not fully reversed.

Epidemiologic studies conducted in the Framingham population in the early 1950's demonstrated LVH according to electrocardiographic criteria in 1.5% of the population; 2% of the population had LVH according to chest X-ray criteria. Recently, a study in second-generation offspring of the original cohort, now at the same age as the original cohort in the early 1950's, showed a decline to 0.2% and 1% respectively. In the recent study, echocardiography was used in addition to electrocardiography and chest X-ray to detect LVH. In the offspring population, 6% had LVH and of the original cohort 22% now had LVH according to echocardiographic criteria. Echocardiography is far more sensitive in detecting LVH than ECG or chest X-ray.

LVH with typical electrocardiographic changes carries an unfavorable prognosis It is found in 45% of all cardiovascular deaths and five-year mortality rates are more than doubled. The prognostic significance of LVH according to echocardiographic criteria cannot be assessed as yet. However, a strong association of LVH on the echocardiogram and ventricular dysrhythmias has already emerged.

These findings suggest that the mortality and morbidity associated with hypertension, valvular heart disease and, to some extent, also with coronary artery disease result largely from the ventricular hypertrophy that accompanies the disease.

At the moment, echocardiography seems to be the best technique available for the detection of LVH. The accuracy of estimation of LV mass with echocardiography has been proven, even in common clinical practice. This technique has been used by a number of investigators to further study the relationship between LVH and hypertension. Results of the Framingham study showed that only a fraction of the population with hypertension develops LVH. Studies by Devereux showed that 25-45% of the population develop LVH due to hypertension, but the majority of the hypertensives do not develop LVH. Other factors including age, sex and hormonal factors play a modulating role, and the mode of therapy with which control of blood pressure is achieved is important with regard to the rate of growth of the heart muscle. Moreover, correlation between LV mass and blood pressure was strongest when blood pressure was measured during active daily life. Blood pressure at rest did not have such a significance for the development of LVH.

The importance of modulating factors for the development of LVH has also been studied by Messerli. Apart from the factors already mentioned, he stresses the importance of volume load as an additional hypertrophogenic factor. Volume load arises from pregnancy, anemia but most commonly from obesity. Hormonal factors, including adrenergic agents, and probably also the renin-angiotensin system, are important as well. Hereditary factors play a role, and particularly the black population seems to be more prone to LVH than whites.

Protein synthesis in hypertrophy is supposedly induced by calcium and cyclic AMP-dependent gene expression. Such a general pathway for the development of hypertrophy is proposed by Mommaerts on the basis of evidence that cAMP-dependent phosphorylation of chromatin-associated basic proteins leads to gene expression. On the analogy of the activation of phosphorylation of the metabolic control protein glycogen phosphorylase probably under control of calcium, further control of gene expression by calcium is likely. If so, a close relation between myocardial energy turnover and free calcium levels in the cell would underly the coupling between cardiac work and growth.

Subtlety of the control mechanisms is underlined by the observation that different kinds of hypertrophy are characterized by differences in excitation-contraction coupling and in contractile properties.

In a study on sarcomere mechanics of trabeculae of the hypertrophied right ventricle from hyperthyroid rat and of hypobaric hypoxia-induced right ventricular hypertrophy, Ter Keurs showed that mechanical recovery is greatly accelerated in hyperthyroidism compared to controls and to hypertrophy from hypobaric hypoxia. Force-sarcomere length relations appeared unaffected, in contrast to an increased maximal velocity of sarcomere shortening in hyperthyroidism compared to controls and a decreased maximal velocity of sarcomere shortening in hypertrophy following hypobaric hypoxia.

A particular aspect of the development of LVH as a result of hypertension may be an impairment of ventricular inotropic responsiveness. Tarazi showed that hypertrophy leads to decreased adrenergic responsiveness with lowered myocardial -adrenergic receptor density. The hypertrophied heart may therefore become more dependent on the Frank-Starling mechanism to meet stress rather than on cardio-adrenergic support. Under these conditions, progressive dilatation may develop, leading to further increase in ventricular stress and progressive deterioration.

From studies on pump function of the heart and matching of the heart with the arterial system it appears that both right ventricle and left ventricle are operating at optimum work output. Elzinga shows that the rate of energy turnover of the heart is not minimal at optimum work output.

A possible mechanism for adaptation of cardiac pump function to the demands of flow and pressure by the circulatory system could be that the heart seeks to work at the optimum of the work output where total energy turnover and calcium turnover? (cf. Mommaerts, ed.) are smallest.

Recent non-invasive studies allow assessment of the function of the hypertrophied ventricle. They revealed an inverse relation between end-systolic stress and overall cardiac performance.

In addition, Fouad found that left ventricular filling rate was reduced in hypertensive patients, even though their cardiac output, ejection fraction, and maximum rate of ejection were still normal. The reduction in filling rate correlated significantly with the echocardiographically determined LV mass. Initial observations on LV dynamics following reversal of hypertrophy suggest that cardiac performance then falls within normal limits again.

The morbidity and mortality associated with LVH arise mainly from myocardial ischemia, which seems to be an inevitable complication of LVH even if the coronary arteries are normal. It has been recognized quite early that myocardial perfusion is compromised in practically all cases of LVH, i.e. the ratio of maximal flow after full vasodilation and normal autoregulated flow is reduced. The cause of this reduction of coronary flow reserve is apparently the failure of the capillaries to increase their number in proportion to the increasing size of the cross-sectional area of muscle mass. Minimal vascular resistance calculated per unit mass therefore increases with increasing mass. Additional factors may play a role in LVH which either raise minimal resistance even further, or increase resting flow. Hoffman points out that high blood viscosity found in congenital heart disease reduces maximal flow while other commonly associated factors, such as anemia, anoxia and tachycardia, increase resting flow in the hypertrophic myocardium. Both reduction of maximal flow and increased resting flow lead to further reduction of flow reserve in the hypertrophied heart. Spaan stresses the importance of intramyocardial pressure for coronary pressure and flow. In hypertrophy caused by aortic valvular stenosis, minimal coronary resistance is higher than in hypertrophy caused by hypertension because intramyocardial vessels in the former case are compressed by the high intramyocardial pressure which is not balanced by a high intravascular pressure. Hypertension, however, tends to increase flow reserve because maximal flow increases more steeply with aortic pressure than does resting flow.

Schipperheyn shows that minimal coronary resistance, intercapillary distance or coronary resistance in the isolated heart indeed increases proportionally to LV mass, as follows from the no-growth rule for capillaries. Only a few exceptions have been described, including cases of congenital hypertrophy. He demonstrates that at high perfusion pressure vasodilation causes formation of edema, which also compresses intramyocardial vessels and further reduces maximal flow, and thus reduces flow reserve.

Many diagnostic tools have been used and developed in the detection of left ventricular hypertrophy. Detection of LVH on the basis of the electrocardiogram is characterized by poor sensitivity and acceptable specificity. This applies both to simple and to elaborate scoring systems for the electrocardiogram.
Kulbertus shows that application of the solid-angle theory of electrocardiography predicts LVH which only appears on the surface electrocardiogram as a result of a critical interplay between wall thickness and chamber dilatation. He furthermore shows the importance of intraventricular conduction defects in the appearance of LVH.
If electrical LVH is present, it should be considered a sign of guarded prognosis.
Development of radionuclide angiography allows assessment of global and regional performance of both right and left ventricles.
Beller emphasizes the importance of application of this technique in studies at rest and during exercise, _e.g._ in evaluation of cardiac function in asymptomatic patients with aortic regurgitation. Diastolic dysfunction appears particularly affected in patients with hypertrophic cardiomyopathy. Tl^{201} scanning allows assessment of regional, _e.g._ right ventricular or septal, hypertrophy.

The recent development of nuclear magnetic resonance (NMR) techniques offers a powerful, completely non-invasive method to study functional and structural properties of the heart. NMR is likely to become the most sensitive approach to quantitate LVH and RVH in the future.

LVH is known to be reversible. This is clearly demonstrated by Drost in patients with severe LVH caused by aortic valvular stenosis. Successful replacement of the stenotic valve leads to almost complete regression of LVH, as follows from electrocardiographic and echocardiographic measurements. Regression can be demonstrated up to 18 months after operation, but appears to be almost completed after six months.

Similar findings are reported by Voogd, who found significant regression of LVH in patients on chronic hemodialysis after correction of volume overload. As discussed by Drayer, LVH related to hypertension can be reversed by medical treatment of the high blood pressure. Reduction of muscle mass is related to the degree of control of blood pressure but reversal of LVH is not always achieved despite successful lowering of pressure. Additional factors play a role, and the type of antihypertensive drug is important. Drugs that reduce sympathetic tone, and probably also converting-enzyme inhibitors and calcium antagonists, induce regression of LVH, while diuretics and vasodilating agents fail to do so.

The hypertrophied ventricle is highly susceptible to ischemic damage. This is due in part to the increased vascular resistance and also to the high oxygen demand of the enlarged heart. The high risk of ischemic damage is especially important for the surgical treatment of valvular heart disease. Van der Laarse shows that after aortic valve replacement in hearts that are usually severely hypertrophic, ischemic damage is commoner and more extensive than after operations on normal hearts. Even continuous selective perfusion of the coronary arteries does not guarantee complete protection of the myocardium from ischemia. Modern techniques employing intermittent cold saline cardioplegia or continuous low-flow cardioplegia with cold saline solution provide excellent protection of the myocardium despite extensive LVH. These procedures have reduced the risk of aortic valve replacement to acceptably low levels.

ACKNOWLEDGMENT

Staff members of MERCK SHARP & DOHME, Holland, suggested to us to organize a post-graduate course on left ventricular hypertrophy, because they recognized the crucial role of myocardial cell growth in the pathogenesis of several heart diseases and hypertension. MERCK SHARP & DOHME made it possible to invite a number of scientists from the United States and European countries to come to Leiden to present their views on the subject. The company's hospitality created an atmosphere that stimulated a fruitful exchange of ideas and new experimental data. For this the editors are truly thankful.

The editors also wish to express their appreciation to MERCK SHARP & DOHME for their support and most efficient help with the preparation of this book.

H.E.D.J. ter Keurs

J.J. Schipperheyn

LIST OF CONTRIBUTORS

- Prof. Dr. G. Beller, University of Virginia Medical Center, Medicine & Pediatrics, Division of Cardiology, Charlottesville, Virginia 22908, U.S.A.

- Prof. Dr. R. Devereux, Box 222, New York Hospital, Cornell Medical Center, 525 East 68th Street, New York, NY 10021, U.S.A.

- Prof. Dr. J.I.M. Drayer, Hypertension Center, W 130, Veterans Administration Medical Center, 5901 East Seventh Street, Long Beach, CA 90822, U.S.A.

- Dr. H. Drost, Department of Cardiology, Leiden University Hospital, Rijnsburgerweg 10, 2333 AA Leiden, The Netherlands

- Prof. Dr. G. Elzinga, Free University, Laboratory for Physiology, Van der Boechorststraat 7, 1081 BT Amsterdam, The Netherlands

- Prof. Dr. F.M. Fouad, Cleveland Clinic Foundation, 9500 Euclid Avenue, Cleveland, OH 44106, U.S.A.

- Prof. Dr. J.I.E. Hoffman, University of California, 1403 H.S.E., San Francisco, CA 94143, U.S.A.

- Dr. H.E.D.J. ter Keurs, Department of Cardiology, Leiden University Hospital, Rijnsburgerweg 10, 2333 AA Leiden, The Netherlands

- Prof. Dr. H. Kulbertus, Hôpital Universitaire Bavière, Institut de Médecine, Dépt. de Clinique et de la Séméiologie Médicales, 66, Bd. de la Constitution, B-4020 Liège, Belgium

- Dr. A. van der Laarse, Department of Cardiobiochemistry, Leiden University Hospital, Rijnsburgerweg 10, 2333 AA Leiden, The Netherlands

- Prof. Dr. F.H. Messerli, Alton Ochsner Medical Foundation, 1516, Jefferson Highway, New Orleans, LA 70121, U.S.A.

- Prof. Dr. W. Mommaerts, Department of Physiology, University of California, 10833 Le Conte Avenue, Los Angeles, CA 90024, U.S.A.

- Prof. Dr. D.D. Savage, Non-Invasive Laboratories, Framingham Heart Study, 118, Lincoln Street, Framingham, MA 01701, U.S.A.

- Dr. J.J. Schipperheyn, Department of Cardiology, Leiden University Hospital, Rijnsburgerweg 10, 2333 AA Leiden, The Netherlands

- Dr. Ir. J.A.E. Spaan, Department of Physiology and Physiological Physics, Leiden University, Wassenaarseweg 62, 2333 AL Leiden, The Netherlands

- Prof. Dr. R.C. Tarazi, Research Division, Cleveland Clinic Foundation, 9500 Euclid Avenue, Cleveland, OH 44106, U.S.A.

- Dr. P.J. Voogd, Department of Cardiology, Leiden University Hospital, Rijnsburgerweg 10, 2333 AA Leiden, The Netherlands

SECTION 1

PREVALENCE AND RISKS OF LEFT VENTRICULAR HYPERTROPHY

2

SUMMARY

Prospective epidemiological studies in Framingham have helped us gain
insight into the prevalence, incidence, pathogenesis, and prognostic
importance of LVH. Highlights of previous Framingham reports regarding
LVH based on ECG's and chest X-rays are reviewed. More recent data for
which M-mode echocardiography has been used, are presented. Data are
based upon an uninterrupted prospective follow-up of 5,209 subjects
selected in the early 1950's. Information on a second generation including 5,134 offspring of the original cohort and offspring spouses was
added in 1971.

Definite ECG-LVH was found in 1.5% of the original Framingham cohort
during the examination in the early 1950's. The prevalence in the offspring-spouse group at their second examination was roughly 0.2%, which
gives some insight into the order of magnitude of the decline of ECG-LVH.
The prevalence of LVH on chest X-ray in the early 1950's was about 2%; it
declined to less than 1% among the offspring subjects when they were
about the same age as the original cohort in the early 1950's.

In the 1979-1982 study, echo-LVH was found in 6% of the offspring study
subjects and in 22% of the older original cohort subjects. The prevalence
was similar in men and women when sex-specific reference values were
used. Eccentric and unclassified LVH were the most common form, septal
hypertrophy was relatively rare. The prevalence and incidence of LVH were
strongly associated with age and level of blood pressure over a period of
time.

ECG-LVH is a lethal marker. Forty-five percent of all cardiovascular
deaths have been preceded by ECG-LVH. Five-year mortality rates for men
and women with ECG-LVH are 35% and 20% respectively, compared to 15% and
10% or less in subjects without ECG-LVH. Risk of cardiac morbidity is
also markedly increased in those with ECG-LVH. Follow-up since the echo
studies has been too brief to assess the prognostic significance of
echo-LVH. However, a strong association of echo-LVH with ventricular
dysrhythmias has already emerged, particularly in subjects over age 40.
The association was independent of blood pressure, ECG-LVH and functional
shortening, an index of systolic function. This suggests that much of the
echo-LVH detected in apparently healthy subjects in the general population may be pathologic, especially in those over age 40.

EPIDEMIOLOGIC FEATURES OF LEFT VENTRICULAR HYPERTROPHY IN NORMOTENSIVE
AND HYPERTENSIVE SUBJECTS

SAVAGE, D.D.[1], ABBOTT, R.D.[2], PADGETT, S.[3], ANDERSON, S.J.[4], GARRISON, R.J.[2]

1. Lecturer Harvard Medical School, Clinic Director and Chief, Noninvasive Laboratories, Framingham Heart Study, NHLBI, NIH
2. Biometrics Research Branch and Epidemiology and Biometry Program, NHLBI, NIH
3. Epidemiology and Biometry Program, NHLBI, NIH
4. Evans Research Foundation, Boston University School of Medicine

INTRODUCTION

Left ventricular hypertrophy (LVH) or increased LV mass is often considered to be a compensatory response to increased hemodynamic loading and abnormal systolic and diastolic stresses at the myocardial fiber level.[1,2] Others have stressed that neurohumoral and genetic factors also may play an important role as determinants of LVH.[3-5] Despite some uncertainty regarding the relative importance of these and possibly other determinants in some settings, most would agree that LVH has important prognostic significance. Prospective epidemiologic studies have helped us gain insight into the prevalence, incidence, pathogenesis, and prognostic importance of LVH. This report reviews some highlights of previous prospective Framingham data regarding LVH based on ECGs and chest X-rays (CXR) and more recent Framingham data for which M-mode echocardiography (echo) (guided by two-dimensional echo) has been used for diagnosis.

The Framingham data are derived from uninterrupted prospective follow-up of 5209 subjects from a population-based sample selected in the early 1950's. A second generation including 5134 offspring of the original cohort and offspring spouses was added to the study group in 1971.

ECG CRITERIA

ECG criteria for definite LVH used in Framingham included an increased R and/or S wave amplitude reflecting potentials primarily from the left ventricle associated with ST-T wave axis opposite in direction to the QRS axis (the "strain" pattern of ST-T changes). By Sokolow-Lyon[6], Gubner-Ungerleides[7], Katz[8], or Romhilt-Estes[9] voltage criteria were used and included one or more of the following: R(1) + S(3) $\geq$ 25 mm; R AvL > 11 mm; single precordial deflections $\geq$ 25 mm ($\geq$ 30 mm in more than one third of those with ECG-LVH); S V1 + R V5 $\geq$ 35 mm; R or S $\geq$ 20 mm in AVF (10 mm = 1 mV).[10] Possible ECG-LVH was considered present if a voltage criterion was present with only minimal T wave changes (relative flattening without the strain pattern).

CXR CRITERIA

CXR criteria for LVH were based on a radiologist's qualitative reading of cardiac enlargement (cardio-thoracic ratio $\geq$ 0.5) and/or left ventricular hypertrophy (a prominent "left ventricular contour").

ECHO CRITERIA

Echocardiographic criteria for LVH have been derived recently in Framingham because of inadequacies of published criteria including:
- their being based on relatively small numbers of subjects; thus being less generalizable;
- their lack of adequate adjustment for the effects of sex, body size (men and women) and age (women); thus giving faulty estimates of LVH prevalence in various sex-age groups;
- their lack of adjustment for the increased variance in the LVH mass as body size increases (among apparently healthy non-obese subjects); thus over-estimating LVH prevalence in large (but non-obese) subjects.

For our criteria we used 1221 apparently healthy subjects from our large free-living population-based sample of about 5000 subjects with adequate echos. The 1221 subjects included subjects with no overt evidence of cardio-pulmonary disease or major systemic illness by history, physical, echo, ECG, or (for most subjects) recent chest X-ray evaluation. Subjects were excluded if their blood pressures exceeded 139/89, if they were taking antihypertensive medications, or if they were obese (weight exceeding the recommended upper limit for height in the 1959 Metropolitan Life Insurance Company table).[14]
Interventricular septal (IVSTd) and LV posterior wall (LVPWTd) thick-

ness in diastole and LV internal dimension (LVIDd) were measured using American Society of Echocardiography recommendations.[15] For dispropor- tionate septal LVH, National Institutes of Health measurement criteria were used.[16] LV mass was calculated using the formula LV mass = 1.05 [(LVIDd + IVSTd + LVPWTd)cubed - (LVIDd)cubed].[17] It was found that body weight (combined with age for women) could be used to predict the echo LV mass for normal subjects (PNLVM) using these equations: for men, PNLVM in grams = 43.62 + 2.18 weight in kg; for women, PNLVM = 44.71 + 1.46 weight + 0.27 age.

Subjects were considered to have echo-LVH if their LV mass exceeded the upper 95% confidence limit calculated as follows: upper 95% confidence limit = PNLVM + 1.96 (standard deviation of LV mass of normal subjects as a function of weight). The relation of LV wall thickness to LV internal radius [relative wall thickness = RWT = (LVPWTd) / (1/2 LVIDd)] was calculated.

Four types of echo-LVH were defined as follows:
- Disproportionate septal LVH: echo-LVH with IVSTd/LVPWTd $\geq$ 1.3;
- Concentric LVH: echo-LVH with RWT $\geq$ 45% without disproportionate septal LVH;
- Eccentric LVH: echo-LVH with RWT < 45%, LVIDd > upper confidence limits and without disproportionate septal LVH;
- Unclassified LVH: echo-LVH in the absence of criteria for other types of LVH.

PREVALENCE AND INCIDENCE OF LVH

Prevalence = incidence of LVH by ECG

Definite ECG-LVH was found in 76 (1.5%) of the 5209 original Framingham cohort (mean age 46 years, range 30-62) during the initial examination in the early 1950's.[10] Prevalence in men and women were similar.

A similar prevalence of possible ECG-LVH was found. The prevalence of definite ECG-LVH in the offspring-spouse group (mean age 44, range 17-77) at their second examination (1979-1982) was roughly 0.2%.[18] These data

give some insight into the order of magnitude of the decline in prevalence of ECG-LVH. This has been concurrent with the emergence of pharmacologic antihypertensive therapy. However, the prevalence should be
viewed only as order of magnitude figures, since the two population
samples are not ideal statistical probability samples and could reflect
some selective bias. In addition, their age compositions, although
similar, are not identical. The increase in prevalence of ECG-LVH with
age in Framingham subjects in both sexes is shown in figures 1 and 2.

As indicated by Kannel, the development of ECG-LVH occurs at a rate
greater than suggested by the prevalence data because of the high associated mortality and the fact that the ECG finding does not necessarily
persist.[10] About 3% of the original Framingham cohort who did not have
definite ECG-LVH at the initial examination, developed it on at least one
of six successive biennial examinations.[10] Another 4.5% without ECG-LVH
at entry developed possible ECG-LVH during this time. Thus, about 10% of
the Framingham subjects had or developed ECG-LVH in the first 12 years of
follow-up.[10] Subjects with possible LVH on the first examination had a
20-fold greater probability of developing definite ECG-LVH on the next
biennial examination compared to subjects who initially had no evidence
of ECG-LVH.[10]

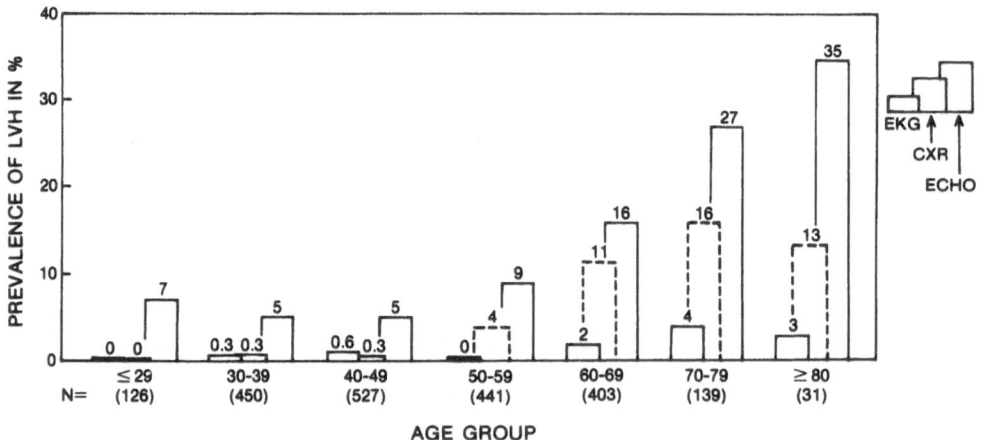

Figure 1. Prevalence of LVH in Framingham males by ECG, CXR, and echo.
Prevalences should be viewed only as order of magnitude since the population samples are not ideal probability samples. Dashed lined bars represent chest X-rays performed two years prior to echo. N's for chest X-rays
and ECG's = 1675 and 1582, respectively.

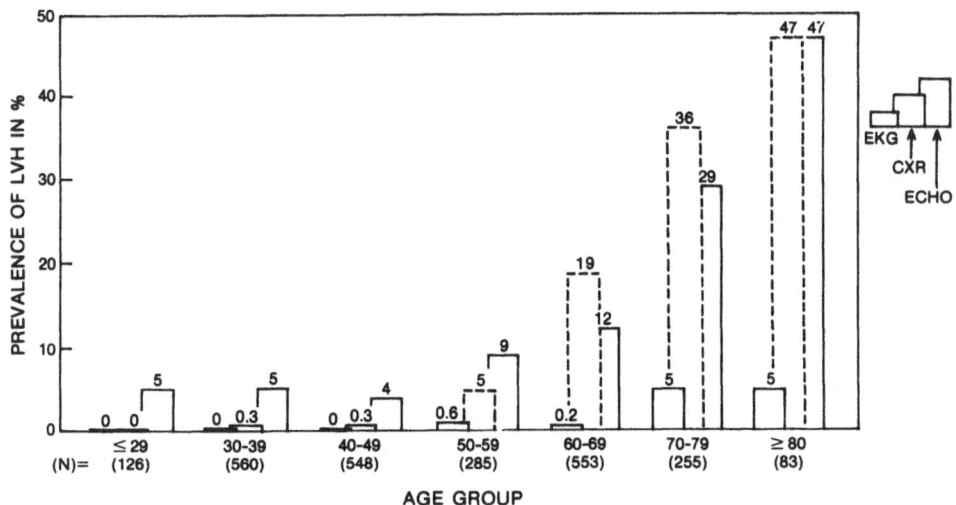

Figure 2. Prevalence of LVH in Framingham females by ECG, CXR, and echo
Dashed lined bars represent chest X-rays performed two years prior to echo. N's for chest X-rays and ECGs = 2082 and 2061, respectively.

Prevalence of LVH by CXR

The prevalence of CXR-LVH in the original Framingham cohort at the initial examination in the early 1950's was about 2%. The prevalence in the survivors 28 years later was roughly 22%. CXR-LVH was found in less than 1% of the offspring study subjects (1979-1982) when they were about the same age as the original cohort in the early 1950's (figures 1 and 2).

Prevalence of LVH by echo

Echo-LVH was found in 514 (10%) of 4972 Framingham subjects. The prevalence of echo-LVH ranged from about 6% in those under age 50 years to up to 33% (men) to 50% (women) in those 80 years and older (table 1, figures 1 and 2). Echo-LVH was found in 220 (6%) of the 3605 offspring study subjects and in 294 (22%) of the 1367 original cohort subjects (when Framingham reference values were used). The prevalence estimates for echo-LVH in the offspring study subjects and the older cohort were 9% and 16% respectively, when published reference values were used.[18]

The prevalence of echo-LVH was similar in men and women when Framingham sex-specific reference values were used for comparison. This was in contrast to the apparent over-estimate (men) and under-estimate (women) of echo-LVH when published (non-sex specific) reference values for echo LVH were used for comparison.[11,18] The degree of echo-LVH was significantly greater in the elderly than in the young. For example, men under age 30 with echo-LVH had average LV masses that were 150 percent of normal values while men over age 80 with echo-LVH had LV masses averaging 192 percent of normal values.

Eccentric and unclassified LVH were the most common forms of echo-LVH in the offspring study subjects. Concentric echo-LVH constituted a somewhat larger proportion of the echo-LVH in the elderly cohort (particularly in women) than in the younger subjects (table 1).

Table 1. Prevalence of various forms of echo-LVH in Framingham subjects

	Total number	Type of LVH N(%)		
		E	C	DS
Original Cohort				
Males	99 of 512 = 19%	52(53)	42(42)	5(5)
Females	195 of 855 = 23%	77(40)	104(53)	14(7)
Offspring-Spouse				
Males	121 of 1715 = 7%	74(61)	42(35)	5(4)
Females	99 of 1890 = 5%	70(71)	27(27)	2(2)

E = eccentric and unclassified LVH, C = concentric LVH
DS = disproportionate septal LVH
* = New Framingham criteria used (see appendix)

Disproportionate septal LVH was found in 0.1 to 0.3% of the offspring study subjects and between 1 and 2% of the elderly cohort.[19] Elderly women had the highest prevalence of disproportionate septal LVH. Systolic anterior mitral leaflet motion (SAM) was found in roughly 30% of elderly subjects with disproportionate septal LVH. None of the subjects under age 60 had both disproportionate septal LVH and SAM.

CORRELATES AND CONCOMITANTS OF LVH

The prevalence and incidence of all forms of LVH were strongly associated with increasing age and level of blood pressure over time. At systolic pressures exceeding 180 mm Hg, ECG-LVH appeared within 12 years in one-half of hypertensive subjects.[10] Although ECG-LVH occurs in the course of various forms of cardiac disease, the level of blood pressure over time appears to be the major determinant of ECG-LVH in the general population.[20]

CXR- and echo-LVH are closely linked to ECG-LVH. In the early years of the study the prevalence of CXR-LVH was about double that of ECG-LVH at any age.[20] More recently, the prevalence of CXR-LVH has exceeded ECG-LVH by 5- to 20-fold in subjects over age 50 (figures 1 and 2). About 16% of those with CXR-LVH subsequently developed ECG-LVH within 10 years of follow-up. LVH by CXR was found in 35-50% of those with ECG-LVH.[20]

Echo is the most sensitive and specific of the three methods for detecting LVH.[18,21] (figures 1 and 2). Echo-LVH mass has been shown to correlate well with actual post-mortem LV mass.[22] The prevalence of ECG-LVH in Framingham subjects ranged from less than 1% in subjects without echo-LVH to about 40% in subjects in the highest quintile of echo-LVH. Thus, virtually all subjects in our population sample with ECG-LVH were detected by echo [using an echo cut-off of 130% of predicted (see appendix)]; but, on average, about 60% or less of subjects with the most severely hypertrophied hearts were detected by ECG (figures 1 and 2).

Tables 2 and 3 review some retrospective blood pressure correlates of echo-LVH. Table 2 shows that the level of blood pressure over time is significantly higher for subjects with all forms of echo-LVH. Disproportionate septal LVH was associated with the lowest long-term blood pressures among those with LVH despite representing the greatest left ventricular mass (and mass index) (table 2). This suggests that mechanisms other than long-term systemic hypertension are also important in disproportionate septal LVH. Table 3 shows that echo may yield valuable information regarding the long-term antecedent blood pressure experience of groups of subjects with similar blood pressures at the time of their echo.

The profile of young male subjects under age 30 who had echo-LVH was one of normotensive, non-obese highly active individuals. This was in contrast to older subjects with echo-LVH who were more likely to be hypertensive and obese.

Table 2. Retrospective blood pressure correlates of various forms of echo LVH*

Type of LVH	N	Age	Systol** BPmmHg	Diastol** BP	LV Mass (g)
None	1178	69+6	128+15	80+8	160+46
E	93	72+7+	139+17+	84+10+	311+96+
C	78	71+7+	137+16+	85+9+	282+58+
DS	19	74+7+	132+15+	79+7	367+101+

E = eccentric and unclassified LVH, C = concentric LVH
DS = disproportionate septal LVH
* = Published [11] LVH criteria used; age is at time of echo
** = Mean and standard deviation of 12 blood pressures for each subject
     over 24 years prior to echo
+ $p < 0.05$ compared to subjects without LVH
All forms of echo-LVH were associated with long-term elevation of systolic blood pressure. Other mechanisms in addition to pressure overload
secondary to long-term elevation of systemic blood pressure are important
in DS-LVH.

PROGNOSTIC SIGNIFICANCE OF LVH

ECG-LVH is a lethal marker. Forty-five percent of all cardiovascular deaths in the Framingham study have been preceded by ECG-LVH. The five year mortality rate in Framingham men who develop ECG-LVH is 35% compared to ~10 to 15% or less expected otherwise.[20] For women, 20% who develop ECG-LVH are dead within five years. For those aged 65 years and older these mortality rates were 50% and 35%, respectively. The excess mortal-ity associated with ECG-LVH is apparently not attributable to associated hypertension since ECG-LVH carried three times the risk of hypertension without the ECG finding. The mortality rate associated with possible LVH was one-half that of definite ECG-LVH. CXR-LVH was associated with one third the cardiovascular mortality rate of ECG-LVH.[20]

Table 3. Past and present systolic blood pressure in male normotensives and hypertensives with and without echo-LVH.*

		normotensive at exam 16			borderline hypertension at exam 16			definite hypertension at exam 16	
	N	Avg SBP (mmHg)		N	Avg SBP (mmHg)		N	Avg SBP (mmHg)	
		at time of echo	over 12 biennial exams		at time of echo	over 12 biennial exams		at time of echo	over 12 biennial exams
echo LVH	28	130+8**	128+15**	22	148+11	140+11**	9	180+23	150+13**
no echo LVH	167	124+10	123+10	152	146+14	133+14	52	170+16	139+13

* Published[11] LVH criteria used
** p < 0.03
Echo appears useful in assessing the antecedent blood pressure experience of groups of subjects with similar blood pressures at the time of echo.

Risk of cardiovascular morbidity is also markedly increased in those with ECG-LVH. ECG-LVH confers a 2 to 9-fold increased risk of strokes, cardiac failure, coronary disease and peripheral arterial disease.[20] Follow-up since our echo studies has been too brief to assess the prognostic significance of echo-LVH. However, a strong association of echo-LVH with complex and frequent ventricular dysrhythmias has emerged in our initial analyses, particularly in subjects over age 40 years. The association of such potentially serious ventricular dysrhythmias with echo-LVH was found in the absence of overt cardiac disease and was independent of blood pressure, ECG-LVH and echo-LVH fractional shortening (a measure of systolic LV function). This suggests that much of the echo-LVH detected in apparently healthy subjects in the general population may be pathological especially in those over age 40.

CONCLUSIONS

The use of echo in the Framingham study has allowed prevalence estimates of various forms of LVH in a free-living population-based sample. Between 5 and 10% of the subjects had echo-LVH in the absence of ECG- or CXR-LVH. ECG-LVH appears to be a late finding in the course of cardiovascular disease. Prevention of associated morbidity and mortality is likely to be most effective if action is taken before the ECG finding appears. Preliminary data suggest that echo might help select those who should be targeted for such action.

APPENDIX

Formulas used to define echo-LVH in Framingham.

If sex = 1 then PSDLVM = 11.18 + 0.36 (WT)

If sex = 1 then PNLVM = 43.62 + 2.18 (WT)

If sex = 1 then VARLVM = (PSDLVM**2)(1.06)
If sex = 1 then COVTERM = [(WT)1.06](-2.20)
If sex = 1 then BOB1TERM = (184.66) + (WT**2)(0.03)
If sex = 2 then PSDLVM = 8.36 + 0.26 (WT)

If sex = 2 then PNLVM = 44.71 + 1.46 (WT) + 0.27 (AGE)

If sex = 2 then VARLVM = (PSDLVM**2)(1.07)
If sex = 2 then COVTERM = [(WT)1.07](-0.8) + AGE (1.07)(-0.27)
If sex = 2 then ROB1TERM = (65.12**2)[(0.02) + AGE**2)](0.01)

95% confidence limit = PNLVM + 1.96 (SQRT)[BOB1TERM + 2(COVTERM) + VARLVM]

If actual echo LV mass > 95% confidence limit then LVH was considered present.

VARLVM, COVTERM, & BOB1TERM = terms used to determine the variance of the LV mass as a function of weight (in kg).

Sex 1 = males, sex 2 = females

Left ventricular hypertrophy is best considered as a continuous variable [i.e., degree of LVH is reflected by a subject's percent of predicted (PPD) LVM].

PPDLVM in % = (measured LVM/PNLVM)100.
PPDLVM ≥ 130% = echo-LVH if a cut point is desirable.

14

REFERENCES

1. Grossman, W.: Cardiac hypertrophy: Useful adaptation or pathologic process?, Am. J. Med., 69, 576, 1980
2. Badeer, H.S.: Biological significance of cardiac hypertrophy, Am. J. Cardiol., 14, 133-138, 1964
3. Frohlich, E.D., Tarazi, R.C.: Is arterial pressure the sole factor responsible for hypertensive cardiac hypertrophy?, Am. J. Cardiol., 44, 959, 1979
4. Laks, M.M., Morady, F.: Norepinephrine - The myocardial hypertrophy hormone?, Am. Heart J., 91, 674, 1976
5. Laks, M.M., Morady, F., Swan, H.J.C.: Myocardial hypertrophy produced by chronic subhypertensive doses of norepinephrine in the dog, Chest, 64, 75, 1973
6. Sokolow, M., Lyon, T.P.: The ventricular complex in left ventricular hypertrophy as obtained by unipolar precordial and limb leads, Am. Heart J., 37, 161, 1949
7. Gubner, R.S., Ungerleider, H.E.: Electrocardiographic criteria of left ventricular hypertrophy, Arch. Intern. Med., 72, 196, 1943
8. Katz, L.N.: Electrocardiography, 2nd edition, Philadelphia, Lea & Febiger, 1946
9. Romhilt, D.W., Estes, E.H.: A point score system for the ECG diagnosis of left ventricular hypertrophy, Am. Heart J, 75, 752, 1968
10. Kannel, W.B., Gordon, T., Offutt, D.: Left ventricular hypertrophy by electrocardiogram. Prevalence, incidence, and mortality in the Framingham study, Ann. Intern. Med., 71, 89, 1969
11. Gardin, J.M., Henry, W.L., Savage, D.D., Ware, J.H., Burn, C., Borer, J.S.: Echocardiographic measurements in normal subjects: evaluation of an adult population without clinically apparent heart disease, J. Clin. Ultrasound, 7, 439, 1979
12. Feigenbaum, H.: Echocardiography, 3rd edition, Philadelphia, Lea & Febiger, 557, 1976
13. Devereux, R.B., Savage, D.D., Drayer, J.I.M., Laragh, J.H.: Left ventricular hypertrophy and function in high, normal and low-renin forms of essential hypertension, Hypertension, 4, 524, 1982
14. Robinson, C.H.: Normal and Therapeutic Nutrition, 14th edition, New York, Macmillan, p. 703, 1972
15. Sahn, D.J., DeMaria, A., Kisslo, J., Weyman, A.: Recommendations regarding quantitation in M-mode echocardiography: results of a survey of echocardiographic measurements, Circulation, 58, 1072, 1978
16. Henry, W.L., Clark, C.E., Epstein, S.E.: Asymmetric septal hypertrophy: Echo-cardiographic identification of the pathognomonic anatomic abnormality of IHSS, Circulation, 47, 225, 1973
17. Troy, B.L., Pombo, J., Rackley, C.E.: Measurement of left ventricular wall thickness and mass by echocardiography, Circulation, 45, 602, 1972
18. Savage, D.D., Garrison, R.J., Kannel, W.B., Castelli, W.P., Anderson, S.J., Stokes, J.III, Padgett, S., Feinleib, M.: Prevalence, characteristics and correlates of echocardiographic left ventricular hypertrophy in a population-based sample - preliminary findings: the Framingham study, Circulation (abst.), 66, II-63, 1982
19. Savage, D.D., Castelli, W.P., Abbott, R.D., Garrison, R.J., Anderson, S.J., Kannel, W.B., Feinleib, M.: Hypertrophic cardiomyopathy and its markers in the general population: the great masquerader revisited: the Framingham study, J. Cardiovasc. Ultrasonography, 2, 41, 1983

20. Kannel, W.B.: Left ventricular hypertrophy in hypertension: prognostic and pathogenetic implications. The Framingham study, The Heart in Hypertension, ed. B.E. Strauer, Springer-Verlag, 123, 1981
21. Savage, D.D., Drayer, J.I.M., Henry, W.L., Mathews, E.C., Ware, J.H., Gardin, J.M., Cohen, E.R., Epstein, S.E., Laragh, J.H.: Echocardiographic assessment of cardiac anatomy and function in hypertensive patients, Circulation, 59, 623, 1979
22. Devereux, R.B., Reichek, N.: Echocardiographic determination of left ventricular mass in man, Circulation, 55, 613, 1977

SUMMARY

An echocardiographic-necropsy correlation study was performed to validate echocardiographic determinations of LV mass. LV dimensions were measured according to the Penn and American Society of Echocardiography (ASE) conventions and used in the cube function and Teichholz regression formulae to calculate LV mass. The results of the study confirm that the Penn-cube function method of determining LV mass is the most accurate one for diagnosis and quantitation of LVH. The accuracy is particularly impressive in view of the diverse echocardiographs and multiple individuals who obtained the tracings.

Echocardiographic measurement of LV mass by the Penn-cube method provides a probe which may be used to study the relationship between hemodynamic overloading in hypertension and development of LVH.

Four echocardiographic studies of patients with hypertension consistently show a high prevalence of increased LV mass among hypertensives. By subtracting the prevalence of LVH among normotensives, one found the "population attributable risk" of LVH due to hypertension to fall in the range of 25 to 45%. Thus, surprisingly a majority of patients with hypertension do not exhibit definite LVH. Prevalence of LVH is strikingly higher among males. The sex difference is not eliminated if one indexes LV mass by body surface area, but reverses if sex-specific upper limits of normal are used. It seems that the level of physical conditioning and hormonal factors play an important role in determining LV mass, also among normotensives.

Echocardiography has been useful in defining factors contributing to the development of LVH among hypertensives. LV mass tends to increase gradually, at a rate of perhaps 5% annually, in patients whose hypertension is not controlled. The mode of therapy by which blood pressure is controlled, may be important with regard to the degree of induced regression of LVH and rate of growth. Non-invasive ambulatory blood pressure monitoring has been used to assess the relationship between blood pressure pattern and the heart. The closest correlation between blood pressure values and LV mass indices was found between diastolic blood pressure during occupational work and end-diastolic relative wall thickness. The correlation between blood pressure measured at rest with LV mass was lower. This observation suggests that blood pressure response to regularly recurring stress may contribute to the development of LVH.

SENSITIVITY OF ECHOCARDIOGRAPHY FOR DETECTION OF LEFT VENTRICULAR HYPER-
TROPHY

DEVEREUX, R.B.; ALONSO, D.R.; LUTAS, E.M.; PICKERING, T.G.; HARSHFIELD,
G.A.; LARAGH, J.H.
Departments of Medicine and Pathology, Cornell University Medical
College, New York, NY, U.S.A.

INTRODUCTION

Myocardial hypertrophy plays an essential adaptive role in many forms of
heart disease, serving as the principal mechanism by which hemodynamic
overloads are offset.[1] Numerous studies have demonstrated that a broad
proportionality exists between the severity of either naturally occurring
or experimentally induced hemodynamic overload and the degree of compensatory hypertrophy.[2-4] Furthermore, it appears that while mild degrees
of hypertrophy can be "physiologic", analogous to that induced in athletes by high levels of physical conditioning, more marked hypertrophy
appears to be "pathologic", e.g. associated with deterioration of myocardial function. The clinical importance of this is indicated by the
finding, in studies which relied on electrocardiographic and roentgeno-
graphic methods, that left ventricular hypertrophy (LVH) was associated
with an impaired prognosis.[5-6]

The studies which established most clearly the clinical significance of
detectable left ventricular hypertrophy relied of necessity on indirect
methods of evaluating the state of the left ventricular muscle. Such
indirect approaches suffer from intrinsic limitations. Electrocardiography relies on electrical phenomena to make inferences about anatomic
variables. It is not surprising that electrocardiographic QRS voltages
bear only a moderate relationship with left ventricular mass.[7-8]

Supported in part by grant HL-18323 from the NHLBI.

Similarly, repolarization abnormalities of LVH - the so-called "strain" pattern - are only reliably present in patients with severe LVH.[9] Therefore, ECG criteria with reasonable specificity (> 90%) are insensitive for the diagnosis of LVH ($\leq$ 50%) and no currently available electrocardiographic method is suitable for estimation of left ventricular mass. A similar situation exists with regard to the chest x-ray, in which measurements of overall cardiac size are used to make inferences about the degree of LVH. The accuracy of standard radiographic techniques has been shown to be similar to the electrocardiogram with regard to both the diagnosis and quantitation of LVH.[10]

More recently, echocardiography has made it possible to visualize directly left ventricular wall thicknesses and chamber dimensions. This capability has been exploited by numerous investigators to assess both LVH and chamber dilatation in a wide variety of disease states. Direct measurements of the thickness of the posterior left ventricular wall and of the interventricular septum have proven useful as indices of myocardial hypertrophy in conditions associated with concentric LVH, including hypertension and aortic stenosis. However, depending on the stimulus to hypertrophy, the pattern of LVH may vary, and patients may also develop eccentric, asymmetric and dilated forms of hypertrophy, all of which are less accurately assessed by a simple measurement of wall thickness.

To deal with this problem, it is desirable to be able to measure overall left ventricular mass, since this represents the total hypertrophy response of the left ventricle. Initially, echocardiographic methods of estimating left ventricular mass were developed which were not directly compared to anatomic LV mass.[11-12] Instead, these echocardiographic methods were validated indirectly, by comparison with angiographic estimates of LV mass, or were simply assumed to be correct, based on the use of reasonable geometric formulae.

DEVELOPMENT OF ECHOCARDIOGRAPHIC METHODS OF MEASURING LEFT VENTRICULAR MASS

Because of the fundamentally unsatisfactory nature of this situation, we undertook a study a number of years ago in which antemortem echocardiographic measurements were compared to postmortem left ventricular weight.[13]

A total of 34 patients were studied, who suffered from a wide range of cardiac and non-cardiac diseases. All had m-mode echocardiograms of excellent technical quality within 120 days of autopsy. Because of uncertainties with regard to the possible effect of alterations in echocardiograph gain settings on the apparent thickness of echoes from endocardial surfaces, we made measurements of left ventricular wall thickness in two ways, either including or excluding the endocardial surfaces. As we reported previously,[13] the best correlation with autopsy left ventricular mass was obtained using wall thickness measurements by the Penn convention, which exclude the thickness of endocardial surfaces, in the cube function formula. Not only was a close correlation ($r = 0.96$, $p < 0.001$) obtained between echocardiographic left ventricular mass by this method and anatomic LV weight, but the technique also exhibited excellent sensitivity (93%) and specificity (95%) in patients with and without LVH. Other previously reported methods of estimating left ventricular mass were shown to be less accurate than the Penn method, both because of intrinsically weaker correlations between echocardiographic and anatomic findings, and because of systemic under-estimation or over-estimation of left ventricular mass. More recently, another commonly used geometric formula for estimating left ventricular volumes, the equation of Teichholz et al.,[14] has also been shown to result in systemic underestimation of left ventricular mass.[15]

Subsequent studies have clarified further the strengths and limitations of echocardiographic measurement of left ventricular mass. Measurement by the Penn method has been shown to correlate well with clinical evidence of LVH,[16] and to remain stable in individual patients despite marked changes in LV geometry, as occur immediately following correction of the LV volume overload of aortic regurgitation.[17] However, despite the accuracy of these m-mode measurements in patients with relatively symmetrical ventricles, potentially important errors may occur in the presence of severely distorted left ventricular shape. Reichek et al.[18] have recently shown this to be the case in a series of patients most of whom had left ventricular aneurysms or other causes of geometric distortion. In these patients Penn convention echocardiographic LV mass measurements diverged from the line of identity with anatomic measurements, although the actual correlation between echocardiographic and anatomic LV mass remained surprisingly close (r = 0.86, p < 0.001).[18] Carefully performed two-dimensional echocardiograms allowed accurate estimation of LV mass even in this series of patients with a high prevalence of abnormally shaped left ventricles (r = 0.93, p < 0.001; sensitivity = 70%; specificity = 100%).

ECHOCARDIOGRAPHIC EVALUATION OF LEFT VENTRICULAR HYPERTROPHY
Current problems

Despite the contribution that echocardiography has already made to clinical investigation of left ventricular hypertrophy, numerous uncertainties persist. Some of these concern methodology: what m-mode echocardiographic measurements conventions and geometric formulae yield anatomically valid measurements of left ventricular mass? When is the accuracy of two-dimensional estimates sufficiently superior to justify its use, in view of the greater difficulty and time required to quantitate two-dimensional echocardiogram? Other uncertainties pertain to the results of the research into LVH which has used echocardiography as a probe. Do all patients with hemodynamic loading conditions develop detectable LVH? What normal limits should be used to determine who has LVH? Can factors be identified, in addition to conventional indices of hemodynamic load, which influence the development of LVH?

In this review we will address these questions using information derived from our studies of cardiac hypertrophy at Cornell University Medical College. We will utilize the research results from a single investigative group in order to focus most clearly on the questions under consideration, without distraction by the possible effects of differences in the approaches and methods used in different institutions. We will provide information about the relationship of echocardiographic to anatomic findings in a series of autopsied patients, and utilize findings in studies of patients with hypertension to analyze the relationship between hemodynamic overload and LVH.

Validity of echocardiographic measurements of left ventricular mass

To provide further insight into the accuracy of currently utilized m-mode echocardiographic methods we will present data obtained from the initial subset of patients in an ongoing echocardiographic-necropsy correlation study. This necropsy series comprised 23 patients with technically satisfactory m-mode echocardiograms performed clinically at the New York Hospital-Cornell Medical Center within 180 days of death. The patients included nine males and 14 females ranging in age from 29 to 76 years; patients suffered a wide variety of cardiac and non-cardiac diseases. Left ventricular mass was determined at necropsy using the standard chamber-dissection technique.[13]

Echocardiograms were performed using standard techniques as previously described from this laboratory.[19-20] SmithKline Ekoline 20A, Picker System C and Irex echocardiographs were employed to make recordings on light-sensitive paper at 50 mm/s paper speed. Studies were performed by three technicians and five cardiology fellows; five were performed in the ward and 18 were obtained in the laboratory. Echocardiograms were coded and read blindly. Only tracings which provided continuous visualization of the endocardial surfaces of the interventricular septum and posterior left ventricular wall throughout the cardiac cycle at the level of the left ventricular minor axis were accepted, similar to our previous echocardiographic-necropsy correlation study.[13] Up to six cycles were measured on each recording. End-diastolic left ventricular measurements were made according to the Penn convention[13] and the recommendations of the American Society of Echocardiography (ASE).[21] The latter measurements differ from Penn convention measurements in two regards: they are made at the onset of the QRS complex instead of at the peak of the R wave, and measurements are made from the leading edge of one interface to the leading edge of the next interface. Thus, the thickness of the endocardial echo arising from the right side of the interventricular septum is included in the ASE measurement of septal thickness, and the thickness of the posterior wall endocardial echo is included in the ASE measurement of posterior wall thickness. These two sets of primary echocardiographic data were utilized in the cube function and Teichholz formulae[13,14] to derive estimates of left ventricular mass.

Relatively close relationships were observed between necropsy left ventricular mass and echocardiographic measurements of left ventricular mass using the cube function formula and either Penn convention measurements (figure 1) or ASE measurements (figure 2).

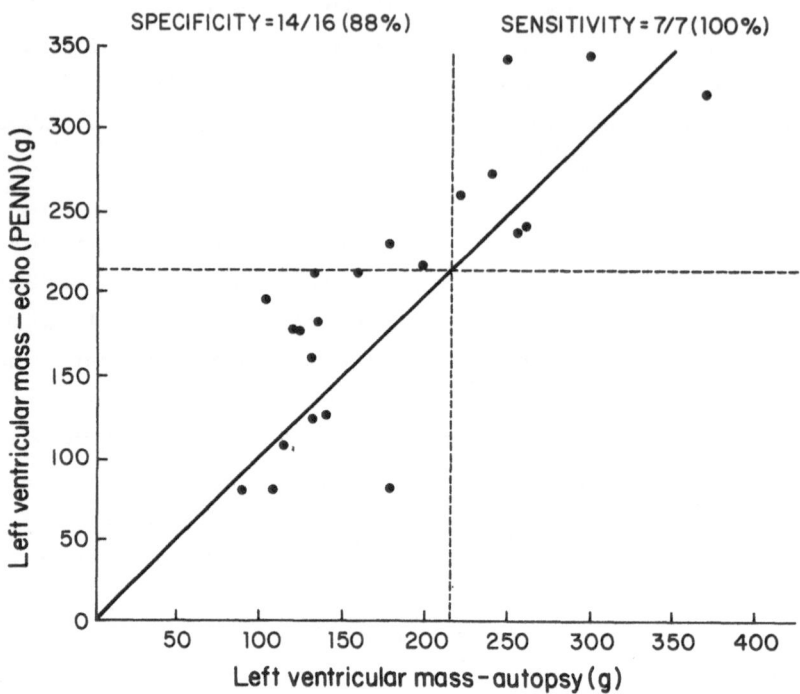

Figure 1. Relationship between necropsy left ventricular mass (horizontal axis) and echocardiographic left ventricular mass by the Penn-cube method (vertical axis) in 23 patients. The overall correlation was moderately close (r = 0.80, p < 0.001). Horizontal and vertical dashed lines represent the upper limit of normal left ventricular mass. The horizontal solid line is the line of identity.

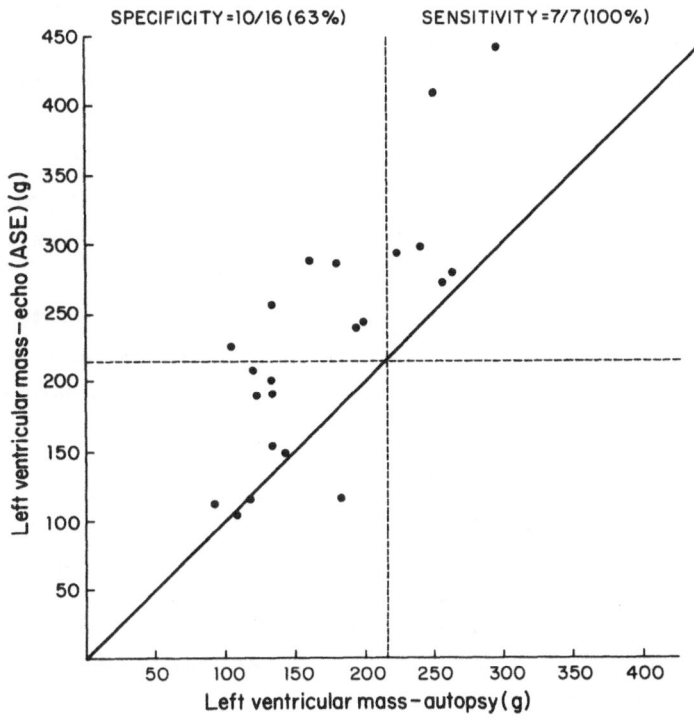

Figure 2. Relationship between necropsy left ventricular mass (horizontal axis) and echocardiographic left ventricular mass by the ASE-cube method described in the text (vertical axis) in 23 patients. The overall correlation was moderately close (r = 0.80, p < 0.001) but specificity was low (10/16 or 63%).

Despite the more limited range of variability of anatomic left ventricular mass (90 to 367 grams) compared to previous echocardiographic-autopsy studies,[13,18] the strength of correlation for both relationships was high (r = 0.80 for both, p < 0.001). An even closer relationship was observed between the two echocardiographic measurements of left ventricular mass in individual patients (r = 0.98, p < 0.001).

However, despite the similarity of the relationships of the results of these two echocardiographic methods to necropsy findings, the Penn-cube and ASE-cube methods differed importantly in both diagnostic accuracy and in the degree to which echocardiographic left ventricular mass estimates faithfully reflected necropsy measurements. As may be seen in table 1, the Penn-cube function method was 100% sensitive in the seven patients with anatomic LVH (LV mass > 215 grams[7,13]) and 88% specific (14/16) in those with normal LV mass, with no significant difference in either group between anatomic and echocardiographic left ventricular mass measurements. In contrast, the ASE-cube function measurements had poor specificity (10/16 or 63%) despite equally high sensitivity. Left ventricular mass by the ASE-cube method significantly exceeded anatomic LV mass, by 25% in the patients with LVH and by 40% in those with normal LV mass.

method	no LVH (n=16)		LVH (n=7)	
	LV mass	specificity	LV mass	sensitivity
autopsy	140 $\pm$ 33	100%*	269 $\pm$ 48	100%*
Penn-cube	160 $\pm$ 52	88%	289 $\pm$ 47	100%
ASE-cube	196 $\pm$ 62**	63%	336 $\pm$ 67+	100%
ASE-Teichholz	121 $\pm$ 28	100%	177 $\pm$ 31**	14%

* By definition sensitivity and specificity are 100% using autopsy measurements. Statistical significance:
** $p < 0.005$ versus autopsy
 + $p < 0.05$ versus autopsy

Table 1. Comparison of echocardiographic left ventricular mass estimates by various methods with necropsy left ventricular mass.

The Teichholz regression equation has been found to provide a useful method of compensating for echocardiographic over-estimation of left ventricular volumes.[14] It has been shown previously that this equation reduced LV mass estimates obtained from Penn convention measurements by approximately 30%.[15] Accordingly, it might be expected to correct the over-estimation of left ventricular mass observed above with ASE-cube function LV mass measurements. Unfortunately, as seen in table 1, use of the Teichholz regression equation with ASE left ventricular measurements also resulted in systematic underestimation of anatomic left ventricular mass. This resulted in very low sensitivity of the method (14%) in patients with LVH (p < 0.01 versus both Penn-cube and ASE-cube methods).

These data confirm that the Penn-cube function method of determining left ventricular mass is sufficiently accurate for diagnosis and quantitation of LVH. The accuracy of this method observed in the present study is particularly impressive in view of the diverse echocardiographs and multiple individuals who obtained the tracings. Other m-mode echocardiographic methods produce results which deviate from anatomic findings sufficiently to preclude their use without adjustment. However, because of the high correlation between estimates of LV mass by Penn-cube and ASE-cube methods, an appropriate regression equation may be developed for use with the latter method.[22]

PREVALENCE OF LEFT VENTRICULAR HYPERTROPHY IN PATIENTS WITH HEMODYNAMIC OVERLOAD

Echocardiographic measurement of left ventricular mass by the Penn-cube method provides a probe which may be used to answer the next question posed at the outset: do all patients with hemodynamic overloading conditions develop detectable LVH? To address this issue, we will use hypertension as a model disease, both because it is the commonest form of hemodynamic loading condition, and because it has been most extensively studied.

Detection of LVH requires definition of an appropriate upper limit of normal so that individuals with larger left ventricular measurements may be recognized. Four echocardiographic studies of patients with hypertension provide data which can be compared to a defined cut-off of left ventricular mass in similarly studied normal subjects.[19,23-26] As depicted in figure 3, the prevalence of increased LV mass was markedly higher among hypertensive patients: 48% versus 2.5%, 47% versus 0.5%, 43% versus 4%, and 26% versus 10%. Several conclusions can be drawn from these data.

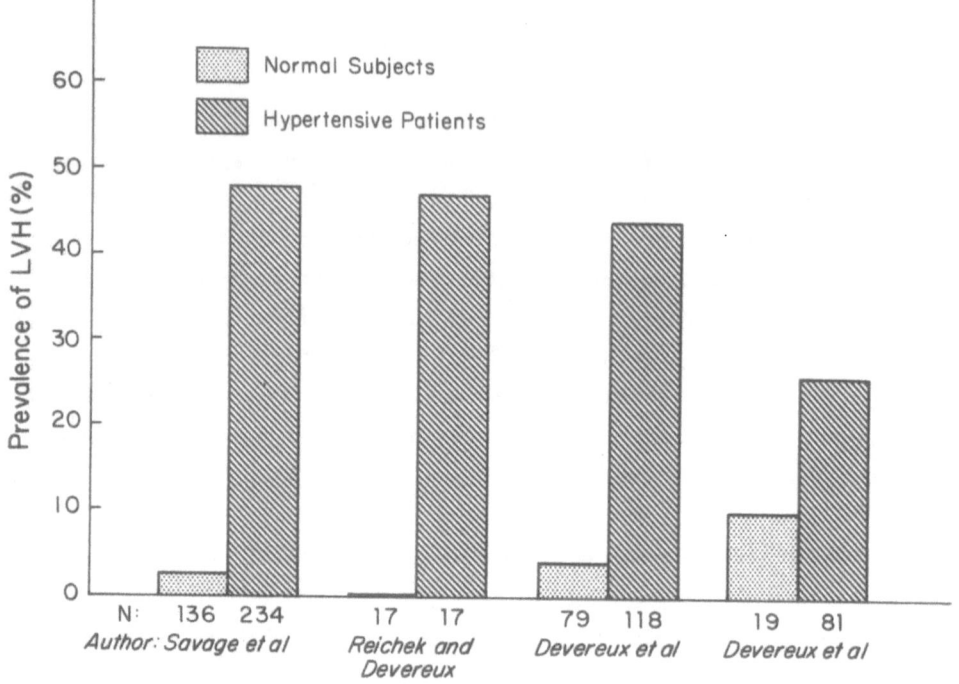

Figure 3. Prevalence of left ventricular hypertrophy in four independent groups of patients with essential hypertension and normotensive
controls.[19,23-26]

First, up to half of patients with hypertension have manifest LVH,
defined as left ventricular mass above specified normal limits. Variations in this percentage probably reflect differences in the severity of
hypertensive cardiovascular disease among patient groups, as well as some
instability of population prevalence estimates related to sampling errors.
Second, these data permit calculation of a more direct measure of the
prevalence of LVH <u>due</u> to hypertension, the "population attributable risk".
This statistic is calculated by subtracting the prevalence of LVH among
normotensive subjects from that in hypertensive patients. The resulting

estimate of the population attributable risk of LVH in patients with hypertension would appear to fall within the range of 25% to 45%, depending on patient characteristics. A third striking conclusion can also be drawn from these data: <u>a majority of patients with hypertension of average severity do not exhibit definite LVH</u>. Further study is needed to elucidate the reasons for this apparent discordance between the presence of hemodynamic overload and a discernable myocardial hypertrophy response. Evidence concerning one possible cause of this discrepancy is presented later in this review.

One patient characteristic appears to influence estimates of the prevalence of LVH to an especially striking degree: the sex of the subjects. If one applies a single upper normal limit for left ventricular mass to both sexes, the prevalence of LVH is strikingly higher among males. This

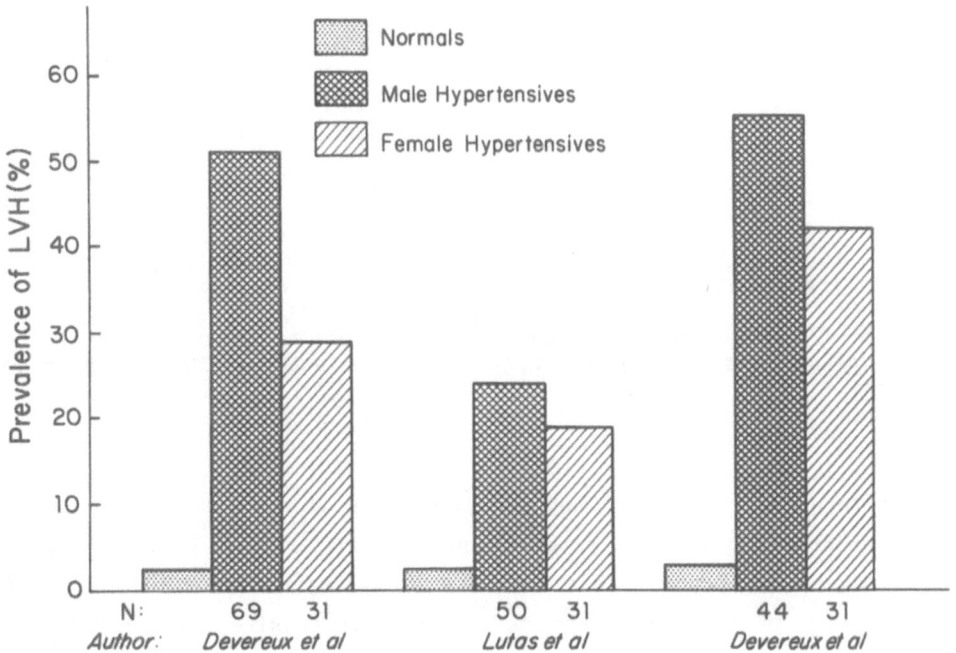

Figure 4a. Prevalence of left ventricular hypertrophy in three independent groups of patients with essential hypertension subdivided by sex.[20,26-27]
Panel A - When upper 95th percentile limits of normal for both sexes pooled (> 119 g/m^2) are used, prevalence of LVH is higher in males.

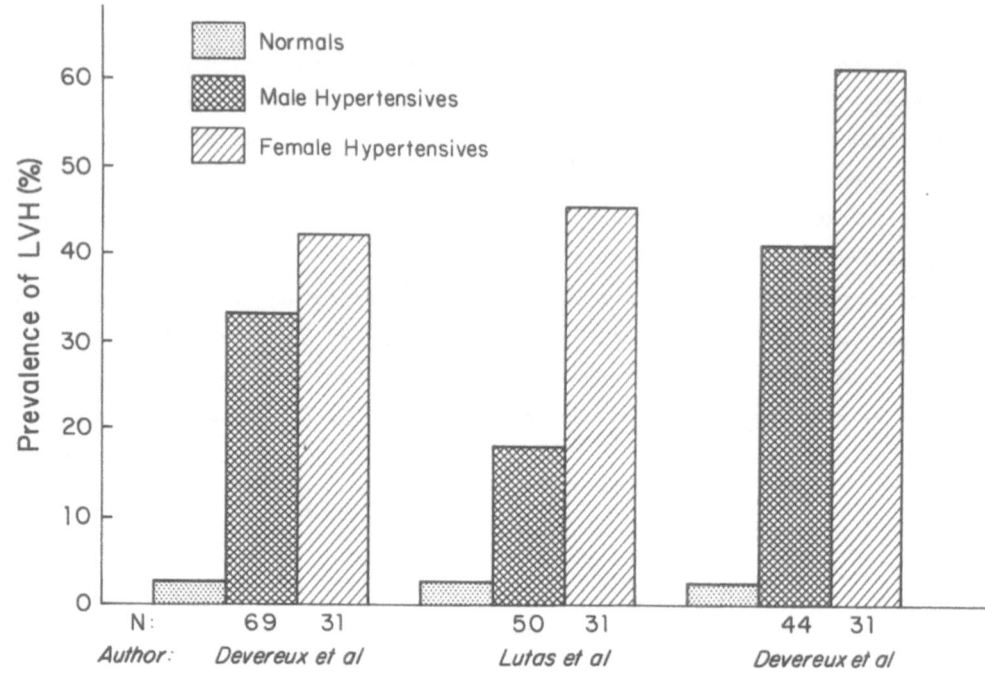

Figure 4b. Prevalence of left ventricular hypertrophy in three independent groups of patients with essential hypertension subdivided by
sex.[20,26-27]
Panel B - When sex-specific upper 95th percentile limits of normal are
used (males 131 g/m^2, females 107 g/m^2) prevalence of LVH is higher in
females.

sex difference is decreased but not eliminated if one indexes LV mass by

body surface area to take into account sex differences in overall body

size. Figure 4a depicts this tendency for a higher prevalence of LVH

among males in three separate series of hypertensive patients[20,26-27]

when this type of definition is used. However, we have observed that left

ventricular mass index differs between normal men and women[28], suggest-

ing that sex-specific normal limits may be more useful for detection of

LVH.[29] If one applies the sex-specific upper limits of normal derived from study of normotensive populations to these same three populations[20,26-27], the prevalence of LVH was consistently lower among hypertensive males (18% to 41%) than hypertensive females (42% to 61%) (figure 4b). The reasons for these sex differences are currently uncertain, but recent evidence that sex differences in left ventricular mass are closely related to differences in lean body mass[30] suggest that the level of physical conditioning and hormonal factors may play important roles.

One final inference from these data concerning the population prevalence of LVH in hypertensive and normotensive subjects may be of considerable importance. If one considers the adult population prevalence of essential hypertension to fall in the range of 10 to 15 per cent, from 50 to 75% of the individuals with LV mass above the upper 95% confidence limits developed from study of normotensive populations will have LVH due to hypertension. An additional proportion will have other cardiovascular conditions capable of inducing LVH, whereas a significant minority - possibly as much as two per cent of the adult population - would be expected to have LV mass above accepted normal limits simply because they fall in the upper tail of the wide normal distribution of LV mass. This fact illustrates why the mere presence of unexplained LVH is not a satisfactory criterion for the diagnosis of hypertrophic cardiomyopathy or any other specific condition.

Role of echocardiography in elucidating factors in the pathogenesis of
left ventricular hypertrophy

In addition to its role in establishing the prevalence of LVH, echocardiography has been useful in defining factors contributing to its pathogenesis. Once again hypertension serves as a useful model disease. One important variable seems to be the duration of uncorrected hemodynamic overload. Thus, a preliminary study in our laboratory indicated that left ventricular mass tended to increase gradually, at a rate of perhaps 5% annually, in patients whose hypertension was not controlled. Furthermore, our own studies and those of other investigators support the hypothesis that the mode of therapy by which blood pressure is controlled may be important with regard to the degree of induced regression of LVH. Thus, preliminary evidence suggests that beta-adrenoceptor blocking agents may be more potent with regard to regression of LVH than other classes of drugs, including diuretics and vasodilators.[31-32] Further study is needed to determine whether such a differential effect of different classes of drugs on regression of LVH is observed consistently, and, if it is, what is its clinical significance.

Finally, the development of accurate non-invasive methods of ambulatory 24-hour blood pressure measurement has made it possible to assess the relationship between blood pressure pattern and the heart. Initial studies performed at Cornell indicated that patients with essential hypertension tended to raise their blood pressures more in response to various stresses than did normotensive subjects.[33] Accordingly, we compared blood pressure measured by automatic portable recorder with echocardiographic indices of LVH in a larger series of patients.[26] In this review we will present our findings in a subset of this population, stratified into normotensive (n=17), borderline hypertensive (n=32) and sustained essential hypertensive (n=32) groups. As depicted in figure 5, a weak albeit statistically significant correlation was observed between

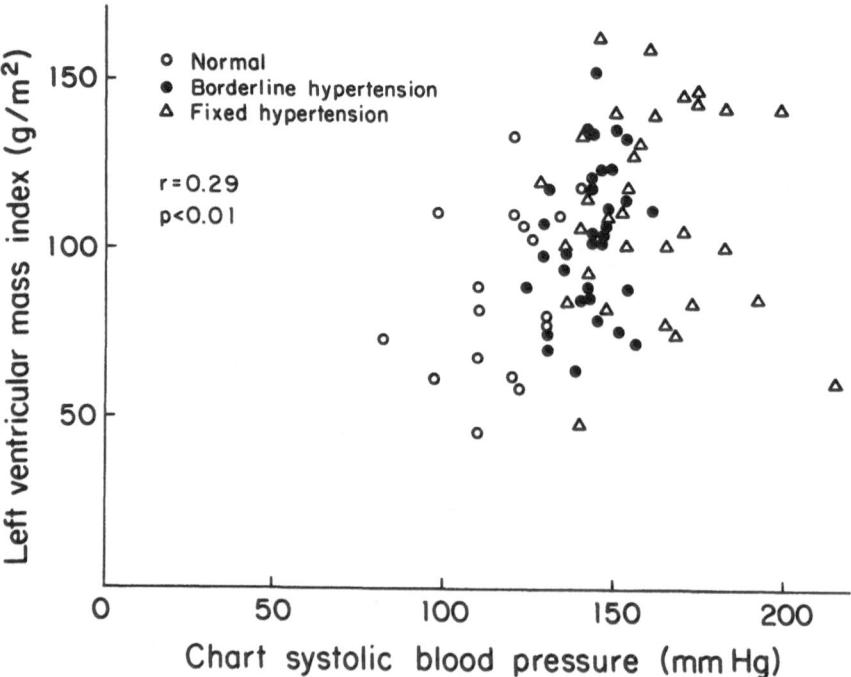

Figure 5. Relation between physicians office measurements of systolic blood pressure (horizontal axis) and left ventricular mass (vertical axis) in 81 patients. See key for patient groups.

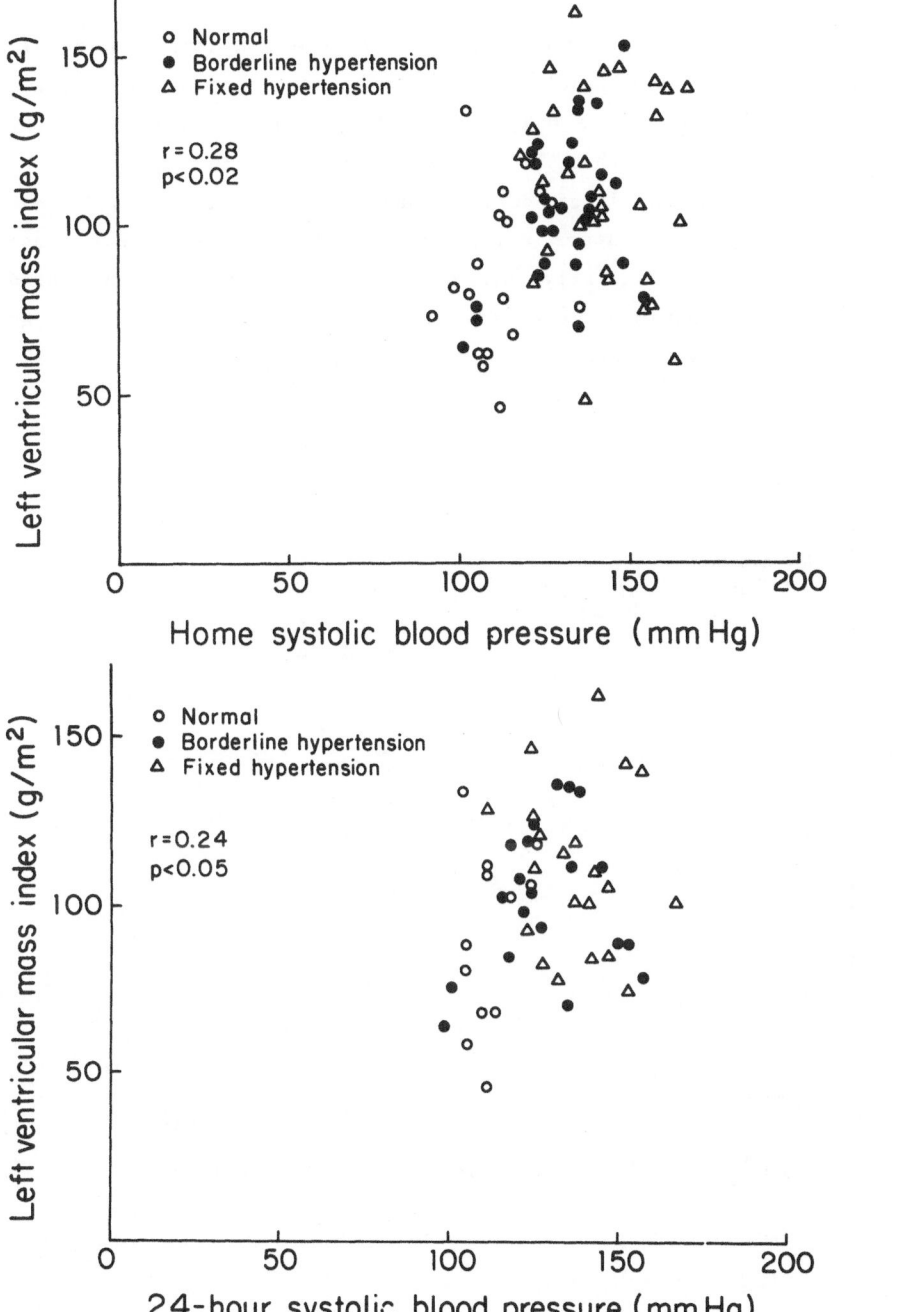

Figure 6. Panel a – Relation between home systolic blood pressure by automatic recorder (horizontal axis) and left ventricular mass (LVM) (vertical axis).
Panel b – Relation between total 24-hour systolic blood pressure and LVM. These relationships are not closer than that between physician blood pressure and LVM. Same key as figure 5.

physician measurements of systolic blood pressure and left ventricular mass. This relationship was not improved by substitution of blood pressure measured at home (figure 6a), during sleep (figure 6b), or over the entire 24 hours (figure 6b). In contrast, as shown in figure 7, the systolic blood pressure level during subjects' occupational work exhibited a significantly closer relationship with left ventricular mass ($r = 0.55$, $p < 0.001$). Similarly, diastolic blood pressure at work showed the closest relationship to end-diastolic relative wall thickness, an index of the severity of concentric LVH ($r = 0.55$, $p < 0.001$) (figure 8).

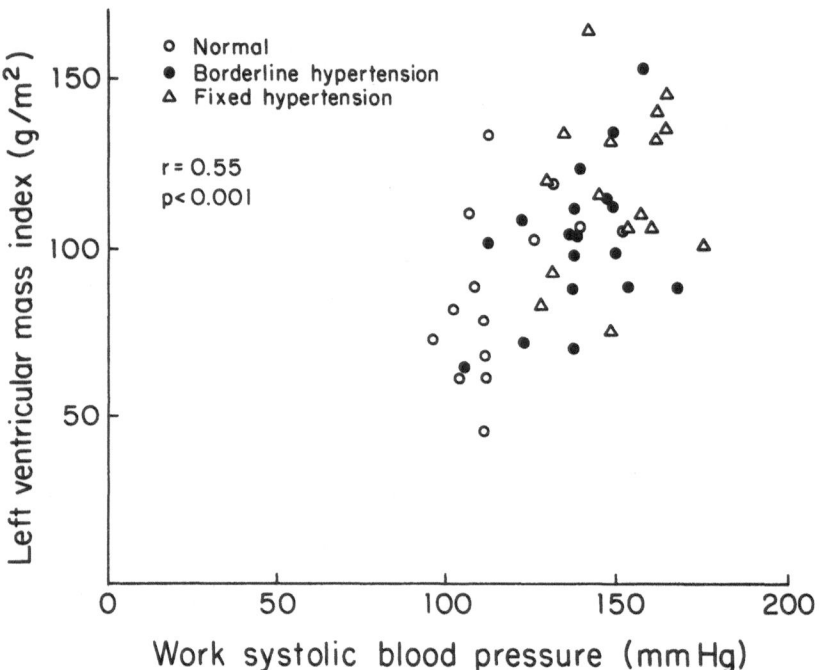

Figure 7. A closer relationship is observed between automatic recorder systolic blood pressure at work (horizontal axis) and LV mass (vertical axis) ($r = 0.55$, $p < 0.001$). Same key as figure 5.

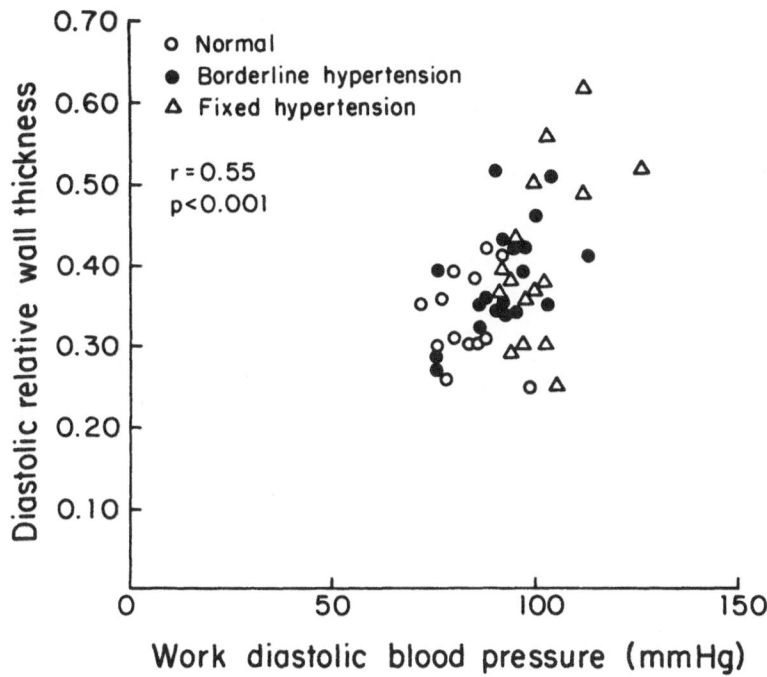

Figure 8. A moderately close relationship (r = 0.55, p < 0.001) was also observed between work diastolic blood pressure (horizontal axis) and LV mass (vertical axis). Same key as figure 5.

These data indicate that blood pressure level during the regularly occurring stress of occupational work is more closely related to the degree of LVH in hypertensive patients than is either the relatively basal blood pressure level at home or during sleep, or blood pressure during the unrepresentative stress of visiting a physician. This observation suggests that blood pressure response to regularly recurring stress may contribute to the development of hypertensive disease. Further study is needed to determine the prognostic significance of stress-induced increases in blood pressure, as well as their relationship to personality pattern and job characteristics.

ACKNOWLEDGMENT

We would like to thank Drs. Nathaniel Reichek, Daniel D. Savage and Jere Mitchell for their contributions to the concepts presented in this review, and Miss Virginia Burns for her assistance in preparation of the manuscript.

REFERENCES

1. Linzbach, A.J.: Heart failure from the point of view of quantitative anatomy, Am. J. Cardiol., 5, 370-382, 1960
2. Badeer, H.S.: Biological significance of cardiac hypertrophy, Am. J. Cardiol., 14, 133-138, 1964
3. Devereux, R.B. and Reichek, N.: Left ventricular hypertrophy, Cardiovasc. Reviews and Reports, 1, 55-68, 1980
4. Meerson, F.Z.: The Failing Heart: Adaptation and Deadaptation, Raven Press, New York, 1983
5. Sokolow, M. and Perloff, D.: The prognosis of essential hypertension treated conservatively, Circulation, 23, 697-713, 1961
6. Spagnuolo, M., Kloth, H., Taranta, A., Doyle, E., Pasternack, B.: Natural history of rheumatic aortic regurgitation. Criteria predictive of death, congestive heart failure and angina in young patients, Circulation, 44, 368-380, 1971
7. Reichek, N. and Devereux, R.B.: Left ventricular hypertrophy. Relation of anatomic, echocardiographic and electrocardiographic findings, Circulation, 63, 1391-1398, 1981
8. Devereux, R.B., Phillips, M.C., Casale, P.N., Eisenberg, R.R., Kligfield, P.: Geometric determinants of electrocardiographic left ventricular hypertrophy, Circulation, 67, 907-911, 1983
9. Devereux, R.B. and Reichek, N.: Repolarization abnormalities of left ventricular hypertrophy. Relation of echocardiographic, hemodynamic and electrocardiographic findings, J. Electrocard., 15, 47-53, 1982
10. Chikaos, P.M., Figley, M.M., Fisher, L.: Correlation between chest film and angiographic assessment of left ventricular size, Am. J. Roentgenol., 128, 367-373, 1977
11. Bennett, D.H., Evans, D.W., Raj, M.V.J.: Echocardiographic left ventricular dimensions in pressure and volume overload, Br. Heart J., 37, 971-980, 1975
12. Troy, B.L., Pombo, J., Rackley, C.E.: Measurement of left ventricular wall thickness and mass by echocardiography, Circulation, 45, 602-610, 1972
13. Devereux, R.B. and Reichek, N.: Echocardiographic determination of left ventricular mass in man. Anatomic validation of the method, Circulation, 55, 613-618, 1977
14. Teichholz, L.E., Kreulen, T., Herman, M.V., Gorlin, R.: Problems in echocardiographic volume determinations: Echocardiographic-angiographic correlations in the presence or absence of asynergy, Am. J. Cardiol., 37, 7-11, 1976
15. Devereux, R.B., Pickering, T.G., Laragh, J.H.: Left ventricular mass in hypertension, Lancet, 1, 1021-1022, 1982
16. McFarland, T.M., Alam, M., Goldstein, S., Pickard, S.D., Stein, P.D.: Echocardiographic diagnosis of left ventricular hypertrophy, Circulation, 57, 1140-1144, 1978
17. Ditchey, R.V., Schuler, G., Peterson, K.L.: Reliability of echocardiographic and electrocardiographic parameters in assessing serial changes in left ventricular mass, Am. J. Med., 70, 1042-1050, 1981

18. Reichek, N., Helak, J., Plappert, T., St. John Sutton, M., Weber, K.T.: Anatomic validation of left ventricular mass estimates from clinical two-dimensional echocardiography: initial results, Circulation, 67, 348-352, 1983

19. Devereux, R.B., Savage, D.D., Drayer, J.I.M., Laragh, J.H.: Left ventricular hypertrophy and function in high, normal, and low-renin forms of essential hypertension, Hypertension, 4, 524-531, 1982

20. Devereux, R.B., Savage, D.D., Sachs, I., Laragh, J.H.: Relation of left ventricular hypertrophy and performance to hemodynamic load in hypertension, Am. J. Cardiol., 51, 171-176, 1983

21. Sahn, D.J., DeMaria, A., Kisslo, J., Weyman, A.: The committee on m-mode standardization of the American Society of Echocardiography: Recommendations regarding quantification in m-mode echocardiography: results of a survey of echocardiographic measurements, Circulation, 58, 1072-1081, 1978

22. Devereux, R.B., Alonso, D.R., Gottlieb, G.J.: Echocardiographic left ventricular mass: Comparison to necropsy findings, Clinical Research, (in press) 1983

23. Savage, D.D., Drayer, J.I.M., Henry, W.L., Matthews, E.C. Jr., Ware, J.H., Gardin, J.M., Cohen, E.R., Epstein, S.E., Laragh, J.H.: Echocardiographic assessment of cardiac anatomy and function in hypertensive patients, Circulation, 59, 623-632, 1979

24. Gardin, J.M., Henry, W.L., Savage, D.D., Ware, J.H., Burn, C., Borer, J.S.: Echocardiographic measurements in normal subjects: Evaluation of an adult population without clinically apparent heart disease, J. Clin. Ultrasound, 7, 439-447, 1979

25. Reichek, N. and Devereux, R.B.: Reliable estimation of peak left ventricular systolic pressure by m-mode echographic determined end-diastolic relative wall thickness: Identification of severe valvular aortic stenosis in adult patients, Am. Heart J., 103, 202-209, 1982

26. Devereux, R.B., Pickering, T.G., Harshfield, G.A., Kleinert, H.D., Denby, L., Clark, L., Pregibon, D., Jason, M., Kleiner, B., Borer, J.S., Laragh, J.H.: Left ventricular hypertrophy in patients with hypertension: Importance of blood pressure response to regularly recurring stress, Circulation, 68 (in press), 1983

27. Lutas, E.M., Reis, G., Devereux, R.B., Alderman, M.H., Crowley, J., Sachs, I., Laragh, J.H.: Left ventricular function in hypertensive and normotensive subjects from a natural population, Clinical Research, 30, 336a, 1982

28. Devereux, R.B., Lutas, E.M., Casale, P.N., Kligfield, P., Eisenberg, R.R., Miller, D.H., Reis, G., Alderman, M.H., Laragh, J.H.: Normalization of left ventricular anatomic measurements, Clinical Research, 178a, 1983

29. Devereux, R.B., Casale, P.N., Kligfield, P., Lutas, E.M., Miller, D.H., Reis, G., Alderman, M.H., Laragh, J.H.: Echocardiographic criteria of left ventricular hypertrophy, Clinical Research, 30, 667a, 1982

30. Devereux, R.B., Hammond, I.W., Lutas, E.M., Alderman, M.H., Spitzer, M.C., Laragh, J.H.: Sex difference in left ventricular mass: Relation to lean body mass, Clinical Research, (in press) 1983
31. Devereux, R.B., Savage, D.D., Sachs, I., Laragh, J.H.: Effect of blood pressure control on left ventricular hypertrophy and function in hypertension, Circulation, 62 (suppl. III), III-36, 1980
32. Devereux, R.B., Case, D.B., Cody, R.J., Sachs, I. Laragh, J.H.: Captopril treatment of hypertension increases low but not normal cardiac index, Clinical Research, 29, 356a, 1981
33. Harshfield, G.A., Pickering, T.G., Kleinert, H.D., Blank, S., Laragh, J.H.: Situational variations of blood pressure in hypertensive patients, Psychosomatic Medicine, 44, 237-245, 1982

SUMMARY

Left ventricular structure can be determined and modulated by a variety of clinical and hemodynamic factors. Any prolonged, consistent change in preload, afterload, or contractility will lead to cardiac structural adaptation.

Arterial pressure remains a primary determinant of ventricular hypertrophy. Recent studies, however, showed only a weak correlation between arterial pressure and LV mass. This is partly accounted for by the complex relationship that exists between arterial pressure and wall stress and also by the presence of additional pathogenetic factors. Adrenergic agents have been shown to modulate the process of hypertrophy. Recently, the renin-angiotensin system has been identified as an additional determinant of left ventricular hypertrophy. Angiotensin II could indirectly stimulate hypertrophy by enhancing sympathetic nervous activity or be directly involved in protein synthesis.

Volume overload in pregnancy, anemia, renal failure and, most commonly, obesity is an additional hypertrophogenic factor increasing wall stress by increasing LV chamber volume. The combination of hypertension and obesity is particularly unfavorable for the heart.

Aging in itself appears to be related to increased LV mass even when blood pressure remains in the normotensive range. The mechanism of this effect is not known, but increased aortic input impedance and degenerative changes in the myocardial wall have been implicated.

Race and other hereditary factors determine the extent of hypertrophy. The black population has been shown to be more susceptible to ventricular hypertrophy at the same blood pressure level. Finally, exercise and the level of activity in daily life seem to be independent factors contributing to the process of hypertrophy. The presence or absence of some of these determinants or modulators has direct implications for the assessment of what constitutes a "normal" left ventricular structure and function in a given patient.

DETERMINANTS AND MODULATORS OF LEFT VENTRICULAR STRUCTURE

MESSERLI, F.H.

Alton Ochsner Medical Foundation, 1516 Jefferson Highway, New Orleans, LA 70121, U.S.A.

INTRODUCTION

"The course of any case of cardiac hypertrophy may be divided into three stages: a) the period of development which varies with the nature of the primary lesion, b) the period of full compensation – the latent stage – during which the heart's vigor meets the requirement of the circulation, and c) the period of broken compensation" (Sir William Osler, M.D.).[1]

Although this description of the pathogenesis of cardiac hypertrophy was published almost a century ago (long before blood pressure was measured in clinical practice), its usefulness has not come of age despite the explosion of knowledge of left ventricular hypertrophy (LVH) occurring over the past two decades. LVH can be defined as an increase in contractile myocardial mass as determined by electrocardiographic or echocardiographic arbitrarily set criteria. It is most commonly caused by a chronically increased afterload such as occurs in arterial hypertension, but it can be idiopathic, result from an increased preload, or represent the adaptation to several of these pathogenetic factors.

In a given patient, usually a single principal incriminating mechanism responsible for cardiac hypertrophy can be identified, but other mechanisms have at least modifying influences. This article reviews a variety of clinical and hemodynamic factors that are known to influence cardiac adaptation to a hypertrophogenic factor (figure 1).

ARTERIAL PRESSURE

Concentric LVH represents the fundamental response of the left ventricle to a chronically increased afterload.[2-9] One might, therefore, suppose that the relationship between arterial pressure and left ventricular mass would be a close one. Indeed, early autopsy studies showed a close cor-

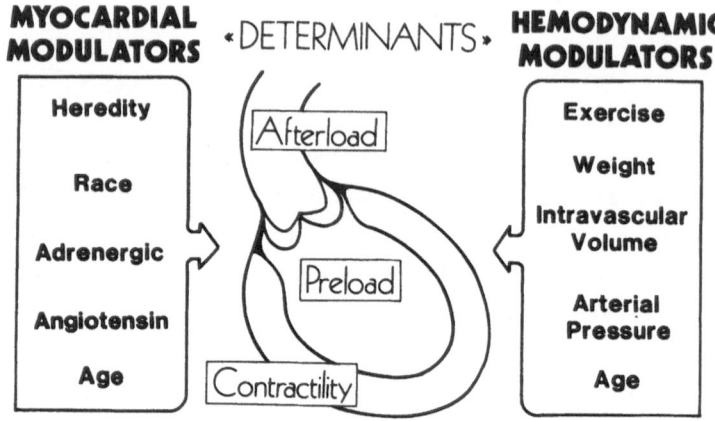

MYOCARDIAL MODULATORS ‹DETERMINANTS› **HEMODYNAMIC MODULATORS**

Heredity	Afterload	Exercise
Race		Weight
Adrenergic	Preload	Intravascular Volume
Angiotensin		Arterial Pressure
Age	Contractility	Age

Figure 1. Determinants and modulators of LVH.

relation between systolic blood pressure and left ventricular mass.[10,11] More recently, echo- and electrocardiographic comparisons indicated a greater scatter between arterial pressure and LV mass.[2,9,12] This is not surprising since arterial pressure levels alone cannot adequately reflect cardiac pressure load.[13] Left ventricular wall stress or aortic impedance might reveal a closer correlation with LV mass.[13-15] Also, it is unlikely that spot blood pressure measurements only would closely correlate with the degree of LVH. Indeed, recent studies have indicated that integrated blood pressure measurements over several hours would provide a better correlation with LV mass than casual measurements.[16,17]

However, even after accounting for inaccuracies of measuring pressure load to the left ventricle, distinctive discrepancies between arterial pressure load and structural adaptation of the left heart persist. As experimental studies have shown, cardiac response to different types of hypertension is not homogeneous.[18,19] Additional pathogenetic factors clearly seem to influence LV structural adaptation.

As Osler points out, LVH appears to be an adaptative process which is well tolerated and clinically silent particularly in its early stages.[1] Cardiac adaptation to a pressure load can be demonstrated echocardiographically in children even before arterial pressure reaches a level that is regarded as abnormal in adults.[20] Initially, the patient may remain asymptomatic, although careful evaluation would detect impaired coronary and ventricular functional reserve[21,22] as well as increased ventricular ectopic activity.[23] No cardiac signs or symptoms can be detected as long as myocardial mass remains below a certain specific level (despite progressive LVH). However, once myocardial mass exceeds this "critical mass", evidence of hypertensive heart disease begins to appear.[24] Unfortunately, this "critical mass" (figure 2) does not cor-

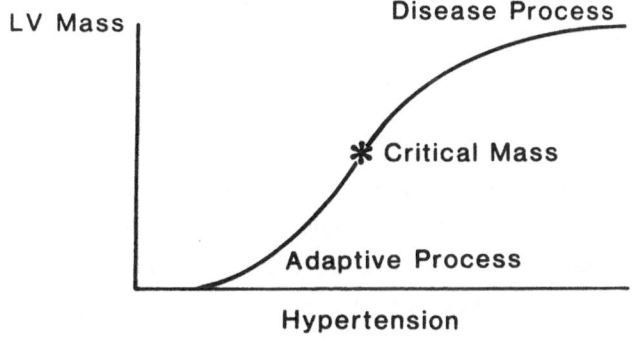

Figure 2. Hypothetical relationship between left ventricular mass and severity of hypertension. (Reprinted with permission from Messerli, F.H., Devereux, R.B.: Left ventricular hypertrophy: Good or evil?, Am. J. Med., in press, 1983)

respond to any established criteria for left ventricular hypertrophy - either electrocardiographic (i.e. Sokoloff or Romhilt Estes point score) or echocardiographic (i.e. posterior wall thickness exceeding 1.1 cm).

Late in the course of stage 2 ("full compensation"), hypertensive heart disease may become symptomatic because of progressive coronary heart disease and ventricular arrhythmias. Eventually, in stage 3 ("broken compensation") congestive heart failure will ensue.

THE ADRENERGIC NERVOUS SYSTEM

The importance of catecholamines in the development of left ventricular hypertrophy was initially suggested by Raab[25] more than three decades ago. Recent work from the Cleveland Clinic has confirmed that adrenergic stimuli or antiadrenergic agents modulate cardiac adaptation to a given pressure load.[26] Left ventricular hypertrophy developed after chronic norepinephrine infusion in rats despite the fact that they were kept normotensive by concomitant alpha-adrenergic blockade.[27] On the other hand, when cardiac beta-adrenergic receptors were blocked, norepinephrine infusion resulted in significantly less hypertrophy even though blood pressure distinctly increased.[27] These elegant experimental data underline the importance of the beta receptor stimulation as a permissive factor in the development of left ventricular hypertrophy. By the same token, antiadrenergic therapy has been shown to be associated with the reduction of left ventricular hypertrophy even in the absence of complete blood pressure control.[28]

THE RENIN ANGIOTENSIN SYSTEM

Converting enzyme inhibition reduces left ventricular mass in some patients with essential hypertension[29,30] as well as in rats with spontaneous or renovascular hypertension without affecting myocardial catecholamine concentration.[31] This identified the renin angiotensin system as another determinant of left ventricular hypertrophy. Angiotensin II could indirectly stimulate the sympathetic nervous system or alternatively be involved in protein synthesis within the myocardial cell.[32]

EXPANDED INTRAVASCULAR VOLUME

Conditions with volume overload such as pregnancy,[33,34] anemia,[35] renal failure,[36,37] and most commonly, obesity,[38] result in a special form of LV adaptation. A high circulating blood volume is associated with an expanded stroke volume, presenting an elevated preload to the left ventricle.[39] An increment in preload results in an LV adaptation that initially consists of an increase in LV chamber volume.[38] According to LaPlace's Law, the wall stress increases in parallel with the diameter. Increased wall stress represents a stimulus for the development of LVH. In hypertension the relative wall thickness distinctly increases, where-as, in contrast, in obesity (and other volume overload states), the radius to wall thickness ratio remains unchanged[40] producing eccentric left ventricular hypertrophy. The combination of hypertension and obesity is particularly unfavorable for the heart (figure 3).

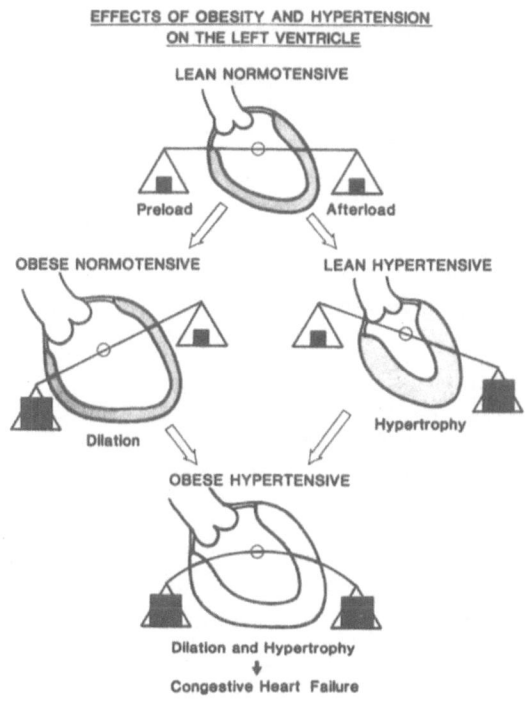

Figure 3. (Reprinted with permission from Messerli, F.H., Lancet, 1, 1166, 1982)

Arterial hypertension increases LV stroke work by an increase in systolic pressure, whereas obesity does so by an increase in stroke volume. The combination of the two evils takes a heavy toll of the left ventricle and commonly leads to premature congestive failure.[41,42]

AGING

Left ventricular posterior wall thickness has been documented to increase with progressive aging even when blood pressure remains in the normotensive range.[43-45] At the same time, no significant chamber enlargement has been found. Gerstenblith et al. reported a positive correlation between LV wall thickness and age in a population free of cardiovascular disease.[44] We recently confirmed the influence of age as a determinant of LV structure in a multivariate analysis in a heterogeneous population of 158 patients. An increase in afterloads such as produced by the presence of arterial hypertension will greatly accelerate this "physiologic" hypertrophy of aging (figure 4).

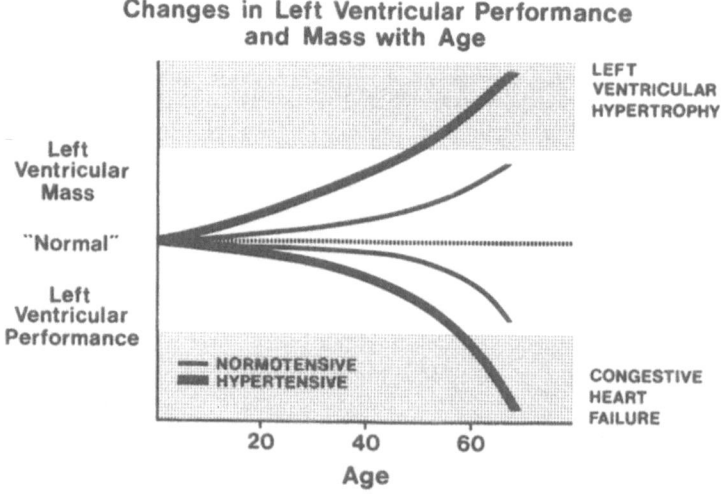

Figure 4. (Reprinted with permission from Messerli, F.H.: Clinical determinants and consequences of left ventricular hypertrophy, <u>Am. J. Med.</u>, in press, 1983)

Several factors could contribute to the LV changes that occur with age in healthy elderly subjects. First, arterial pressure increases throughout life even within the normotensive limits and therefore remains a major determinant of LV wall thickness. Second, changes in peripheral resistance as well as in arterial compliance will increase aortic input impedance regardless of the level of arterial pressure. Third, as occurs with other organs, functioning tissue is gradually replaced by inactive tissue, thereby stimulating the remaining contractile muscle cells to hypertrophy. Moreover, subclinical degenerative disorders such as amyloidosis, hemochromatosis, etc., could further contribute to the thickening of the left ventricle. Although these age-dependent changes only increase LV wall thickness by about 25 percent over five decades, they have to be taken into account when defining "normal" or "abnormal" LV structure.

RACE AND FURTHER HEREDITARY FACTORS

A genetic predisposition to develop cardiac hypertrophy and vascular changes in the presence of minimal pressure elevation has been documented experimentally.[45-47] Similarly, a strong family history of essential hypertension could conceivably facilitate the development of cardiovascular changes at pressure loads that are marginally elevated or that are elevated only for a relatively short period of time. We have recently found that some teenagers who had only borderline hypertension had significantly increased LV wall thickness and mass as well as increased relative wall thickness.[20] However, these studies do not clearly dissociate cause from mechanism. Black patients seem to have more cardiac involvement at similar levels of arterial pressure than white patients.[48,49] Thus, a greater increase in voltages on the electrocardiogram, and rate of cardiac enlargement on chest x-ray have been documented in blacks than in whites after adjusting for age and arterial pressure.[49] However, black and white patients have been found to have similar systemic hemodynamics (with the exception of heart rate, renal blood flow and renal vascular resistance).[50] Recent data from our laboratories have demonstrated a higher left ventricular mass in black patients that were matched with regard to mean arterial pressure, sex, and age with white patients. The adaptative process of the left ventricle may reach a pathologic stage earlier in black patients than in white patients.

EXERCISE

Endurance exercise such as running, bicycling, and swimming has been found to produce LV chamber enlargement.[53] Several studies have shown an increase in left ventricular chamber volume of about ten percent, and wall thickness occasionally also increases by about one millimeter.[53-55]

Repeated isometric exercise has been shown to increase relative LV wall thickness, and it seems to affect the septum more than the posterior wall.[53,56] A wall thickness ratio of about 1.3 mimicking hypertrophic cardiomyopathy has been documented in weight lifters.[53,56]

The question that comes to mind is whether such cardiac adaptation to exercise would be beneficial or detrimental for the patient. Scheuer et al.[56] (figure 5) have recently studied the combined effects of cardiac overload imposed by arterial hypertension and exercise in an 8- to 10-week swimming program in male and female rats. Not surprisingly,

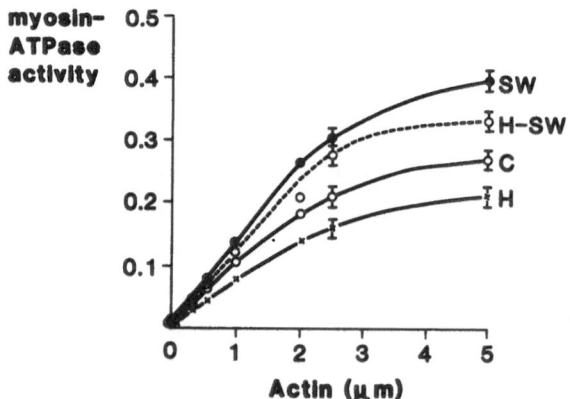

Figure 5. Actin-activated Mg^{2+}-myosin ATPase activity as a function of actin concentration. Results are mean $+SE$ of four samples. C = control, SW = swimmer, H = hypertensive, H-SW = hypertensive swimmer. (Modified with permission from Scheuer et al., J. Clin. Invest., 70, 1303, 1982)

they found hypertension to be associated with the development of cardiac hypertrophy which was more pronounced in hypertensive swimmers. In contrast, cardiac contractile protein ATPase activities were enhanced in normotensive swimmers and depressed in hypertensive sedentary animals and normal to increased in hypertensive swimmers. Myocardial contractility has been shown to parallel, in general, the myosin ATPase activity. Despite the fact that LVH is exaggerated by superimposed physical training, the decrease in myocardial contractility accompanying pathologic hypertrophy might be improved by regular physical training.

REFERENCES

1. Osler, W.: The Principles and Practice of Medicine, New York, D. Appleton & Co., 1982
2. Gaasch, W.H.: Left ventricular radius to wall thickness ratio, Am. J. Cardiol., 43, 1189-1194, 1979
3. Dunn, F.G., Chandraratna, P., deCarvalho, J.G.R., Basta, L.L., Frohlich, E.D.: Pathophysiologic assessment of hypertensive heart disease with echocardiography, Am. J. Cardiol., 39, 789-795, 1977
4. Savage, D.D., Drayer, J.I.M., Henry, W.L., Mathews, E.C. Jr., Ware, J.H., Gardin, J.M., Cohen, E.R., Epstein, S.E., Laragh, J.H.: Echocardiographic assessment of cardiac anatomy and function in hypertensive patients, Circulation, 59, 623-632, 1979
5. Cohen, A., Hagan, A.D., Watkins, J., Mitas, J., Schvartzman, M., Mazzoleni, A., Cohen, I.M., Warren, S.E., Vieiveg, W.V.R.: Clinical correlates in hypertensive patients with left ventricular hypertrophy disguised with echocardiography, Am. J. Cardiol., 47, 335-341, 1981
6. Schlant, R.C., Felner, J.M., Blumenstein, B.A., Heymofield, S., Gilbert, C.A., Shulman, N., Tuttle, E.P.: Echocardiographic studies of left ventricular anatomy and function before and after treatment of essential hypertension, Am. J. Cardiol., 39, 296, 1977 (abstract)
7. Devereux, R.B., Reichek, N.: Left ventricular hypertrophy, Cardiovasc. Rev. Rep., 1, 55-68, 1980
8. Rowlands, D.B., Glover, D.R., Ireland, M.A., McLeay, R.A.B., Stallard, T.J., Watson, R.D.S., Littler, W.A.: Assessment of left ventricular mass and its response to antihypertensive treatment, Lancet, 1, 467-470, 1982
9. Messerli, F.H., Sundgaard-Riise, K., Ventura, H., Dunn, F.G., Oigman, W., Frohlich, E.D.: Clinical and hemodynamic determinants of left ventricular hypertrophy, Arch. Intern. Med. (in press), 1983
10. Evans, G.: a contribution to the study of arteriosclerosis, with special reference to its relation to chronic disease, Quart. J. Med., 14, 215-282, 1921
11. Linzberg, A.J.: Hypertrophy, hyperplasia and structural dilatation of the human heart, Adv. Cardiol., 18, 1-14, 1976
12. Devereux, R.B., Savage, D.D., Sachs, I., Laragh, J.H.: Relation of hemodynamic load to left ventricular hypertrophy and performance in hypertension, Am. J. Cardiol., 51, 171-176, 1983

13. Tarazi, R.C., Levy, M.N.: Cardiac response to increased afterload, Hypertension, 4 (suppl. II), II-8 - II-18, 1982
14. Grossman, W., Jones, D., McLaurin, L.P.: Wall stress and patterns of hypertrophy in human left ventricle, J. Clin. Invest., 56, 56-64, 1975
15. Milnor, W.R.: Arterial impedance as ventricular afterload, Circ. Res., 36, 565-569, 1975
16. Devereux, R.B., Pickering, T.G., Harshfield, G.A., Sachs, I., Jason, M., Kleinert, J.D., Laragh, J.H.: Relation of hypertensive left ventricular hypertrophy to 24-hour blood pressure, Circulation, 64, (suppl. IV), IV-321, 1981 (abstract)
17. Drayer, J.I.M., Weber, M.A., DeYoung, J.L.: BP as a determinant of cardiac left ventricular mass, Arch. Intern. Med., 143, 90-92, 1983
18. Sen, S., Tarazi, R.C., Khairallah, P.A., Bumpus, F.M.: Cardiac hypertrophy in spontaneously hypertensive rats, Circ. Res., 35, 775-781, 1974
19. Sen, S., Tarazi, R.C., Bumpus, F.M.: Reversal of cardiac hypertrophy in renal hypertensive rats: medical vs. surgical therapy, Am. J. Physiol., 240, H409-H412, 1981
20. Culpepper, W.S. III, Sodt, P.C., Messerli, F.H., Ruschhaupt, D.G., Arcilla, R.A.: Cardiac status in juvenile borderline hypertension, Ann. Intern. Med., 98, 1-7, 1983
21. Strauer, B.E.: Hypertensive Heart Disease, New York, Bohn, Heidelberg, Springer-Verlag, 26, 1980
22. Marcus, M.L.: Left ventricular hypertrophy and coronary heart disease, Am. J. Med. (in press), 1983
23. Messerli, F.H., Glade, L.B., Elizardi, E.G., Dreslinski, G.R., Dunn, F.G., Frohlich, E.D.: Cardiac rhythm, arterial pressure, and urinary catecholamines in hypertension with and without left ventricular hypertrophy, Am. J. Cardiol., 47, 480, 1981 (abstract)
24. Messerli, F.H., Devereux, R.B.: Left ventricular hypertrophy: Good or evil?, Am. J. Med. (in press), 1983
25. Raab, W.: Hormonal & Neurogenic Cardiovascular Disorders, William & Wilkins Co., Baltimore, 1953
26. Sen, S.: Regression of cardiac hypertrophy: Experimental animal model. Symposium on left ventricular hypertrophy, Am. J. Med. (in press), 1983
27. Yamori, Y., Tarazi, R.C., Ooshima, A.: Effect of -receptor-blocking agents on cardiovascular structural changes in spontaneous and nonadrenaline-induced hypertension in rats, Clin. Sci., 59, 457s-460s, 1981
28. Fouad, F.M., Nakashima, Y., Tarazi, R.C., Salcedo, E.E.: Reversal of left ventricular hypertrophy with methyldopa, Am. J. Cardiol., 49, 795-801, 1982
29. Nakashima, Y., Fouad, F.M., Tarazi, R.C., Bravo, E.L.: Left ventricular function with reversal of left ventricular hypertrophy in hypertensive patients, J. Am. Coll. Cardiol., 1, 598, 1983 (abstract)
30. Dunn, F.G., Oigman, W., Ventura, H., Kobrin, I., Messerli, F.H., Frohlich, E.D.: Enalapril improves systemic and renal hemodynamics and regresses left ventricular mass in essential hypertension, J. Am. Coll. Cardiol., 1, 611, 1983

31. Sen, S., Tarazi, R.C., Bumpus, F.M.: Effect of converting enzyme inhibitor (SQ 14225) on myocardial hypertrophy in spontaneously hypertensive rats, Hypertension, 2, 169-176, 1980

32. Khairallah, P.A., Kanabus, J.: Angiotensin and myocardial protein synthesis. In: Cardiac Hypertrophy in Hypertension: An NHBI Symposium, edited by R.C. Tarazi and J.B. Dunbar, Raven Press, New York, 1983 (in press)

33. Katz, R., Karliner, J.S., Resnik, R.: Effects of a natural volume overload state (pregnancy) on left ventricular performance in normal human subjects, Circulation, 58, 434-441, 1978

34. Larkin, H., Gallery, E.D.M., Hunyor, S.N., Gyory, A.Z., Boyce, E.S.: Haemodynamics of hypertension in pregnancy assessed by M-mode echocardiography, Clin. Exper. Pharmacol., 7, 463-468, 1980

35. Gerry, J.L., Baird, M.G., Fortuin, N.J.: Evaluation of left ventricular function in patients with sickle cell anemia, Am. J. Med., 60, 968-972, 1976

36. Scharf, S., Wexler, J., Longnecker, R.E., Blaufox, M.D.: Cardiovascular disease in patients on chronic hemodialytic therapy, Prog. Cardiovasc. Dis., 22, 343-356, 1980

37. Ikaheimo, M., Linnaluoto, M., Huttunen, K., Takkunen, J.: Effects of renal transplantation on left ventricular size and function, Br. Heart J., 47, 155-160, 1982

38. Messerli, F.H.: Cardiovascular effects of obesity and hypertension, Lancet, 1, 1165-1168, 1982

39. Messerli, F.H., Sundgaard-Riise, K., Reisin, E., Dreslinski, G.H., Dunn, F.G., Frohlich, E.D.: Disparate cardiovascular effects of obesity and arterial hypertension, Am. J. Med., 74, 808-812, 1983

40. Messerli, F.H., Sundgaard-Riise, K., Reisin, E., Dunn, F.G., Dreslinski, G.R., Ventura, H., Oigman, W., Frohlich, E.D.: Left ventricular adaptation to obesity, Am. J. Cardiol., 49, 977, 1982

41. Gordon, T., Kannel, W.B.: Obesity and cardiovascular disease: the Framingham study, Clin. Endocrinol. Metab., 5, 367-374, 1976

42. Alexander, J., Pettigrove, J.R.: Obesity and congestive heart failure, Geriatrics, 22, 101-106, 1967

43. Lakatta, E.G.: Alterations in the cardiovascular system that occur in advanced age, Fed. Proc., 38, 163-167, 1979

44. Gerstenblith, G., Weisfeldt, M.L., Lakatta, E.G.: Age changes in myocardial function and exercise response, Prog. Cardiovasc. Dis., 19, 1-21, 1976

45. Hallback, M.: Interaction between central neurogenic mechanisms and changes in cardiovascular design in primary hypertension. Experimental studies in spontaneously hypertensive rats, Acta Physiol. Scand. (suppl. 424), 5-29, 1975

46. Weiss, L., Lundgren, Y.: Chronic antihypertensive drug treatment in young spontaneously hypertensive rats: Effects on arterial blood pressures, cardiovascular reactivity and vascular design, Cardiovascular Res., 35, 775-781, 1974

47. Cutilletta, A.G., Benjamin, M., Culpepper, W.S., Oparil, S.: Myocardial hypertrophy and ventricular performance in the absence of hypertension in spontaneously hypertensive rats, J. Mol. Cell. Cardiol., 10, 689-703, 1978

48. Gillum, R.F.: Pathophysiology of hypertension in blacks and whites. A review of the basis of racial blood pressure differences, Hypertension, 1, 468-475, 1979

49. McDonough, J.R., Garrison, G.E., Hames, C.G.: Blood pressure and hypertensive disease among negroes and whites, Ann. Intern. Med., 61, 208-228, 1964
50. Messerli, F.H., DeCarvalho, J.G., Christie, B., Frohlich, E.D.: Essential hypertension in black and white subjects. Hemodynamic findings and fluid volume state, Am. J. Med., 67, 27-31, 1979
51. Dunn, F.G., Oigman, W., Sundgaard-Riise, K., Messerli, F.H., Ventura, H., Reisin, E., Frohlich, E.D.: Racial differences in cardiac adaptation to essential hypertension determined by echocardiographic indexes, Am. J. Cardiol., 1, 1348-1351, 1983
52. Morganroth, J., Maron, B.G., Henry, W.L., Epstein, S.E.: Comparative left ventricular dimensions in trained athletes, Ann. Intern. Med., 82, 521-524, 1975
53. DeMaria, A.N., Neumann, A., Lee, G., Fowler, W., Mason, D.T.: Alterations in ventricular mass and performance induced by exercise training in man evaluated by echocardiography, Circulation, 57, 237-244, 1978
54. Adams, T.D., Yanowitz, F.G., Fisher, A.G., Ridges, J.D., Lovell, K., Pryor, T.A.: Noninvasive evaluation of exercise training on college-age men, Circulation, 64, 958-965, 1981
55. Menapace, F.J., Hammer, W.J., Ritzer, T.F., Kessler, K.M., Warner, H.F., Spann, J.F., Bove, A.: Left ventricular size in competitive weight lifters: An echocardiographic study, Med. Sci. Sports Exercise, 14, 72-75, 1982
56. Scheuer, J., Maltrotra, A., Hirsch, C., Capasso, J., Schaible, F.T.: Physiologic cardiac hypertrophy corrects contractile protein abnormalities associated with pathologic hypertrophy in the rat, J. Clin. Invest., 70, 1300-1305, 1982

SECTION 2

ETIOLOGY AND FUNCTIONAL ASPECTS AT THE CELLULAR LEVEL

52

SUMMARY

The fundamental relation between myocardial work conditions and ener-
getics can be expressed as:

$$E = A + f(P,t) + \alpha.\overline{\Delta L} + W \qquad (1)$$

in which E is energy; A is energy involved in activation; f(P,t) is
energy that is a function of force and of time of its maintenance;
$\alpha.\overline{\Delta L}$ is that which is liberated in proportion to the shortening distance
$\overline{\Delta L}$; and W that which is turned into actual work.

Different contraction modes, in which the various terms of eq. (1) are
brought out at different levels of energy usage per cycle, lead to
different degrees of phosphorylation of at least one example of a meta-
bolic control protein, glycogen phosphorylase. The activation of phos-
phorylase appeared strictly proportional to the energy per contraction
cycle. Analysis of possible metabolic regulators suggests that only the
varying amount of calcium liberated during excitation-contraction coup-
ling at varied work load can account for control of phosphorylation of
glycogen phosphorylase b and other Ca^{++}-stimulated processes.

One consequence of this conclusion, directly applicable to hypertrophy,
is that calcium may control biochemical mechanisms for protein synthesis
presumably at the level of DNA-transcription. An important precedent was
recently set by Murdoch, Rosenfeld and Evans (1982), who found that
cyclic AMP stimulates the expression of the prolactin gene in cultured
pituitary cells by inducing phosphorylation of the chromatin-associated
basic protein. It is plausible that calcium modulates the cyclic AMP-in-
duced protein kinase that stimulates gene expression as well. It must be
emphasized that protein phosphorylase regulation varies from enzyme to
enzyme so that extrapolation of observations should be done with cau-
tion. This is also evident from the fact that myosin synthesis in
cardiac hypertrophy involves synthesis with a different preference for
isoforms of this protein. Thus, in hypertrophy we are not only dealing
with the total extent of protein synthesis but also with yet subtler
choices between the transcriptions for closely similar genes.
From these observations a general pathway for the control of cardiac
growth emerges in which calcium and cyclic AMP are involved in aspects
of DNA-transcription and synthesis, and this may provide the link
between cardiac work and growth.

RELATIONSHIP BETWEEN CARDIAC WORK AND CARDIAC GROWTH:
SOME GENERAL THOUGHTS ON CARDIAC HYPERTROPHY

MOMMAERTS, W.F.H.M.

Department of Physiology and Heart Association Cardiovascular Research Laboratory, The University of California, Los Angeles

INTRODUCTION

This presentation has a double title. The first one was suggested by the Organizing Committee, the second was my own addition. They both address the same problem. The former states the question explicity, the second serves as a reminder that the literature is too vast and too hetero-geneous, as well as uneven, to be reviewed in its entirety, and that there is a need for an attempt to bring out the several diverse princi-ples of general portent, and in their natural connections.

It is difficult to detach the question of the relationship between cardiac work and hypertrophy from that between cardiac work and metab-olism. After important early approaches to the latter especially by Starling[1] and Lovatt Evans[2], this problem appeared to have settled down a quarter century ago after a set of investigations from the laboratory of Stanley Sarnoff[3]. The methodology, notably including improved surgical and support techniques, seemed to have reached a definitive level, and no changes seemed to be expected in the conclusion that 'pressure work' showed a far greater demand upon the O_2-consumption associated with it than did 'volume work'. This conclusion was comforting because, on the chronic scale, cardiac hypertrophy suggested the same relation to cardiac work in its two indicated forms, at least with respect to the thickness of the ventricular wall. We all lived comfortably with this until the recent work by my young colleague, Dr. Jacob Vinten-Johansen[4,5], showed a dependence of the O_2-consumption primarily upon cardiac work no matter in what form. This is not the place to discuss the differences between the newer and the older work: it may be a matter of yet further refined techniques, or both may have their own ranges of validity and thus may not be in factual conflict, once all experimental factors are fully understood. At the same time, none may be completely right because metabolism, and also hypertrophy, may not just depend on one factor only. This contrast is actually indicated by the results of the myothermal and biochemical investigations which have occupied us since about 1951. These have been summarized[6] by the four-term equation:

$$E = A + f(P,t) + \alpha.\bar{\Delta}L + W \qquad \text{eq. (1)}$$

in which E is the energy in thermal or other units; A is the energy involved in the activation, _i.e._, excitation-contraction coupling; $f(P,t)$ indicates that which is a function of the force generated and of the time of its maintenance; $\alpha.\bar{\Delta}L$ that which is liberated in proportion to the shortening distance, $\bar{\Delta}L$; and W that which is turned into actual work. This is a phenomenologic equation in which some of the terms may be interdependent.

For a favorable object (i.e., the frog sartorius or semitendinosus muscle), it has taken us several decades to establish and validate the equation by both myothermal and biochemical studies. Although there may be experimental transients during which out-of-phase processes may seemingly suggest unaccounted energies, we can now say that all the terms in the four-term model derive in the balance directly from the splitting of ATP, indirectly of PC, and ultimately from the energy of metabolism.

A difficulty has been that, even if A is relatively constant, the other terms vary independently of one another. In cardiac muscle, there are additional complications, notably that A is much more variable due to the principle of variable excitation-contraction coupling which was discovered as the result of another set of our investigations[7]. No equivalent formula can hence be documented for cardiac contraction, though the work started with us by Gibbs[8,9], supports the notion that the same general principles apply to cardiac activity as well. Thus, to return to our initial dilemma, one would conclude that cardiac metabolism depends on contractile activity in some adherence to the equation, even if one may be able to stage the experiments so as to bring out one factor in particular. We will rest the case at this point, but keep it in mind when facing the question how, in order to determine normal or enhanced growth, the cardiac tissue contains information about its energy turnover in such a way that this becomes translated into a regulation with respect to biosynthetic activity.

To introduce the latter concept, let me refer to our early work with Kölbel[10] in which we showed that the induction of left ventricular hypertrophy by aortic constriction in rats involves an increase in both

the amount of ribosomes, and their translational activity in terms of
their synthesis of podyphenylalanine under the direction of the artificial messenger, polyuridylate. This our early work, which seems to be the
first attempt to connect cardiac hypertrophy to isolated molecular
mechanisms, had a peculiarity which deserves to be recalled: the control
operation, in which all aspects of the surgery were identically performed
but for the actual closure of the aortic constriction ring, showed large
blank increases, not only in the heart but also in the liver. One would
tentatively ascribe this to the surge in growth hormone production in
response to the surgical trauma. The effect necessitates appropriate
control experiments. The current work by Markert et al. on a humoral
factor involved in the induction of hypertrophy is of interest in suggesting participation of as yet unidentified growth substances[11,12],
translating the instant information regarding metabolic determinants into
enhanced growth.

Since the time of our early inquiry, vastly more has become known about
the mechafisms of gene expression and protein synthesis. Indeed, this has
become one of the principal scenes of present-day scientific endeavor.
We shall have to relate the problem of cardiac hypertrophy to the problem
of what factors determine organ size in general, and to the molecular
mechanisms executing those controls in terms of regulated protein synthesis. Nor is it certain that the mechanisms are uniformly the same for all
aspects of cardiac growth. For example, it is held that ventricular
hypertrophy is a matter of increased transcription of a constant amount
of DNA[13] but atrial hypertrophy one of increased DNA synthesis[14].

One important partial aspect of molecular-biological inquiry is that
dealing with regulatory proteins which control the occurrence of metabolic reaction by means of the phosphorylation of key-enzymes, the
activity of which is sensitive to such phosphorylation or its reversal.
The original discovery with respect to muscle was that of the distinction
between the inactive (b) and the active (a) forms of glycogen phosphorylase[15], carried out by a Ca^{++}-activated phosphorylase kinase[16], which in
turn is transformed by phosphorylation from a low into a high activity
form by another protein kinase which requires cyclic-AMP[17]. You will all
be aware of the tremendous amplification which followed upon Sutherland's
discovery of cyclic AMP[18], which led to the recognition of many such
cascades of protein kinases, with Ca^{++} and cyclic nucleotides as frequent

activators, and of protein phosphatases with the opposite effects, which enter into well-nigh all functional and enzymatic regulatory systems; each example has its own peculiarities leading to such a multitude of biological effects. Of all these, the regulation of glycogen phosphorylase is and remains the prototype.

Therefore, when I attempted to explore whether such cascade systems might be regulated in parallel with the energy output of muscles, it seemed natural to resort to the use of glycogen phosphorylase activation as a model system, not only for reasons of historical perspective, but also since any connections to be uncovered might be expected to relate rather directly to questions of metabolic control[19].

The experimental system was as follows: thoroughly rested frog muscles, in which the phosphorylase-a content was undetectably low, were given 40 brief tetanic contractions, and the resulting formation of phosphorylase-a was assayed. This phosphorylative activation was found to occur at a constant level of phosphorylase kinase, hence this process did not depend on a stimulatory contribution on the part of cyclic AMP; although, the prevalent level of the kinase could be measurably decreased by prolonged treatment with guanethidine prior to the experiment, as a reminder of the widely applicable rule of the adrenergic origin of activation by cyclic AMP. The muscles were randomly grouped in four categories with respect to the conditions of contraction, of which the energy turnovers per cycle were measured myothermally. These levels corresponded to about 1, 2, 3 and 3.5 mcals per gram muscle. These different values were obtained, respectively, by (i) stimulation of muscles stretched to mean sarcomere lengths beyond I- and A-filament interdigitation, thus displaying essentially the factor A in the four-component equation; (ii) isotonic contractions of very lightly loaded muscles, essentially yielding $A + \alpha . \Delta L$, and thus corresponding to 'volume work' in the cardiological sense; (iii) isometric contractions at standard length, expressing $A + f(P,t)$; and (iv) isotonic contractions at an optimal load for giving maximal isotonic work, thus involving a maximal isotonic combination of $A + f(P,t) + \alpha . \Delta L + W$, and perhaps corresponding to what would be typical 'pressure work'. It was found that the ensuing phosphorylase-phosphorylation was strictly proportional to the energy turnover per cycle (figure 1).

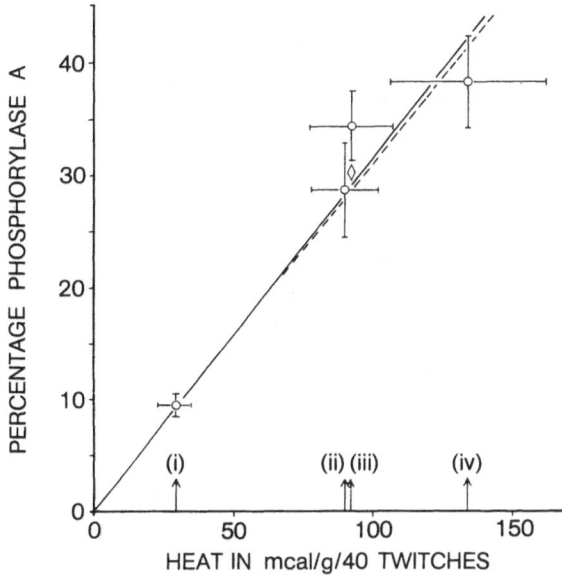

Figure 1: The linear regression between the energy turnover per cycle (abscissa) and the per cent phosphorylase-a activation (ordinate).

No explanation was explicitly given at the time, because this seemed premature. We knew then of no metabolic products, say ADP transients for the sake of argument, which could be contributory activators for any of the reaction steps involved (actually only one, the action of the phosphorylase kinase present). In the meantime, a large number of such substrates, products, or intermediary regulators have been discovered, fructose-2,6-(bis)phosphate being latest[20,21]. None of these substances can explain the findings. Thus, eight years after the original work, we can say that to the best of our knowledge, no such activators occur under the circumstances. We revert, therefore, more convincingly now to the one mechanism considered in the original paper: the pulsatile activation of phosphorylase-kinase by Ca^{++} ions passingly released in each excitation-contraction cycle in response to stimulation. But the consequence, or the prerequisite rather, is then that these Ca^{++} pulses vary in their magnitude and/or their persistences, in correlation with the contraction parameters which determine the magnitudes of the four terms in the equation.

This seemed a strange thought, at first. It is not, of course, an infraction of the all-or%none principle, this allows modification of the responses under the influence of functional determinants. But no mechanism was discernible at the time. Now, however, the first precedent-setting examples are beginning to appear.

I refer, first of all, to a study by Allen and Kurihara[22] which appeared just in time to support my contention (which also has vast implications for the energetics of contraction and the foundations of eq. (1), but that point will not be pursued on this occasion). These authors assessed the magnitude of the calcium burst upon stimulation of mammalian cardiac muscle fibers which were injected with aequorin, a Ca^{++}-sensitive photoemitter protein. Upon an imposed and maintained stretch, the active contractile tension increased instantly in consequence of the length-tension diagram, but then continued to increase slowly[23], reminiscent perhaps, though slower, of the oft forgotten Anrep effect[24]. The peaks of the Ca^{++}-pulses likewise increased slowly, in parallel with the slow rise in contractile strength. This was not, perhaps, surprising; indeed, effects of this sort had been surmised for some time, if discretely, by workers in the field. The second finding, however, was that when a quick-release was allowed during a contraction, an immediate increase in detectable Ca^{++}-concentration was observed. The authors concluded that their observations can 'be explained if the binding constant of troponin for calcium is a function of developed tension'. The latter assumption has a basis in earlier work by Bremel and Weber[25] on myosin-actin-troponin systems in vitro, when rigor-links were induced to be formed by removal of the ATP; whereas Fabiato and Fabiato[26] and Hibberd and Jewell[27] found that an increased sarcomere spacing causes an alteration in the pCa^{++}-tension relation. Recent work by Ter Keurs et al.[28] also bears upon this question.

Following the quoted work by Bremel and Weber[25], the molecular basis of the effects has been studied especially by Fuchs[29-31]. Briefly, the results are as follows: isolated troponin-C has four binding sites for Ca^{++}. In a glycerol and detergent-extracted muscle fiber preparation, only three binding sites are available when the sarcomeres are stretched beyond A- and I-filament overlap; the three isolated binding sites are non-interacting. All four become accessible at maximal filament interdigitation. At that point, also, the affinities change in such a way as to suggest the appearance of cooperativity. Isolation of force development as a separate detereinant leads to additional questions, which are still in flux. See also recent abstracts by Fuchs and Planchak[32] and Solaro and Rocklin[33].

While the details of the newly emerging viewpoint cannot yet be perceived, let us discuss one among possible connections. The primary purpose of the calcium cycle is to release this ion from the sarcoreticulum to combine with troponin-C, thus relieving the troponin-tropomyosin inhibition of the contractile apparatus. If the fact of shortening has such conformational connotations as to change the Ca^{++} binding by troponin-C, more or less Ca^{++} would at constant release be available to activate the phosphorylase kinase. Mechanisms such as these may be expected to yield an explanation. Whatever the mechanism, our experimental findings on phosphorylase activation set the precedent of demonstrating the possibility that regulatory protein phosphorylations can be elicited by factors that are proportional to the energy flux. In this case, variable availability of Ca^{++} presumably constitutes the mechanism; in others, cyclic nucleotides may amplify the possibilities.

Can this thought be extended to processes related not to acute metabolic control, but to the regulation of protein synthesis? Ionic influences upon DNA synthesis are already becoming clearly indicated. As to DNA transcription, a precedent seems to be offered by the phenomenon of catabolite repression by glucose in coli bacilli[34,35]. Enzyme formation for catabolism is suppressed in the presence of glucose, which lowers this microbe's cyclic AMP. However, addition of cyclic AMP (or removal of glucose) leads to the induced transcription of DNA-regions for catabolic enzymes. Cyclic AMP acts in this system by combining with a catabolite gene-activator protein, and this complex binds to certain areas of the DNA in proximity to the attachment of RNA polymerase in the process of gene transcription. This is not the occasion to review the rapidly increasing literature on this type of problem, but we simply notice that phenomena akin to what we discussed can interact with aspects of genetic expression, so as to selectively or generally activate the synthesis of groups of proteins. These are the first hints of novel sets of phenomena. It seems likely that in eukaryotic cells, control mechanisms will be discovered at the transcriptional and perhaps translational levels as well. An important precedent has recently been published by Murdoch et al.[36].

Using a cell-line derived from rat pituitary cells, these authors studied the expression of the gene for prolactin synthesis. This is relatively dormant, untal it is stimulated by the addition of lipidpermeable cyclic-AMP analogs, or also under the influence of the diterpene, forskolin, which selectively stimulates the catalytic subunit of adenylate cyclase so this leads to a long-lasting increase in intracellular cyclic-AMP. Expression of the gene was studied both by determining the expression of the product, prolactin, and in terms of prolactin messenger-RNA as detected by cloned prolactin DNA-probe hybridization techniques. The main point, for our present purpose, is the discovery that under these conditions, there occurs a phosphorylation of a specific chromatin-associated basic protein of molecular weight 23 k dalton, different from any known histone, which is of low but nevertheless significant abundance, one per cent of the mass of the majority-type histone. This is regarded as a regulator of gene transcription, which acts upon a limited set of transcription sites as they interact with type II RNA-polymerase. Ca^{++} ions were not invoked in this important study, but the authors emphasize that a kinase cascade may be involved, thus leaving this possibility open for our consideration. It certainly is plausible that the cyclic-AMP-induced protein kinase, in physiological situations, is modulated by Ca^{++}, as suggested by our phosphorylase work.

Important insights into the regulation of gene expression for contractile proteins begin to emerge from studies in cell cultures, as reviewed by Buckingham and Minty[37]. In such cultures, muscle-specific proteins, preceded by their m-RNA's, become prominent when myoblasts withdraw from the cell division cycle, and fuse into myotubes. This correlation is, however, not precise, and can be disconnected by reducing the Ca^{++} in the medium, which prevents biosynthesis. While its role in the latter is not clearly shown, workers in the field entertain the view that intracellular Ca^{++} and Mg^{++} are both essential for protein synthesis[38]. The latter is not subject to wide natural fluctuations while, as argued in this presentation, the former is.

There is yet another matter which deserves mention. Cardiac hypertrophy not only involves the synthesis of more protein in more or less harmonious proportions, but also, as shown for myosin[39,40], expresses a different preference for isoforms of this protein. In another context, we have studied selective isogene expression for myosin as determined by the innervation of skeletal muscle[41,42] and by thyroid hormone in the myocardium[43], and we have just announced the role of thyroid hormone in the controd of developmental myosin gene-switches, presumably exerted via the nervous system[44]. Thus, we are not only dealing with the total extent of protein synthesis, but also with yet subtler choices between the transcriptions for closely similar genes.

We may summarize our considerations in the following picture. Different contraction modes, at different levels of energy usage per cycle, lead to different degrees of phosphorylation of at least one example of a metabolic control protein, glycogen phosphorylation. The analysis of this finding leaves only one possible explanation: different time integrals of the Ca^{++} pulses occurring in conjunction with excitation-contraction coupling, but also available for other Ca^{++} stimulated processes. One consequence, directly applicable to ventricular hypertrophy, is an increase in the biochemical mechanisms for protein synthesis, presumably controlled at the level of DNA-transcriptaon. Indications begin to appear that Ca^{++} as well as cyclic AMP are involved in aspects of DNA-transcription and synthesis. Thus, a general pathway for the control of cardiac growth is beginning to appear.

If one is baffled by the seeming multitude of these mechanisms and their interactions, the sobering thought is that, while vital processes are explicitly based in molecular events, even the simplest physiological phenomena involve interactions between molecular mechanisms which become very complex indeed.

REFERENCES

1. Starling, E.H.: The Law of the Heart (The Linacre Lecture) London: Longmans, Green & Co., 1918, reprinted in: Starling on the Heart Chapman, C.B., Mitchell, J.E., editors and authors of commentary, London: Dawsons of Pall Mall, 121–147, 1965

2. Evans, C.L.; Matsuoko, Y.: The effect of various mechanical conditions on the gaseous metabolism and efficiency of the mammalian heart, Journal of Physiology (London) 49: 378–405, 1915

3. Sarnoff, S.J.; Berglund, E.: Ventricular function. I. Starling's Law of the Heart studied by means of simultaneous right and left ventricular function curves in the dog, Circulation 9: 706–718, 1954

4. Vinten-Johansen, J.; Barnard, R.J.; Buckberg, G.D.; Becker, H.; Duncan, H.W.; Robertson, J.M.: Left ventricular O_2 requirements of pressure and volume loading in the normal canine heart and inaccuracy of pressure-derived indices of O_2 demand, Cardiovascular Research 16: 439–447, 1982a

5. Vinten-Johansen, J.; Duncan, H.W.; Finkenberg, J.G.; Hume, M.C.; Robertson, J.M.; Barnard, R.J.; Buckberg, G.D.: Prediction of myocardial O_2 requirements by indirect indices, American Journal of Physiology 243 (Heart Circ. Physiol. 12): H862–H868, 1982b

6. Mommaerts, W.F.H.M.: Energetics of muscular contraction, Physiological Reviews 49: 427–508, 1969

7. Mommaerts, W.F.H.M.: The variable contractile force of the heart, Acta Cardiologica 20: 277–296, 1965

8. Gibbs, C.L.: Cardiac energetics, in: The Mammalian Myocardium, Langer, G.A.; Brady, A.J. editors, New York: Wiley, 105–133, 1974

9. Gibbs, C.L.; Mommaerts, W.F.H.M.; Ricchiuti, N.V.: Energetics of cardiac contractions, Journal of Physiology (London) 191: 25–46, 1967

10. Kolbel, F. Mommaerts, W.F.H.M.: Ribosomen des hypertrophierten Herzmuskels: ^{14}C-Phenylalanin-Einbau in vitro, in: Heart Failure, Pathophysiology and Clinical Aspects. International Symposium, Reindell, H.; Keul, J.; Doll, E., editors, Stuttgart: Georg Thieme Verlag, 189–194, 1968

11. Hammond, G.L.; Lai, Y.K.; Markert, C.L.: The molecules that initiate cardiac hypertrophy are not species-specific, Science 216: 529–531, 1982

12. Hammond, G.L.; Wieben, E.; Markert, C.L.: Molecular signals for initiating protein synthesis in organ hypertrophy, Proceedings of the National Academy of Sciences (USA) 76: 2455–2459, 1979

13. Meerson, F.Z.; Alekhina, G.M.; Aleksandrov, P.N.; Bazardjan, A.G.: Dynamics of nucleic acid and protein synthesis of the myocardium in compensatory hyperfunction and hypertrophy of the heart, American Journal of Cardiology 22: 337–348, 1968

14. Rumyantsev, P.P.; Kassem, A.M.: Cumulative indices of DNA synthesizing myocytes in different compartments of the working myocardium and conductive system of the rat's heart muscle following extensive left ventricle infarction, Virchows Archiv B--Cell Pathology 20: 329–342, 1976

15. Cori, G.T.; Cori, C.F.: The enzymatic conversion of phosphorylase a to b, Journal of Biological Chemistry 158: 321–332, 1945

16. Krebs, E.G.; Fischer, E.H.: The phosphorylase b to a converting enzyme of rabbit skeletal muscle, Biochimica et Biophysica Acta 20: 150–157, 1956

64

17. Walsh, D.A.; Perkins, J.P.; Krebs, E.G.: An adenosine 3',5'- mono-phosphate-dependent protein kinase from rabbit skeletal muscle, Journal of Biological Chemistry 243: 3763-3765, 1968
18. Sutherland, E.W.: Rall, T.W.: Fractionation and characterization of a cyclic adenine ribonucleotide formed by tissue particles, Journal of Biological Chemistry 232: 1077-1091, 1958
19. Mommaerts, W.F.H.M.; Vegh, K.: Homsher, E.: Activation of phosphorylase in frog muscle as determined by contractile activity, Journal of General Physiology 66: 657-669, 1975
20. Hers, H.-G.; Schaftingen, E. van: Fructose 2,6-bisphosphate 2 years after its discovery, Biochemical Journal 206: 1-12, 1982
21. Hue, L.: Role of fructose 2,6-biphosphate in the stimulation of glycolysis by anoxia in isolated hepatocytes, Biochemical Journal 206: 359-365, 1982
22. Allen, D.G.; Kurihara, S.: The effects of muscle length on intracellular calcium transients in mammalian cardiac muscle, Journal of Physiology (London) 327: 79-94, 1982
23. Parmley, W.W.; Chuck, L.: Length-dependent changes in myocardial contractile state, American Journal of Physiology 224: 1195-1199, 1973
24. Anrep, G. von: On the part played by the suprarenals in the normal vascular reactions of the body, Journal of Physiology (London) 45: 307-317, 1912
25. Bremel, R.D.; Weber, A.: Cooperation within actin filament in vertebrate skeletal muscle, Nature, New Biology 238: 97-101, 1972
26. Fabiato, A.; Fabiato, F.: Myofilament-generated tension oscillations during partial calcium activation and activation dependence of the sarcomere length-tension relation of skinned cardiac cells, Journal of General Physiology 72: 667-699, 1978
27. Hibberd, M.G.; Jewell, B.R.: Length-dependence of the sensitivity of the contractile system to calcium in rat ventricular muscle, Journal of Physiology (London) 290: 30P-31P, 1979
28. Keurs, H.E.D.J. ter; Rijnsburger, W.H.; Heuningen, R. van; Nagelsmit, M.J.: Tension development and sarcomere length in rat cardiac trabeculae, Circulation Research 46: 703-714, 1980
29. Fuchs, F.: Cooperative interactions between calcium-binding sites on glycerinated muscle fibers. The influence of cross-bridge attachment, Biochimica et Biophysica Acta 462: 314-322, 1977a
30. Fuchs, F.: The binding of calcium to glycerinated fibers in rigor. The effect of filament overlap, Biochimica et Biophysica Acta 491: 523-531, 1977b
31. Fuchs, F.; Fox, F.: Parallel measurements of bound calcium and force in glycerinated rabbit psoas muscle fibers, Biochimica et Biophysica Acta 679: 110-115, 1982
32. Fuchs, F.; Planchak, R.: (abstract) Is Ca^{2+}-troponin affinity force-dependent? Biophysical Journal 41: 262a, 1983
33. Solaro, R.J.; Rocklin, M.S.: (abstract) "Freezing" of cardiac myofibrils in the "on" and "off" state by cross-linking with glutaraldehyde, Biophysical Journal 41: 265a, 1983
34. Crombrugghe, B. de; Chen, B.; Anderson, W.; Nissley, P.; Gottesman, M; Pastan, I.: Lac DNA, RNA polymerase and cyclic AMP receptor protein, cyclic AMP, lac repressor and inducer are the essential elements for controlled lac transcription, Nature, New Biology 231: 139-142, 1971

35. Zubay, G.; Schwartz, D.; Beckwith, J.: Mechanism of activation of catabolite-sensitive genes: a positive control system, Proceedings of the National Academy of Sciences (USA) 66: 104-110, 1970

36. Murdoch, G.H.; Rosenfeld, M.G.; Evans, R.M.: Eukaryotic transcriptional regulation and chromatin-associated protein phosphorylation by cyclic AMP, Science 218: 1315-1317, 1982

37. Buckingham, M.E.; Minty, A.J.: Contractile protein genes, in: Eukaryotic Genes, their Structure, Activity and Regulation, Maclean, N.; Gregory, S.; Flavell, editors, London; Boston: Butterworths (to be published), 1983

38. Ranu, R.S.: Regulation of protein synthesis in rabbit reticulocyte lysates: effect of Ca^{2+}, Mg^{2+}, and Mn^{2+} on self-phosphorylation and heterophosphorylation catalyzed by the heme-regulated and double-stranded-RNA-activated protein kinases, Bioscience Reports 2: 813-817, 1982

39. Lompre, A.-M.; Schwartz, K.; d'Albis, A.; Lacombe, G.; Thiem, N. van; Swynghedauw, B.: Myosin isoenzyme redistribution in chronic heart overload, Nature 282: 105-107, 1979

40. Mercadier, J.J.; Lompre, A.-M.; Wisnewsky, C.; Samuel, J.L.; Bercovici, J.; Swynghedauw, B.; Schwartz, K.: Myosin isoenzymic changes in several models of rat cardiac hypertrophy, Circulation Research 49: 525-532, 1981

41. Mommaerts, W.F.H.M.; Seraydarian, K.; Suh, M.; Kean, C.J.C.; Buller, A.J.: The conversion of some biochemical properties of mammalian skeletal muscles following cross-reinnervation, Experimental Neurology 55: 637-653, 1977

42. Buller, A.J.; Mommaerts, W.F.H.M.; Seraydarian, K.: Enzymic properties of myosin in fast and slow twitch muscles of the cat following cross-innervation, Journal of Physiology (London) 205: 581-597, 1969

43. Mommaerts, W.F.H.M.; Seraydarian, K.; Marusich, M.; Vegh, K.: The role of thyroid hormone in the selection of myosin heavy-chain isogene expression, Journal of Muscle Research and Cell Motility (in preparation), 1983

44. Mommaerts, W.F.H.M.: Fetal maturation of myofibrillar proteins, abstract for the 10th Conference of Fetal Breathing Movements and other Fetal Measurements, Malmo, June 1983

SUMMARY

*The purpose of this study was to analyze whether and to what extent (i)
the force-interval relationship, (ii) the force-sarcomere length relationship and (iii) the force-velocity relationship are modified in acute
hypertrophy. Mechanical properties of trabeculae that were dissected from
the right ventricle of rats were studied. Three experimental models were
used: (i) 3-4 months' old Wistar rats with normal blood pressure served
as controls; (ii) hyperthyroid Wistar rats of 3-4 months of age were
studied after two weeks of triiodothyronine injections (50 μg daily);
(iii) rats of the same age after 2-4 weeks of hypobaric hypoxia which
leads to hypertrophy of the right ventricle as a result of pulmonary
hypertension at elevated cardiac output. The muscles were studied in a
bath, which was rapidly perfused with modified oxygenated Krebs Hense-
leit solution at 25 °C at pH 7.4. Force was measured with a strain
gauge. Muscle length was measured and controlled with a servomotor.
Sarcomere length was measured and controlled by means of laser diffraction techniques. Mechanical recovery curves in controls and hearts
following hypobaric hypoxia showed a rapid rise in the first 600 ms
followed by a slow rise to plateau level that was attained at 60 seconds. Mechanical recovery in hyperthyroid muscles showed only the rapid
phase of recovery. Force at test intervals between 800 ms and 100 s was
100% of steady-state value. Both passive force (F), sarcomere length (SL)
relations and active F-SL relations, studied at external calcium concentration = 2.5 mM were comparable for the three groups. No difference in
stress development between the three groups was observed. The influence
of Ca^{++} on the shape of F-SL relations in controls and trabeculae of
T_3 rats was identical. The F-SL curve at Ca^{++} = 2.5 mM in trabeculae
following hypobaric hypoxia was slightly steeper than in controls.
Maximal shortening velocity of the sarcomeres (V_0) was 13.6 ± 3.0 μm/s
(mean ± 1 SD) in controls; 17.9 ± 2.1 μm/s in T_3 rats; and 8.62 ± 2.0
μm/s in muscle of hypobaric hypoxia rats. Results suggest 1) increased
capacity and transport rate of Ca^{++} in structures coupling excitation
with contraction in T_3 hypertrophy compared to controls and hypertrophy
resulting from hypobaric hypoxia; 2) no appreciable effect of hypertrophy
on length dependence of activation; 3) changes of V_0 in the hypertrophy
states correlate with reported changes in myosin isoenzyme composition.*

MYOCARDIAL CELL PROPERTIES AND HYPERTROPHY

KEURS, H.E.D.J. TER, MULDER, B.J.M., SCHOUTEN, V.J.A.

Department of Cardiology, Leiden University Hospital,
Rijnsburgerweg 10, 2333 AA Leiden, the Netherlands

INTRODUCTION

Pure cardiac hypertrophy can be defined as an increased cardiac mass that results from stimulated growth of myocardial cell organelles to adjust cardiac pump function to circulatory demands. Such a definition postulates a control system or a set of control systems, which sense and process the parameter(s) to be controlled and possess an effector path to correct deviation of the processed parameter from setpoint value.

Many fragments of the control system(s) that operate by means of induction of cardiac hypertrophy are known. The importance of 1) work load, 2) the energy charge of myocardium, 3) stretch of myocytes, 4) humoral factors as stimulus--or pathway--in the control loop[3] have been intensely studied.[34]

Although it is not yet easily possible to reconstruct the control system or to put an upper limit to the number of control systems, many important aspects have been revealed in the past decade. For example, the time constants of development and regression of hypertrophy are now known to be short.[10,11] The observation that significant hypertrophy may develop experimentally within a day, however surprising, is in line with studies with H3 leucine in man suggesting a daily protein turnover rate of approxmately 7%.[36] The very fact that hypertrophy provides the cardiovascular system with a rapid and reversible response to altered circulatory conditions suggests a rapidly operating control system. If, on the other hand, adjustment of pump function cannot be attained by cardiac hypertrophy, damage and degeneration of cardiac cells commence. Definition of the factors that control or accompany transition of pure regulatory cardiac growth into growth combined with degeneration or even into growth that is enhanced by concurrent degeneration is a question of considerable importance to proper diagnosis and treatment of patients.

68

Such a definition requires study of structure and function of the heart in various models of hypertrophy to assess impact of growth on function of myocytes per se, and to assess the additional contribution of cell degeneration to biochemical metabolic electrophysiological and mechanical properties of hypertrophied myocardium. In this chapter we will compare functional properties of hypertrophic myocardium with normal myocardium.

Basic factors controlling cardiac pump function: end-diastolic and end-systolic volume; force interval relations; the effect of regulatory control systems on calcium handling by the cell and on sensitivity of the contractile proteins to calcium can be illustrated by means of figure 1.

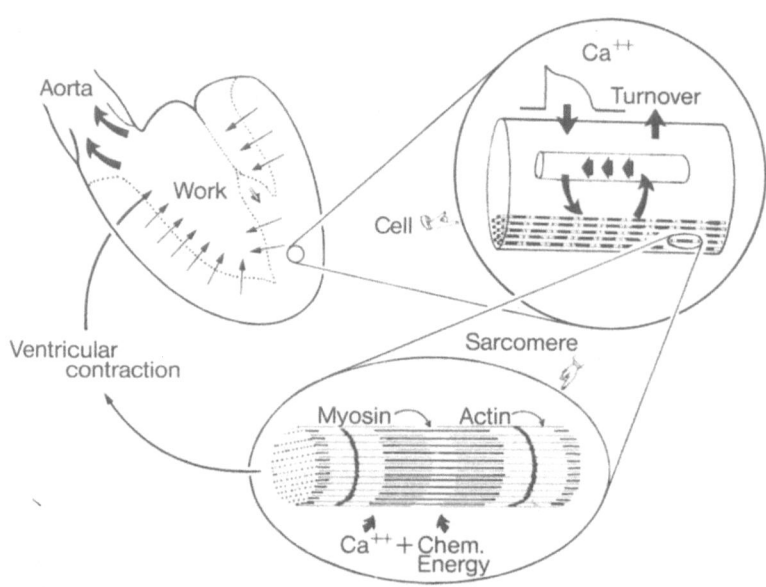

Figure 1. Diagram of the contribution of myocardial cell properties to pump function of the heart. Cardiac work is determined by contraction of the myofibrils and by their number. Contractile performance of the myofibrils is determined by their enzyme properties which control conversion of chemical energy into work in the presence of calcium. The cytoplasmic calcium concentration determines the fraction of active force generators and is itself controlled by the excitation-contraction coupling process. See text for further details.

The contractile response of myocytes to activation by calcium loss is governed by structures that are responsible for calcium handling and for contraction. The close proximity of these structures allows rapid exchange of calcium and a rapid contractile response. The response of the contractile machinery depends on the intracellular calcium concentration and therefore on the calcium levels that occur in myocytes. Figure 1 shows the main structures in a myocardial cell schematically: the membranous elements; the sarcolemma that regularly invaginates the cell by its T tubuli, which make contact with an intracellular tubular system: the sarcoplasmic reticulum. The membranes of T tubuli and sarcoplasmic reticulum come into extremely close contact with every myofibril and form functional units with the latter.

Ultrastructural studies[9] have shown that hypertrophied non-degenerated cardiac muscle cells may be qualitatively normal in man in many respects except for size. Enlargement of Golgi complexes and nuclei is found as well as an increased number of ribosomes. Proliferation, dilatation and tortuosity of T tubules and increased foldings of sarcolemmal membranes with an increased number of multiple intercalated discs indicate changes of the structures subserving the excitation-contraction coupling process. Myofibrils show formation of new sarcomeres.[28] The effect of ventricular hypertrophy on the relative volume and surface area of different components of the cell depends on the causal factor, e.g. load vs hyperthyroidism.[31]

The sequence of events during excitation-contraction coupling in these structures is diagrammatically indicated in figure 1. Calcium influx during the plateau phase of the action potential both adds calcium to intracellular stores and triggers release of calcium from specialized compartments of the stores, i.e. mainly the terminal cisternae of the sarcoplasmic reticulum (SR). The released calcium activates the contractile proteins. Rapid reuptake of calcium by the sarcoplasmic reticulum and extrusion through the cell membrane initiates relaxation and preserves calcium homeostasis in the cell. Calcium that has been resorbed by the SR is transported back to the release compartment in the course of approximately one second. In this way a constant fraction of the amount of calcium that is released during any contraction becomes available for release during the next beat. The remainder is supplied by the calcium that has entered during the action potential of the preceding beat. The transport time, necessary for filling the release compartment, depends on functional properties of the SR and determines the force-interval relations in the heart. The transport process can be studied by measuring the recovery of force development of test contractions at varied intervals following a control contraction.

Mechanical properties of activated myocardial cells depend upon properties of the myofibrils. The myofibrils are organized in a ladder-like structure of identical units: the sarcomeres. The structure of sarcomeres is schematized in figure 1. The borders of the sarcomeres are formed by the Z lines that consist of a transverse protein network from which many actin filaments protrude longitudinally in both directions. Myosin filaments are suspended between actin filaments from opposing Z bands and contribute by virtue of their regular arrangement to the cross-striated appearance of the cell under the microscope. Myosin and actin[18] slide freely along each other, but minimal and maximal length are restrained in the mammalian heart. Stretch of the sarcomeres in the myocardium beyond 2.4 μm is limited probably because myosin filaments are connected to Z lines by elastin fibers. Shortening of sarcomeres is probably limited to 1.65 μm by the myosin molecule, which at this sarcomere length collides with the Z band and resists deformation during contractions of short duration.[12] The working range of the functional unit therefore lies between sarcomere lengths of 1.6 and 2.4 μm. It has recently been shown that the active force-sarcomere length relation that underlies the Frank-Starling mechanisms of the heart is based on length-dependent sensitivity of the contractile proteins to calcium.[15,20,26] Hypertrophy may affect sensitivity of the contractile proteins to calcium and cyclic AMP.[40]

Knowledge about changes of enzymatic properties of organelles in hypertrophied cells has increased rapidly over the past years. Particularly attention has been focussed on myosin ATPase (see for reviews [37]). Three isoenzymes have been described, designated V_1, V_2 and V_3 by Hoh et al.[17]

The relative amounts of V_1, V_2 and V_3 are sensitive to factors which cause hypertrophy, e.g. hypertrophy in hyperthyroid state leads to exclusive presence of V_1 isoenzyme.[17,29] Hypertrophy due to increased afterload is characterized by increased amounts of V_3 isoenzymes.[30] ATPase activity of myosin directly relates to its isoenzyme composition.[32] High concentrations of V_1 isoenzyme with a high ATPase rate correlate with a high rate of rise of force[5] and with increased energetic cost of maintenance of force as result of a high rate of crossbridge cycling.[1,27] Moreover, it has recently been shown that myosin in heart muscle containing predominantly V_1 isoenzyme is activated under the influence of CAMP[40], whereas slow myosin is not. The control mechanisms activating slow myosin are still unknown.

Another aspect of changes in the composition of myosin isoenzymes is that the maximal velocity of shortening correlates closely with the myosin ATPase activity.[2,5] The prediction that different types of hypertrophy are characterized by their maximal velocity of shortening has been confirmed in various studies.[4,7,38,39]

Information about mechanical properties of hypertrophied heart muscle on the level of sarcomeres is not yet available.

Therefore we studied aspects of the excitation-contraction coupling process and of contraction in rat heart. Hypertrophy was induced by hyperthyroidism or by increased afterload to the right ventricle resulting from hypobaric hypoxia. Particularly, mechanical recovery, the relation between force and sarcomere length, force-velocity relations and specially maximal velocity of shortening in the two forms of hypertrophy were compared with age-matched control rats.

METHODS

Experimental animals

Hypertrophy in hyperthyroid rats. Six Wistar rats received subcutaneous injections of 50 μg of triiodothyronine (T$_3$; Sigma) per 100 g of body weight daily for 14 days, and were used for experiments 18-24 hours after the last dose.[8] Weight of the hearts in which both left and right ventricle were grossly hypertrophied was 1.4 g + 0.15 g; 22 age-matched Wistar rats served as controls. Heart weight of controls was 1.1. g + 10%.

Hypertrophy in hypobaric hypoxic rats. One group of six rats was submitted to hypobaric hypoxia by 16 hours overnight exposure to a similated altitude of 6000-7000 m (0.5-0.4 atm of air). Exposure to hypoxia lasted 2-4 weeks. Such exposure is known to induce hypertrophy of the right ventricle [10,35], whilst no significant change in body weight compared to controls was found.[34]

Preparation and mounting procedures. Twelve-week-old Wistar rats were anesthetized with ether. The heart was rapidly removed and transferred to a dissection chamber. The aorta was cannulated and perfused with oxygenated physiological salt solution at a flow rate of 5 ml/min. The right ventricle and atrium were opened, and the free wall of the right ventricle was exposed. Papillary muscles were removed. Trabeculae attached to the atrioventricular (AV) ring and the free wall of the right ventricle were selected. Ventricular tissue and atrial tissue were carefully dissected from the AV ring, freeing part of the tricuspid valve, the AV ring, and the trabecula. The part of the ventricular wall to which the trabecula was attached, was dissected. The trabecula was next transferred to an experimental chamber mounted on the stage of an inverted Zeiss microscope (fig. 2). The specimen was remounted repeatedly so that all cell strands throughout the cross-section of the muscle had equal lengths at all muscle lengths. The dimensions of the trabeculae reported here were as follows: thickness, 80 + 15 (SD) μm; width, 200 + 50 μm; n = 15. They were unbranched and uniformly shaped for nearly their whole length of more than 2.5 mm.

The microscopic image of the muscle area that was illuminated by the laser beam was observed with the use of an inverted microscope and television system (Sony video monitor model PVM-90CE) (fig. 2). Translation of the muscle region under study, which in all experiments was located at a short distance (0.5-1 mm) from the stationary force transducer end, always occurred in three directions. The region of study was selected on the basis of its minimal motion. If translation during contractions exceeded 100 μm in any direction or if rotation exceeded five degrees, another region was chosen or the muscle was repositioned. Muscles were discarded if these conditions could not be met.

Perfusion solutions. Solutions used during dissection and during experiments consisted of the following components in mM: NAcl, 115; KCl, 5; MgCl, 1.2; NaH$_2$PO$_4$, 2.0; Na$_2$SO$_4$, 1.2; CaCl$_2$, 2.5; glucose, 10. The solutions were equilibrated with 95% O$_2$ and 5% CO$_2$; the pH in the perfusion chamber was 7.41; PCO$_2$, 5.3 kPA; PO^2, 80 kPa. The volume of the chamber was 2 ml and the flow rate through it 2 ml/min. Temperature of the fluid in the chamber was kept constant at 25.0 ^oC. Under these conditions, stable responses were observed for experiments lasting six hours and longer.

Measurements of force and muscle length. Force was measured with a strain gauge force transducer (Akselskjapet and Statham GI-225), which was connected through a stainless steel hook (100 μm diameter) to the muscle.

The opposite end of the muscle was connected to a servomotor (Cambridge Technology Dual Mode Servo) via stainless steel hooks. The servomotor system has been described recently. Its behavior is summarized in a table of dynamic properties (table 1).

Sarcomere length measurement. We have made use of diffraction methods as described earlier and as illustrated in figure 2.

The trabecula diffracts the incident light of a laser beam into a zero-order band and multiple symmetrical higher order band pairs. The spacing d. which exists between the first order bands is uniquely related to sarcomere length SL, a relation given by SL = K λ/d, where K is constant, and λ is the wave length of the laser light (0.6328 μm).

Sarcomere length was computed electronically with the aid of a computation circuit modified after Iwazumi from the intensity distribution of the first order band after correction for the contribution of scattered light of the zero order. Intensity distribution of one first order was

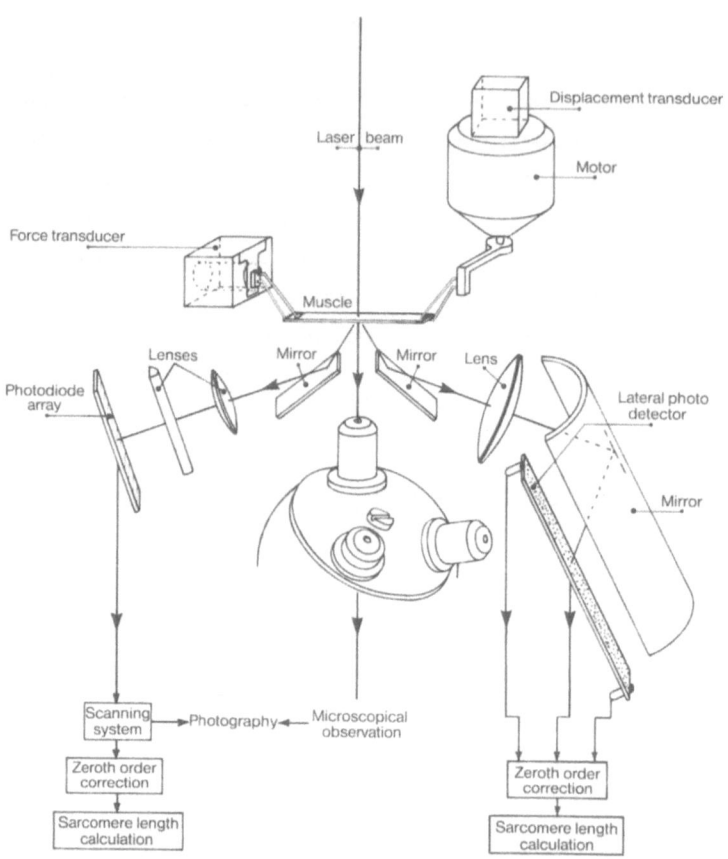

Figure 2. Diagram of experimental set-up. Muscle and entering laser beam were observed through the microscope. Two surface mirrors deflect the light of the first-order diffraction pattern onto two photo detector systems. The positions of the median and mean of the first-order light intensity distributions are converted to median and mean sarcomere length respectively. Force is measured with a capacitive force transducer. Muscle length is measured and controlled by a servomotor system with length transducer.

Table 1. Dynamic properties.

Servomotor system		
noise	1	μm
frequency response (-3 dB)	350	Hz
linearity	2	%
step-response time 90%	1.4	ms
compliance	0.6	μm/mN
drift	1	μm/°C ambient temperature

Force transducer system		
compliance	1	μm/mN
noise	0.05	mN
sensitivity	1.5	mV/mN
resonance frequency (submersed, preparation attached)	2.4	kHz
drift	0.2	mN/0 °C
linearity (0-100 mN)	> 0.1%	

scanned four times per ms by a photodiode array (Reticon 256 EC). The intensity of the zero order, close to the first order, was measured during each scan and its distribution under the first order peak was approximated by an exponential decay. The simulated zero-order intensity was subtracted from the intensity distribution under the first order. The position of the median of the first order intensity distribution was calculated. The position signal was converted to a voltage, proportional to sarcomere length, with the aid of a non-linear amplifier which had the same transfer function as the above equation. Calibration of the calculating circuitry was performed with test gratings before every experiment. The calibration error proved smaller than 1%. Resolution of the measurement was limited by noise to 20 nm nominally in cardiac trabeculae.

The other first order of the diffraction pattern was deflected onto a position-sensitive photodetector (United Detector Technology LSC 4). The difference and sum of detector output currents are directly related to first and zero moment of the distribution of light impinging upon the detector respectively. The zero and first moment of the zero-order intensity distribution were calculated with the aid of photodiodes, placed at both ends of the detector, and a network which simulated a parabolic decay of the zero-order light. The curvature of the simulated decay could be adjusted with one parameter. After subtraction of the approximated zero-order distribution, the ratio of first and zero moment of the intensity distribution of the first order band were calculated. This yielded the position of the center of gravity of the first-order light distribution, which was converted to sarcomere length with the use of the same transfer function as used in the photodiode array system. Calibration of both systems was carried out in similar fashion. Frequency response of the lateral photodetector was 23 Hz and the error due to noise and drift 30 nm typically. Non-linearity of the system was 10 nm maximally. The error due to intensity variations of a factor x5 was less than 1 nm.

Sarcomere length control and force control systems. Sarcomere length in the observed region was controlled by imposing muscle length changes through the servomotor system. The methods used and their limitations have been described recently.[14] In short, both negative feedback of the sarcomere length signal into the servosystem from either diffractometer system, and feed-forward control of sarcomere length by imposing carefully adjusted stretches and releases to the muscle, were used.

In order to achieve a measurement of the relation between force and velocity of shortening, following a quick release at a selected moment during contraction and at a given sarcomere length, either force control or controlled release of sarcomere was used.

Force control could be imposed upon a muscle that contracted at constant muscle length or at constant sarcomere length by exchange of the feedback loop that was in operation for the loop carrying the force signal. Interchange was imposed by a gating pulse from a timing device (Digitimer

4030) that was fed into a specially designed field effect transistor-operated gated switch.[14] This procedure allowed control of force from the start of the gating pulse until either the end of contraction or the end of the pulse. However, force control was unstable at zero force. Therefore, we used sarcomere length control for measurement of velocity of sarcomere shortening at zero load.

Modification of the set point during sarcomere length feedback allowed shortening of sarcomeres at a preselected rate and moment of onset. Sarcomere shortening with either control mode was chosen so that force development upon release remained constant for at least 200 ms.

Force-sarcomere length relations

The trabeculae were stimulated at a rate of 0.2 Hz by two platinum electrodes parallel to the muscle. Stimulus intensity was 50% above threshold, and the stimulus duration was 5 ms. The data were obtained from contractions in a medium containing a calcium concentration of 2.5 mM. The muscle was kept at reference length (sarcomere length, 2.10 μm) for six contractions between series of test contractions. Peak force for relations between tension and sarcomere length was derived from the third contraction of each test series. The results from the first and second contractions were similar. Test lengths were chosen in random order. Tension developed during the test contractions was highly reproducible with this procedure.[19,21]

RESULTS

Mechanical recovery

Mechanical recovery was studied at SL = 2.15 m by introducing extrasystoles at varied intervals (see fig. 3 A and B) following steady-stated stimulation at a basic rate of 0.2 Hz. Twitch duration in trabeculae controls and hypobaric hypoxia rats was similar (600 ms). Twitch duration of hyperthyroid preparations was shorter, i.e. 300-450 ms. Mechanical recovery was expressed as % F_{max} of the test beat relative to F_{max} of the control as a function of the test interval. Recovery consisted in controls (n = 20) (fig. 4) of a rapid phase during which force increased to 85% in 2 s followed by a slow rise to a maximum at 120 s. Mechanical

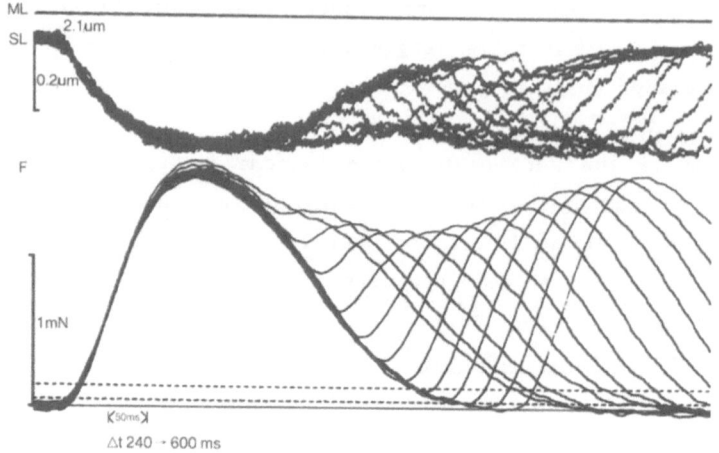

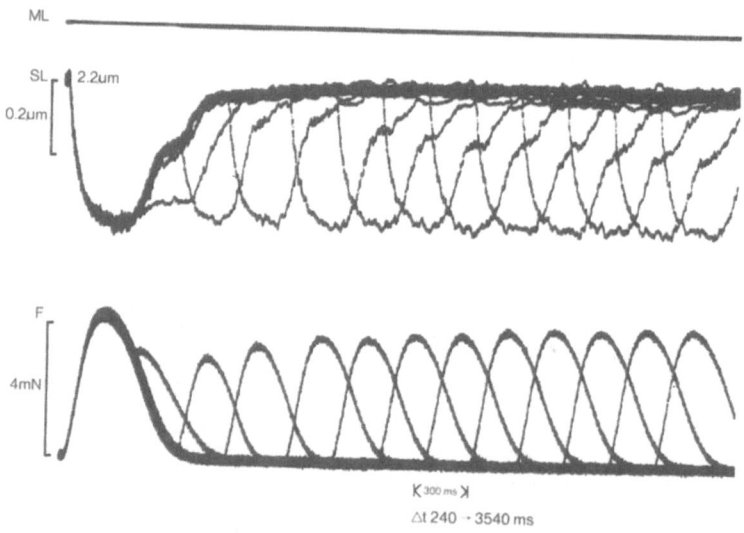

Figure 3. Typical rapid mechanical recovery immediately following a twitch (A) in hyperthyroid rat; (B) slower increase of peak force during the four seconds after a twitch in cardiac trabecula from hypobaric rat. In both experiments the basic rate of stimulation was 0.2 Hz, Ca_o was 5 mM.

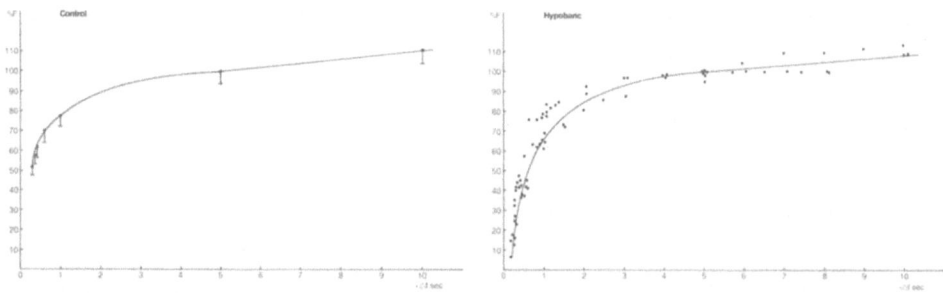

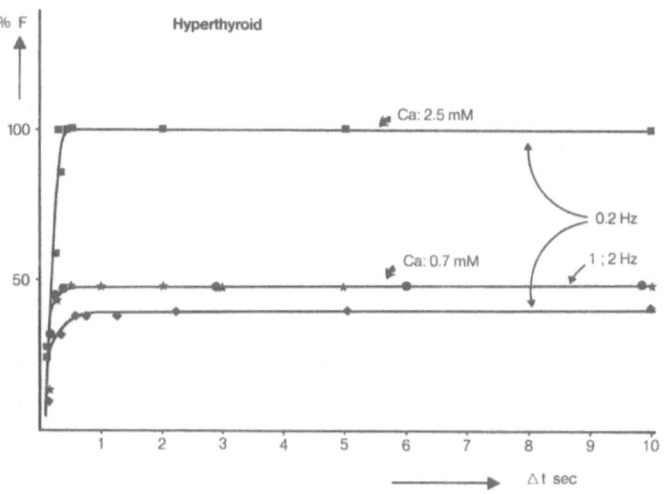

Figure 4. Mechanical recovery plotted as peak force as a function of the test interval following contractions at a regular rate (F = 100%). A and B show that at Ca 2.5 mM and 0.2 Hz mechanical recovery in controls (n = 20) and in hypobaric hypoxia (n = 4) rats is identical. C shows that 1) the initial recovery of force development is much more rapid than in B and A and reaches a plateau at Δt = 450 ms irrespective of external calcium concentration (squares Ca_o = 2.5, all other symbols at 0.7 mM Ca_o) and of basic rate of stimulation (squares and diamonds 0.2 Hz; asterisks and circles 1 and 2 Hz, respectively); 2) the slow rise of force which lasts up to 100 s in controls is abolished in hypertrophied heart of hyperthyroid rat.

recovery of hypertrophy following hypobaric hypoxia was identical to that of controls (fig. 4). In contrast, trabeculae from hypertrophied heart after thyroid hormone stress showed only an accelerated rapid recovery phase. F_{max} reached 100% at 600 ms and then remained constant for 100 seconds.

Force-sarcomere length relations

Figure 5 shows the relation between actively developed stress and sarcomere length derived from 12 trabeculae of control hearts. Externally developed force is zero at a sarcomere length of about 1.60 μm and rises continually with sarcomere length. Although the curve is derived from auxotonic contractions, no difference was found with isotonic or sarcomere-isometric contractions as described previously.[13,14,21]

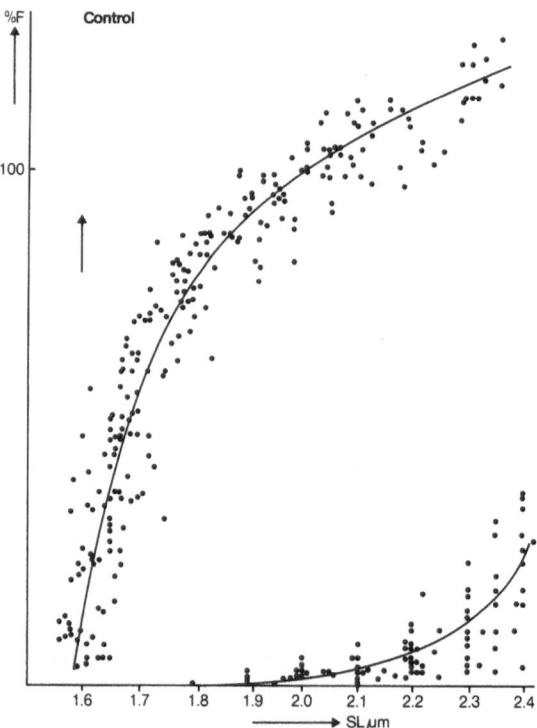

Figure 5 A. The relation between the active and passive tension in the muscle and sarcomere length measured during isometric contraction. Active tension is expressed as total tension minus passive tension borne at the sarcomere length which is measured at peak tension. Pooled data from 12 muscles at $1Ca^{2+}I_o$ = 2.5 mM. Passive tension data are indicated (small dots).

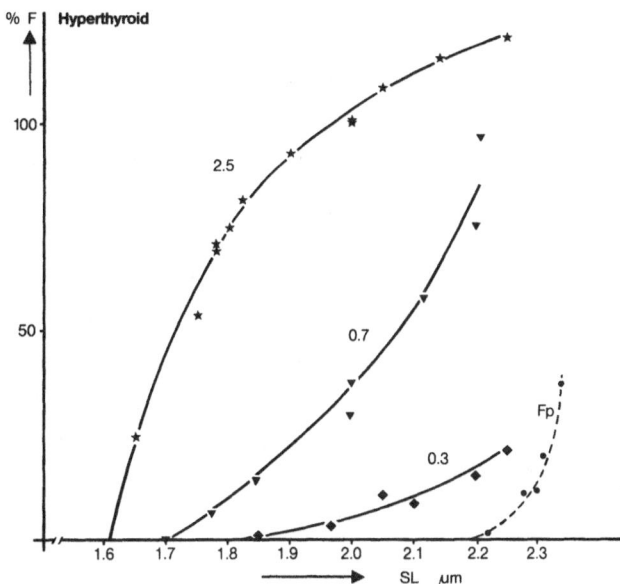

Figure 5 B. Typical passive F-SL relations (filled circles) and active F-SL relations in Ca_O 2.5 mM (asterisks); Ca_O 0.7 mM (triangles) and Ca_O 0.3 mM (diamonds) in a trabecula (2 mm long, 70 μm thick, 180 μm wide; stress at SL = 2.0 μm, Ca_O = 2.5 mM, 100 mN/mm^2) from hyperthyroid rat.

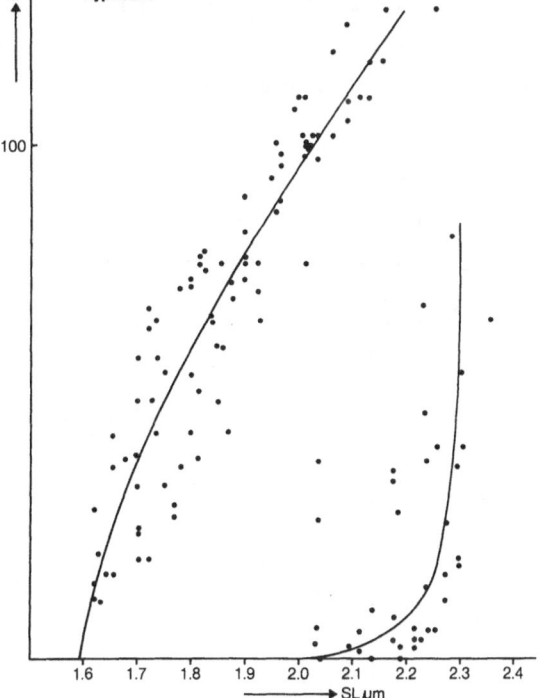

Figure 5 C. Passive and active F-SL relations of five trabeculae from hypertrophic hearts from hypobaric hypoxic rats.

Similar relations measured in hyperthyroid hearts also showed monotonic increase of active stress with sarcomere length (see fig. 5), whereas the passive force-length relation seemed steeper at long sarcomere lengths. The same held for stress-sarcomere length relations of trabeculae from hypertrophic hearts induced by hypobaric hypoxia (see fig. 5).

Differences between force-sarcomere length relations of the three groups were small at Ca_O 2.5 mM. The effect of variation of Ca_O was tested in trabeculae of hyperthyroid rats (fig. 5). The changes in shape of the F-SL curve with varied Ca_O were identical to those found in control trabeculae.[13,20, 21,26] The F-SL curve in trabeculae of hypobaric hypoxia rats was slightly steeper at Ca_O = 2.5 mM than in controls and hyperthyroid rats.

Force-velocity relations

With the use of the isovelocity technique[6,23] (fig. 6), hyperbolic F-V relations (fig. 7) were obtained at Ca_O = 2.5 mM, SL = 2.0 m and at time of peak force in controls and have been reported in detail.[6,24] For the purpose of this study V_O (fig. 8) was compared between the three groups. V_O for controls was 13.6 + 3.0 μm/s (n = 16, mean + 1 SD); V_O for hyperthyroid trabeculae was 17.9 + 2.1 μm/s (n = 4, mean + 1 SD); V_O was 8.62 + 2.0 μm/s for trabeculae from five hypobaric hypoxia rats.

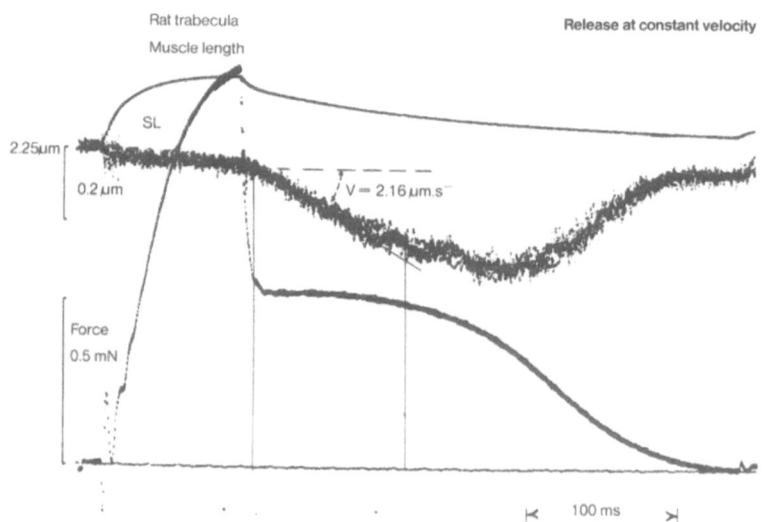

Figure 6 A illustrates the isovelocity release method (see text) to measure F-V relations

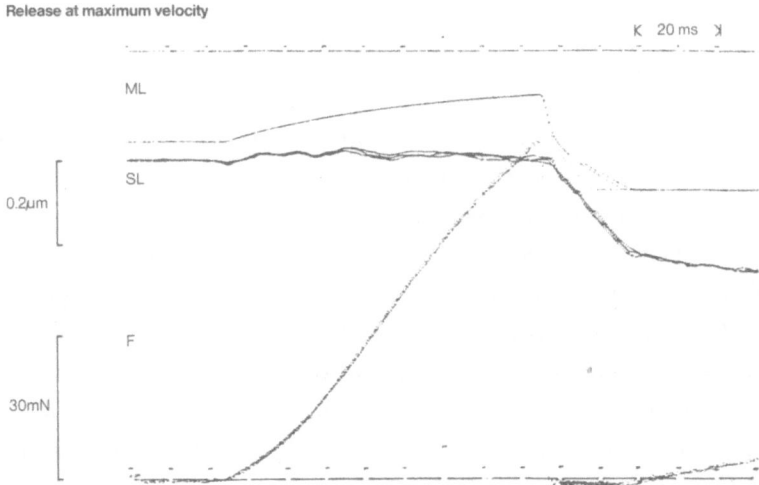

Release at maximum velocity

Figure 6 B. Unloaded shortening velocity (V_o) as preselected SL and
time during the twitches that start at constant SL. Calibrations are
indicated.

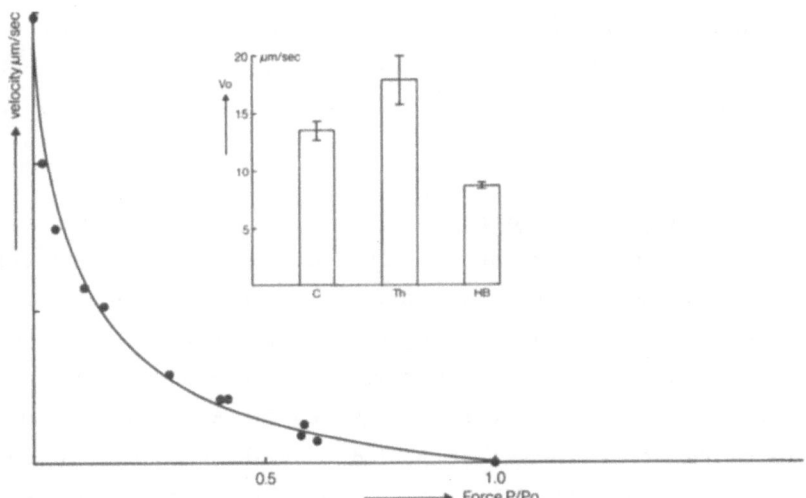

Figure 7. The fit of Hill's relation (P_o - P)b = (p + a)V to F - V data
of isovelocity releases as illustrated in figure 5. Inset: directly
measured V_o in controls (C) is significantly lower (P < 0.02) than in
trabeculae from hyperthyroid (Th) animals and significantly higher (P <
0.001) than in trabeculae from hypoxic hypobaric rats.

DISCUSSION

Force-interval relations

Hypertrophy induced by hypobaric hypoxia did not modify the F-Δt relation from that of controls. This finding contrasted with the impressive acceleration of mechanical recovery in T3-induced hypertrophy. F-Δt relations in T3 specimens moreover showed no slow increase of F over 100s following contraction described in the normal rat (Wohlfart.[42] This behavior was found at all Ca$_O$ tested over a wide range of stimulus rates (0.2-2 Hz). Thus, masking of the slow component of recovery by saturation of one of the steps leading to force generation in T3 rats is virtually excluded. The above observation also argues against the possibility that the slow phase of recovery in normal heart is due to diffusion and binding of calcium to cell organelles that are not involved in excitation-contraction coupling. It is more likely that both the rapid and slow phase are representative of steps in transport of calcium by sarcoplasmic reticulum and sarcolemma. T3-stimulated hypertrophy probably accelerates these steps both by modulation of Ca pump activity and by selectively stimulated growth of the SR.[31] Absence of selective growth of SR in load-induced hypertrophy [31] and unchanged mechanical recovery would be consistent with such a tentative hypothesis. Shortening of the twitch with conservation of high stress (up to 100 mN.mm^{-2}) developed by T3 trabeculae is also consistent with a rapidly working SR of large capacity.

Force-sarcomere length relations

Force-sarcomere length relations in T3 hypertrophy were identical to those of controls. This observations both held at high Ca$_O$ and at decreased Ca$_O$. The effect of varying Ca$_O$ consisted in a change of the shape of the F-SL curve from convex toward the ordinate at Ca$_O$ = 2.5 mM to concave at Ca$_O$ 0.3 mM. Identical F-SL curves are found in skinned trabeculae which are activated at varied controlled calcium concentrations.[15,26] This suggests that the shape of the F-SL curves can be completely explained by properties of the myofibrils and that the F-SL relation results from the influence of SL on the sensitivity of the contractile proteins to calcium. A model relating length-dependent response to calcium was described by one of us.[25] In current concepts of activation of contraction it is assumed that binding of calcium to troponin (TNI) activates contractile force generation. The absence of any effect of T_3 hypertrophy on the shape of the force–sarcomere length relation suggests that TNI properties are unchanged by T_3 hypertrophy. This is in full agreement with conclusions based upon biochemical studies that suggest no changes in calcium binding and phosphorylation of TNI following T_3 stress.[40] Modification of myosin regulation of contraction by cAMP[40] plays a role following T_3 stress, but would escape notice in these experiments as thorough perfusion and superfusion of the heart and muscle with saline probably rinsed out all β-adrenergic transmitter.

Similar tentative conclusions may be drawn in regard to hypobaric hypoxia trabeculae although the F-SL was only studied at Ca_o = 2.5 mM. The observed F-SL relation in these preparations at Ca_o = 2.5 mM was slightly less convex than in controls. This could be caused by increased sensitivity of TNI or decreased levels of intracellular calcium during the twitch.[25] Further analysis of the effect of Ca_o on the F-SL relating hypobaric hypoxia rats is mandatory before interpretation of these curves can be meaningful.

Force–velocity relations and V_o

Force–velocity relations in cardiac muscle measured with the isovelocity technique obey the same rules as found in skeletal muscle and predicted by Hill[16] on the basis of heat measurements in tetanized skeletal muscle. The F-V relations and the dependence of directly measured V_o in normal trabeculae of rat have recently been described.[24] In the present study, a striking increase of V_o was found in T_3 trabeculae and an even larger decrease of V_o was found in hypobaric hypoxia rat myocardium

Full F-V relations were not studied, so no statement about the coefficients of the hyperbola $(P_o - P)b = (P + a)V$ in hypertrophy can be made. V_o (= bP_o/a) is correlated with the ATPase activity of myosin[2] and has been reported to be determined by the isoenzyme composition of myosin.[7] The increase in V_o that we found is consistent both with data in literature on measurement of velocity in T_3-stressed cardiac muscle and with the reported increase in V_1 myosin isoenzyme.[29] It is surprising, however, that V_O increased in animals which were only four to five months old and therefore still possess a large fraction V_1 isoenzyme. Increase of V_O in T_3 trabeculae is in line with the observed decrease of twitch duration and increased dF/dt. The effects of both enhanced SR activity and a faster myosin ATPase rate would in this respect be additive, and would allow an increased power output that is expected to meet an increased demand for flow by the organism. This would, however, occur at the expense of efficiency of the system.[1]

Slowing of the contractile apparatus as we have observed in hypobaric hypoxic trabeculae would optimize the heart for increased stress development at high efficiency. Such behavior would be accounted for by an enhanced fraction V_3 myosin isoenzymes in load-induced hypertrophy. Whether this is present in hypobaric hypoxia hypertrophy remains to be tested.

REFERENCES

1. Alpert, N., Mulieri, L.: Heat, mechanics and myosin ATPase in normal and hypertrophied heart muscle, Fed. Proc., 41: 192-198, 1982.
2. Barany, M.: ATPase activity of myosin correlated with speed of muscle shorterning, J. Gen. Physiol., 50: 197-216, 1967.
3. Beznak, M., Korecky, B., Thomas, G.: Regression of cardiac hypertrophy of various origin, Can. J. Physiol. Pharmacol., 47: 579-586, 1969.
4. Buccino, R.A., Spann Jr, J.F., Pool, P.E., Sonnenblick, E.H., Braunwald, E.: Influence of the thyroid state on the intrinsic contractile properties and energy stores of the myocardium, J. Clin. Invest., 46: 1669-1682, 1967.
5. Carey, R., Bove, A., Coulson, R., Spann, J.: Correlation between cardiac myosin ATPase activity and velocity of muscle shortening, Biochem. Med., 21: 235-245, 1979.
6. Daniels, M., Donselaar, W. van, Keurs, H.E.D.J. ter, Noble, M.I.M., Wohlfart, B.: Sarcomere-force-velocity relations in rat myocardium, J. Physiol., 324: 23P, 1982.
7. Ebrecht, G., Rupp, H., Jacob, R.: Alterations of mechanical parameters in chemically skinned preparations of rat myocardium as a function of isoenzyme pattern of myosin, Bas. Res. Cardiol., 77: 220-234, 1982.
8. Everts, M.E., Hardeveld, C. van, Keurs, H.E.D.J. ter, Kassenaar, A.A.H.: Force development and metabolism in perfused skeletal muscle of euthyroid and hyperthyroid rats, Horm. Metabol. Res (in press), 1983.
9. Ferrans, V.J.: Human cardiac hypertrophy: structural aspects, Eur. Heart J. 3/suppl. A: 15-27, 1982.
10. Genovese, A., Chiariello, M., Ferro, G. Cacciapvoh, A.A., Condorelli, M.: Myocardial hypertrophy in the rat. Correlation between two experimental models, Jap. Heart J., 21: 511-517, 1980.

11. Genovese, A., De Alfieri, W., Latte, S., Chiariello, M., Condorelli, M.: Regression of myocardial hypertrophy in the rat following removal of acute or chronic hypobaric hypoxia, Eur. Heart J. 3/suppl. A: 161-164, 1982.
12. Gordon, A.M., Huxley, A.F., Julian, F.J.: The variation in isometric tension with sarcomere length in vertebrate muscle fibers, J. Phys. iol., 184: 170-192, 1966.
13. Gordon, A.M., Pollack, G.H.: Effects of calcium on the sarcomere length-tension relation in rat cardiac muscle, implications for the Frank-Starling mechanism, Circ. Res., 47: 610-619, 1980.
14. Heuningen, R. van, Rijnsburger, W.H., Keurs, H.E.D.J. ter: Sarcomere length control in striated muscle, Am. J. Physiol., 242: H411-H420, 1982.
15. Hibberd, M.G., Jewell, B.R.: Calcium- and length-dependent force production in rat ventricular muscle, J. Physiol., 329: 527-540, 1982.
16. Hill, A.V.: Heat of shortening and the dynamic constants of muscle, Proc. Roy. Soc. ser. B, 126, 136, 1938.
17. Hoh, J.F.Y., McGrath, P.A., Hale P.T.: Electrophoretic analysis of multiple forms of rat cardiac myosin: effects of hypophysectomy and thyroxine replacement, J. Mol. Cell Cardiol., 10: 1053-1076, 1977.
18. Huxley, H.E., Hanson, J.: Changes in the cross-striation of muscle during contraction and stretch and their structural interpretation, Nature, 173: 973-976, 1954.
19. Jewell, B.R., Rovell, J.M.: Influence of previous mechanical events on the contractility of isolated cat papillary muscle, J. Physiol. (London), 235: 715-740, 1976.
20. Kentish, J.C., Keurs, H.E.D.J. ter, Noble, M.I.M., Ricciardi, L., Schouten, V.J.A.: The relationship between force, calcium concentration and sarcomere length in skinned muscle from rat ventricle, J. Physiol., P-paper (in press), 1983.
21. Keurs, H.E.D.J. ter, Rijnsburger, W.H., Heuningen, R. van, Nagelsmit, M.J.: Tension development and sarcomere length in rat cardiac trabeculae, Circ. Res., 46: 703-714, 1980a.
22. Keurs, H.E.D.J. ter, Rijnsburger, W.H., Heuningen, R. van: Restoring forces and relaxation of rat cardiac muscle, Eur. Heart J. 1/suppl. A: 67-80, 1980b.
23. Keurs, H.E.D.J. ter, Wohlfart, B.: Influence of calcium concentration on maximal velocity of sarcomere shortening in rat trabeculae, J. Physiol., 330: 41P, 1982.
24. Keurs, H.E.D.J. ter, Noble, M.I.M., Wohlfart, B.: Velocity of sarcomere shortening in rat cardiac muscle: relationship to force, sarcomere length, Ca^{++} and time. Submitted to J. Physiol., 1983.
25. Keurs, H.E.D.J. ter: Calcium and contractility. In: Cardiac Metabolism (in press). Eds: Noble, M.I.M., Drake, A., Wiley and Sons (London) Publishers, 1983.
26. Keurs, H.E.D.J. ter, Kentish, J., Noble, M.I.M., Ricciardi, L., Schouten, V.J.A.: The relation between force, sarcomere length and calcium in rat heart muscle (in press), 1983.
27. Kissling, G., Rupp, H., Malloy, L., Jacob, R.: Alterations in cardiac oxygen consumption under chronic pressure overload: significance of the isoenzyme pattern of myosin, Bas. Res. Cardiol., 77: 255-269, 1982.

88

28. Legato, M.J.: Sarcomereogenesis in human myocardium, <u>J. Mol. Cell Cardiol.</u>, 1: 425–437, 1970.
29. Martin, A.F., Pagani, E.D., Solaro, R.J.: Thyroxine-induced redistribution of isoenzymes of rabbit ventricular myosin, <u>Circ. Res.</u>, 50: 117–124, 1982.
30. Mercadier, J.J., Lompré, A.M., Wisnewsky, C., Samuel, J.L., Bercovici, J., Swynghedauw, B., Schwartz, K.: Myosin isoenzyme changes in several models of rat cardiac hypertrophy, <u>Circ. Res.</u>, 49: 525–532, 1981.
31. Page, E., McCallister, L.P.: Quantitative electron microscopic description of heart muscle cells; application to normal, hypertrophied and thyroxin-stimulated hearts, <u>Am. J. Cardiol.</u>, 31: 171–181, 1973.
32. Pope, B., Hoh, J.F.Y., Weeds, A.: The ATPase activities of rat cardiac myosin isoenzymes, <u>FEBS Letters</u>, 118: 205–208, 1980.
33. Rabinovitch, M., Zak, R.: Biochemical and cellular changes in cardiac hypertrophy, <u>Am. Rev. Med.</u>, 23: 245–262, 1972.
34. Rabinovitch, M., Gamble, W., Nadas, A.S., Miettinen, O.S., Reid, L.: Rat pulmonary circulation after chronic hypoxia: hemodynamic and structural features, <u>Am. J. Physiol.</u>, 236: H818–H827. 1979.
35. Rau, E., Meyer, D.K.: Diurnal rhythm of incorporation of L-(3H) leucine in myocardium of the rat. In: <u>Biochemistry and pharmacology of myocardial hypertrophy, hypoxia and infarction</u>, pp. 105–110, 1976, Eds. Harris, P., Ring, R.J., Fleckenstein, A., Baltimore University Park Press.
36. Rennie, M.J., Vaughan, J.M.M., Sugden, P.H., Bennett, G., Nead, W.W., Ford, C., Halliday, D.: Protein synthesis in human atrial and ventricular muscle measured by stable isotope labelling, <u>Eur. J. of Clin. Invest.</u>, 13: A 26, 1983.
37. Scheuer, J., Bhan, A.K.: Cardiac contractile proteins, adenosine triphosphatase activity and physiological function, <u>Circ. Res.</u>, 45: 1–12, 1979.
38. Schwartz, K., Lecarpentier, Y., Martin, J.L., Lompré, A.M., Mercadier, J.J., Swynghedauw, B.: Myosin isoenzyme distribution correlates with speed of myocardial contraction, <u>J. Mol. Cell Cardiol.</u>, 13: 1071–1075, 1981.
39. Wikman Cofelt, J., Reform, H., Hollosi, G., Rouleau, L., Chuck, L.: Parmley, W.W.: Comparative force-velocity relation and analysis of myosin of dog atria and ventricles, <u>Am. J. Physiol.</u>, 243, H391–397, 1982.
40. Winegrad, S., McClellan, G., Tucker, M., Lin, L.: Cyclic AMP regulation of myosin isoenzymes in mammalian cardiac muscle, <u>J. Gen. Physiol.</u>, 81: 749–765, 1983.
41. Wohlfart, B., Noble, M.I.M.: The cardiac excitation-contraction cycle, <u>Pharmacol. Ther.</u>, 16: 1–43, 1982.
42. Wohlfart, B.: <u>Interval-strength relation of mammalian myocardium interpreted as altered kinetics of activator calcium during the cardiac cycle</u>, Thesis, Lund, 1982.

SECTION 3

ETIOLOGY AND FUNCTIONAL ASPECTS OF THE HYPERTROPHIED HEART

SUMMARY

Whether left ventricular hypertrophy is a useful compensatory process or whether it bears, in its very development, the seeds of future cardiac decompensation, is still not completely clear. Two functional consequences of ventricular hypertrophy resulting from systemic hypertension are discussed, which may play a role in long-term deterioration of cardiac function. Reduction of inotropic responsiveness to adrenergic stimulation can reduce effective cardioadrenergic support and by making the heart more dependent on the Frank-Sterling mechanism, may initiate a vicious circle of dilation and ultimately decompensation.

Reduced coronary vascular reserve was shown to occur whenever the degree of left ventricular hypertrophy was inappropriate for the level of arterial pressure. The reduced ability in some types of left ventricular hypertrophy to increase coronary flow adequately under stress, may interfere with cardiac function and intensify the effect of incidental coronary artery disease.

SOME FUNCTIONAL CONSEQUENCES OF LEFT VENTRICULAR HYPERTROPHY IN HYPERTENSION

Tarazi, R.C.

Research Division, Cleveland Clinic Foundation, Cleveland, Ohio

INTRODUCTION

Hypertension was the most common antecedent of left ventricular hypertrophy (LVH) and of congestive heart failure in the prospective studies of the Framingham community[1-3]. Yet our understanding of the factors responsible for the evolution from hypertension to hypertrophy and eventual cardiac failure is far from complete[4,5]. The common assumption was that LVH developed partly as a compensatory process in direct response to the increased arterial pressure[6,7] and that decompensation recurred either because of some incidental myocardial or coronary artery disease or because of a sudden exacerbation of hypertension[8]. Neither of these suppositions proved quite correct[9,10].

A large body of evidence has been developed over the past few years to the effect that LVH in hypertensive patients is not closely related to arterial pressure levels[10-13] but that both its development and regression are modulated by other influences as well, particularly cardioadrenergic factors[14]. Further, different investigators also suggested that ventricular hypertrophy might not be wholly beneficial or compensatory but might carry within itself the seeds of future failure[15]. The factors responsible for that evolution are many, including incidental heart disease, the renal disorders of hypertension[16], disorders of coronary perfusion, exhaustion of the myocardium[6] and even the side-effects of some antihypertensive medications[17]. In the following discussion, I will limit myself to two possible contributory factors, alterations in inotropic responsiveness of the hypertrophied ventricle and a disturbance of the balance between coronary perfusion pressure and LV mass.

This study was supported in part by the National Heart, Lung and Blood Institute (NHLBI-6835) and the American Heart Association, Northeast Ohio Affiliate, Cleveland, Ohio.

1) Adrenergic responsiveness of left ventricular hypertrophy (LVH)

Sympathetic stimulation is one of the major mechanisms that help the heart meet with an increased load[18,19]; the ability of the myocardium to respond to that stimulation has been termed the "cardiac contractile reserve"[20] to differentiate it from other "reserve mechanisms" such as the increased performance induced by the Frank-Starling relationship. In order to determine adrenergic responsiveness of the myocardium in hypertensive LVH, we determined in rats the inotropic response of the heart to isoproterenol, as measured from the increase in rate of LV pressure development normalized at pressure 40 mm Hg (LV $dP/dt/P_{40}$). There was a definite reduction compared with appropriate controls, in inotropic responsiveness both in renal hypertensive rats (RHR)[20] and in spontaneously hypertensive rats (SHR)[21]. This finding was subsequently confirmed in isolated hearts (Langendorff preparation), suggesting that the reduced beta-adrenergic responsiveness did not result from changes in cardiovascular control systems operative in the total animal[22]. In both in vivo and in vitro studies, an inverse relationship was found between the degree of LVH and the inotropic response of the ventricle to beta-adrenergic stimulation (fig. 1). That reduction was reversible; control

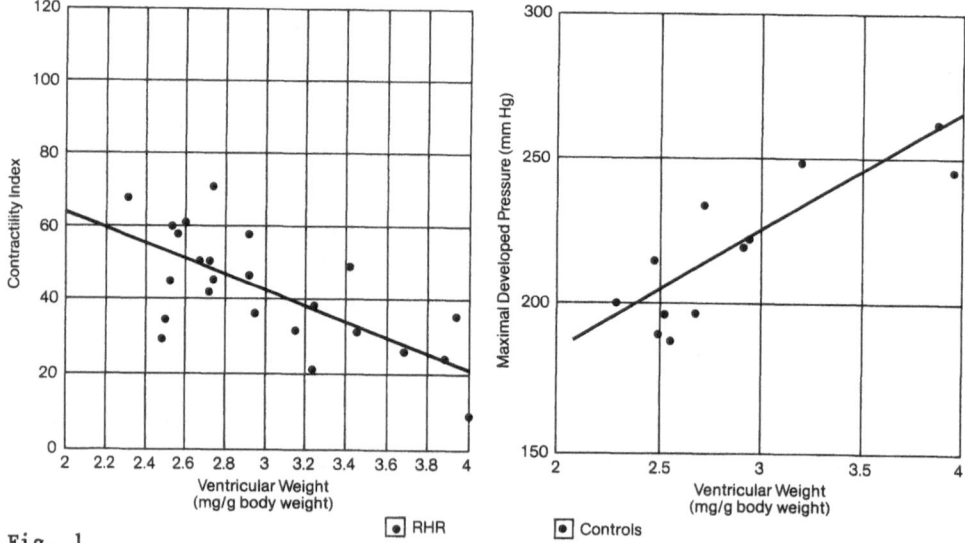

Fig. 1

The inotropic response to isoproterenol was inversely related to ventric-ular weight (left diagram), whereas the response to transient aortic occlusion (maximal developed pressure) was directly related to ventric-ular weight (right diagram) (derived from ref. 20).

of hypertension and regression of LVH by converting enzyme inhibitors or by nephrectomy restored inotropic responsiveness to isoproterenol[23]. From these observations, a series of questions converged. Firstly, was this reduction specific for adrenergic stimuli? Secondly, what was its basis? In answer to the first question, Dr. Ayobe and I[22] studied the response of the isolated heart to changing concentrations of extracellular calcium. No difference in ventricular response was found either at 37 °C or at 20 °C between controls and hypertensive rats over the whole range of calcium concentrations investigated (0.8 to 2.7 mM). Similarly, the inotropic response of the isolated heart to scillaren (a cardiac glycoside to which the rat's heart is relative sensitive) was not different in LVH from normotensive controls[22]. Thus, left ventricular responsiveness was not depressed as a whole by LVH in RHR, but the reduction in inotropic responsiveness was apparently restricted to beta-adrenergic stimulation. The second question regarding the mechanism of reduced adrenergic responsiveness was investigated in the same model of hypertension (two-kidney, one clip hypertension, Goldblatt) (RHR) in two ways: by determining myocardial beta-adrenergic receptors[22] and by investigating the contractile response to agents that stimulate adenylate cyclase without involving the beta-adrenergic receptors (Fouad and Shimamatsu, unpublished observations). Our initial results confirmed those reported previously from many centers; beta-adrenergic receptor density was found to be reduced in hypertrophied hearts from different models of hypertension by most investigators[22,24-27] although not by all[28,29] (table 1). The affinity constant of the receptors (K_d) was not usually changed. Ayobe et al.[23] further documented that regression of hypertrophy was associated with a return of beta-receptor density toward normal.

In a second study, differential regression of LVH and of hypertension was induced by altering the time of survival allowed after nephrectomy of the clipped kidney of RHR. The RHR studied four days after nephrectomy had already a significant reduction in blood pressure but still showed LVH with reduced density of beta-receptors. In those studied 40 days after nephrectomy, LVH had regressed and beta-receptors had returned to normal[23]. Thus, it seemed as if "hypertrophy" itself, and not "hypertension", was associated with reduction in ventricular beta-receptor density and presumably with diminished inotropic responsiveness of the heart to activation of the beta-adrenergic complex.

TABLE 1

MYOCARDIAL BETA-ADRENERGIC RECEPTORS IN LEFT VENTRICULAR HYPERTROPHY

authors	model	receptor no.	affinity
Woodcock et al.[24]	SHR	↓	N
Limas and Limas[25]	SHR	↓	N
Woodcock et al.[26]	1K-DOCA-salt	↓	N
Woodcock and Johnston[27]	1K-1C	↓	N
Tarazi and Ayobe[22]	2K-1C	↓	N
Giachetti et al.[28]	Grollman ligatures	N	↓
Limas[29]	abdominal aorta banding	↑	N

(from ref. 14)

2) Mechanism(s) of reduction in inotropic responsiveness to beta-adrenergic stimulation

The frequent finding of diminished ventricular beta-receptor density in different hypertensive models (table 1) as well as the significant, albeit modest, correlation between the response of max $dP/dt/P_{40}$ to isoproterenol and the density of ventricular beta-receptors (B_{max}), would suggest that the reduction of responsiveness of LVH was due to decrease of ventricular beta-receptors. However, it is not likely that the decrease in receptors will explain by itself all aspects of the reduced inotropic response:

(a) because of the relative small correlation ($r = 0.4$) between B_{max} and inotropic responsiveness to isoproterenol[22] and

(b) because of the reduced responsiveness of hypertrophied ventricles to both glucagon (Fouad and Shimamatsu, unpublished observations) and the vasoactive intestinal peptide[30]. Other components of the adenylate cyclase system[31] could also be involved.

In fact, Kumano et al.[32] have described a number of alterations in the chain of events stretching from the beta-receptor to activation of adenylate cyclase. They found that stimulation of the nucleoregulatory protein by sodium fluoride or by $Gpp(NH)_p$ was blunted in the hypertrophied heart of RHR whereas stimulation of the catalytic subunit by forskolin remained normal. In a subsequent study, they found that these alterations extend to involve more steps in this chain, as the duration of hypertension progresses.

Whatever their ultimate mechanism, the net effect of these abnormalities is to reduce the effectiveness of adrenergic support to the heart, leading to a diminished contractile reserve[20]. The functional consequences of the reduction are better understood in comparison with the mechanical response of the hypertrophied heart.

3) Ventricular response to aortic occlusion

In response to transient ($\leqslant$ 3 s) complete aortic occlusion, the left ventricle develops the maximum force of which it is capable[33,34]. Our experience with the hypertrophied hearts of RHR[20] as well as that of Pfeffer et al. with SHR[34] showed that the maximum pressure developed by these isovolumic contractions of the left ventricle was directly correlated with LV weight. However, this increased force and greater pressure development in LV hypertrophy occurred at the expense of an increased left ventricular end-diastolic pressure (fig. 2). The increased force of contraction appeared, therefore, to involve the Frank-Starling mechanism with minimal contribution from sympathetic activation because of the very short duration of the test[33].

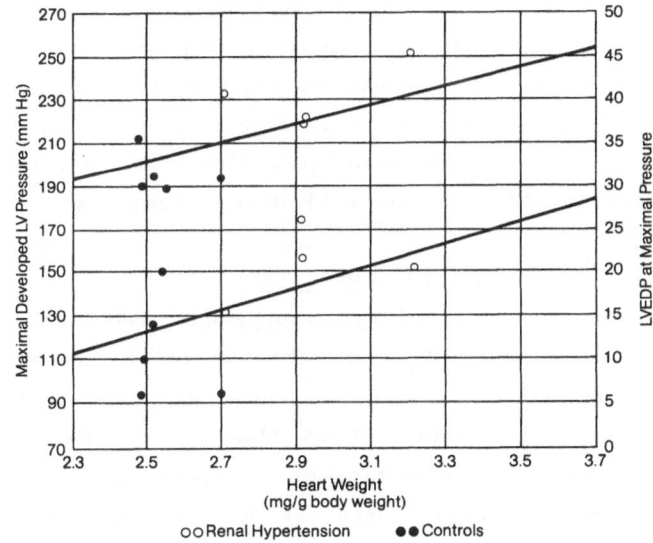

Fig. 2

When rats with renovascular hypertension were subjected to transient aortic occlusion, they responded with an increased left ventricular pressure during systole, as compared with normotensive controls. In both groups there was a direct correlation between maximal developed pressure and ventricular weight, but the higher systolic pressure of the hypertrophied ventricle in the hypertensive rats was associated with a higher left ventricular end-diastolic pressure (LVEDP).

The contrast between the two consequences of LVH is illustrated in figure 1; on the one hand, inotropic responsiveness to adrenergic stimulation decreases as ventricular weight increases and on the other, the maximum force of the left ventricle increases with increasing muscle mass. The stage thus appears to be set for a progressive encroachment on cardiac performance. A hypertrophied left ventricle can continue to perform quite well despite systemic hypertension but it becomes more dependent on the Frank-Starling mechanism. This is consonant with the repeated observation of slightly elevated left arterial and left ventricular end-diastolic pressures in hypertensive rats[35]. Since the passive pressure-volume relationship early in the development of hypertensive hypertrophy was unchanged, both in our experience[20] and that of others[36], this must mean that the heart is operating at a slightly higher end-diastolic volume. A vicious circle now begins; greater volume means greater wall stress; this means greater hypertrophy and less responsiveness to adrenergic stimuli and still more dependence on the Frank-Starling mechanism with greater dilation. In time, heart failure develops from the the early reduction in beta-inotropic responsiveness associated with left ventricular hypertrophy. This hypothesis certainly does not preclude the participation of other mechanisms such as alterations in myosin ATPase[15] or abnormalities in myocardial perfusion. However, it can help explain the long latent period before the development of heart failure in most types of hypertension. In fact, the decline in cardiac performance which develops in older SHR ($>$ 18 months) was associated with increased ventricular dilation and a reduction in their LV mass/volume ratio[37].

4) Coronary flow and left ventricular hypertrophy (LVH)

In the following paragraph, the effect of hypertrophy on coronary flow will be discussed. For discrimination between sub-endocardial flow and sub-epicardial flow, the reader is referred to the chapter by Prof. Hoffman. In all our experiments, coronary blood flow was measured in conscious non-anesthetized rats by radioactive microspheres (15 μ) injected into the left atrium. The method used was described in detail elsewhere[40]; injections into the left atrium are important to ensure adequate mixing of the microsphere for proximal vascular beds such as the coronary system[41]. The results were similar to those of many investigators before us and showed that coronary blood flow in ml/g ventricle is normal in hypertensive hearts. Coronary reserve, however, can be decreased; the phenomenon is graded, and the reduction of the coronary vasodilatory capacity usually occurs only when hypertrophy is severe[38,39]. The diminution in coronary vascular reserve has also been reported in hypertensive patients without coronary arterial disease[42,43]. Whether it plays a role in the genesis of failure is not yet clear, but it could become particularly significant when coronary arterial disease complicates any hypertensive condition[44].

Of particular importance were the results observed in maximum coronary blood flow when the degree of LVH was inappropriate for the level of arterial pressure[45]. This dissociation of "systemic pressure" from "hypertrophy" was achieved by treatment of RHR for different periods of time by a converting enzyme inhibitor. A group of renovascular hypertensive rats was treated for one week only; their blood pressure was well controlled by that but LV hypertrophy was still present. Another group was treated for 14 weeks and then treatment was stopped for a few days; blood pressure returned to hypertensive levels but the ventricle remained small. In the rats with normalized blood pressure but hypertrophied hearts, coronary vascular reserve was low. In those with high blood pressure and small hearts, coronary vascular reserve was close to normal (table 2).

TABLE 2

DISSOCIATION BETWEEN ARTERIAL PRESSURE AND LEFT VENTRICULAR MASS BY THERAPY IN RENOVASCULAR HYPERTENSIVE RATS: EFFECT ON CORONARY FLOW

group	duration (wk)	d/c	MAP (mm Hg)	LV weight (mg/g)	rest	after carbochome
A (n=9)	1	0	115 $\pm$ 11	2.9 $\pm$ 0.3	411 $\pm$ 80	554 $\pm$ 113
A (n=9)	14	1	153 $\pm$ 12	2.4 $\pm$ 0.2	446 $\pm$ 83	878 $\pm$ 232
p value			< 0.01	< 0.01	NS	< 0.01

Group A treated for one week, blood pressure controlled, left ventricle still hypertrophied.

Group B treated for 14 weeks, treatment was then stopped and blood pressure went back up but the left ventricle weight which had regressed to normal remained low.

MAP = mean arterial pressure; LV weight = left ventricular weight; d/c = discontinued

(Derived from ref. 45)

Thus, coronary flow reserve appeared to be a direct correlate of the ratio of coronary perfusion pressure (systemic pressure) to left ventricular mass (fig. 3). If confirmed, this conclusion would carry important clinical implications. In markedly hypertrophied hearts with low

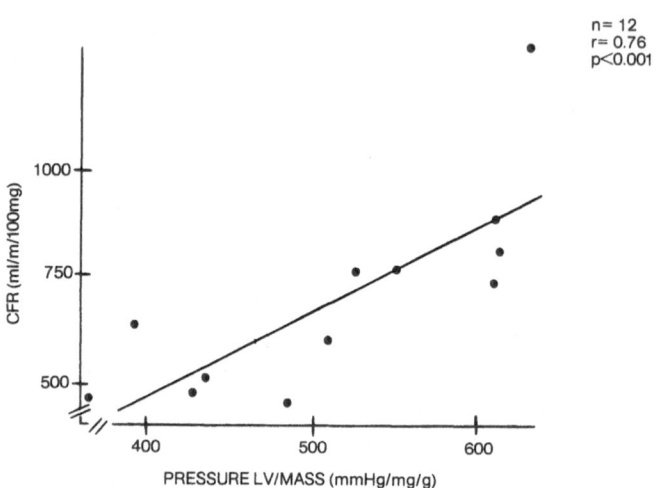

Fig. 3

Correlation between coronary flow reserve and the ratio of coronary pressure to left ventricular mass (see text). n = 12, r = 0.76; p < 0.01 (derived from ref. 38).

systemic perfusion pressure, such as aortic stenosis, the coronary reserve must be much less than in hypertrophied hearts with high systemic pressure, hence the common incidence of coronary insufficiency. As regards hypertension, we may need to reevaluate the role of drugs that control blood pressure well but do not reverse hypertrophy[46]. It is still not clear whether regression of hypertrophy will influence cardiac performance significantly[46] but persistence of hypertrophy despite normalization of arterial pressure may impair coronary vascular reserve and deserve close follow-up. Moreover, apart from the hemodynamic importance of balancing systemic pressure and LV mass, recent advances raise the possibility that hypertensive vascular hypertrophy may, indeed, be reversed by appropriate therapy[47].

In summary, the cardiac response to hypertension is a complex multifaceted process. Left ventricular hypertrophy can play a useful compensatory role for the increased pressure load (see chapter by Fouad), but it can also entail alterations in myocardial inotropic responsiveness or biochemical composition. An imbalance between the level of hypertension and the degree of LVH may lead to impaired coronary blood reserve.

REFERENCES

1. Kannel, W.B.: Role of blood pressure in cardiovascular morbidity and mortality, Prog. Cardiovasc. Dis., 17: 5-24, 1974
2. Kannel, W.B., Castelli, W.P., McNamara, P.M., McKee, P.A., Feinleib, M.: Role of blood pressure in the development of congestive heart failure, N. Engl. J. Med., 287: 782-787, 1972
3. Kannel, W.B., Sorlie, P.: Left ventricular hypertrophy in hypertension: Prognostic and pathogenetic implications (The Framingham study), in: The Heart in Hypertension, ed. by Strauer, B.E., Berlin/Heidelberg: Springer-Verlag, 223-233, 1981
4. Pfeffer, M.A., Pfeffer, J.M.: Cardiac hypertrophy in the spontaneously hypertensive rats: Adaptation or primary myopathy, in: Perspectives in Cardiovascular Research, Cardiac Hypertrophy in Hypertension, ed. by Tarazi, R.C. and Dunbar, J.B., New York: Raven Press, 8, 193-200, 1983
5. Tarazi, R.C.: The progression from hypertrophy to heart failure, Hosp. Pract. 18: 101-122, 1983
6 Meerson, F.Z.: Hyperfunction, Hypertrophy and Heart Failure, Monograph no. 26. Am. Heart Association, New York, 1979
7. Grossman, W., Jones, D., McLaurin, L.P.: Wall stress and patterns of hypertrophy in the human left ventricle, J.Clin. Invest., 56: 56-64, 1975
8. Friedberg, C.K.: The heart in hypertension and renal disease, in: Diseases of the Heart, Philadelphia: W.B. Saunders,Co., 1474, 1966
9. Ibrahim, M.M., Tarazi, R.C.: The heart in hypertension, in: Cardiovascular Clinic, Cleveland Clinic Consultations, ed. by Vidt, D.G., Philadelphia: F.A. Davis, 7, 1: 121-132, 1975
10. Tarazi, R.C., Ferrario, C.M., Dustan, H.P.: The heart in hypertension, in: Hypertension: Physiopatholgy and Treatment, ed. by Genest, J., Koiw, E. and Kuchel, O., New York: McGraw-Hill, Inc. 738-754, 1977
11. Frohlich, E.D., Tarazi, R.C.: Is arterial pressure the sole factor responsible for hypertensive cardiac hypertrophy? Am. J. Cardiol., 44: 959-963, 1979
12. Hartford, M., Wickstrand, J., Wallentin, I., Ljungman, S., Wilhelmsen, L., Berglund, G.: Non-invasive signs of cardiac involvement in essential hypertension, Eur. Heart J. 3: 75-87, 1982
13. Abi-Samra, F., Fouad, F.M., Tarazi, R.C.: Determinants of left ventricular hypertrophy and function in hypertensive patients: An echocardiographic study, Am. J. Med. 1983 (in press)
14. Tarazi, R.C., Sen, S., Saragoca, M., Khairallah, P.A.: The multifactorial role of catecholamines in hypertensive cardiac hypertrophy, Eur. Heart J. 3: 103-110, 1983
15. Hoar, P.F., Siverick, K.T., Hamrell, B.B., Alpert, N.R.: The ATPase activity and Ca^{2+} affinity of myosin B from hypertrophied nonfailing cat hearts, in: Cardiac Hypertrophy, ed. by Alpert, N.R., New York: Academic Press, 333-344, 1971
16. Mickerson, J.N.: Heart failure in hypertensive patients, Am. Heart J. 65: 267-274, 1963
17. Fouad, F.M., Tarazi, R.C.: Cardiac and hemodynamic effects of enalapril, Hypertension, 1983 (in press)
18. Braunwald, E., Ross, J. Jr., Sonnenblick, E.H.: Mechanisms of Contraction of the Normal and Failing Heart, 2nd ed. Boston: Little Brown & Co. 292-306, 1976
19. Tarazi, R.C., Levy, M.N.: Cardiac responses to increased afterload, Hypertension 4: suppl. II: II-8 - II-18, 1982

20. Saragoca, M., Tarazi, R.C.: Left ventricular hypertrophy in rats with renovascular hypertension. Alterations in cardiac function and adrenergic responses, Hypertension, 3 (suppl. II) II-216 - II-221, 1981

21. Saragoca, M., Tarazi, R.C.: Impaired cardiac contractile response to isoproterenol in the spontaneously hypertensive rats, Hypertension, 3, 380-385, 1981

22. Ayobe, M.H., Tarazi, R.C.: Beta-receptors and contractile reserve in left ventricular hypertrophy, Hypertension, 5 (suppl. I) I-192 - I-197, 1983

23. Ayobe, M.H., Tarazi, R.C., Khairallah, P.A.: Alterations of beta-adrenergic receptors with development and reversal of cardiac hypertrophy, J. Mol. Cell. Cardiol., 14: 23, 1982 (abstract)

24. Woodcock, E.A., Funder, J.W., Johnston, C.I.: Decreased cardiac beta-adrenoceptor in hypertensive rats, Clin. Exp. Pharmacol. Physiol., 5: 545-550, 1978

25. Limas, C., Limas, C.J.: Reduced number of beta-adrenergic receptors in the myocardium of spontaneously hypertensive rats, Biochem. Biophys. Res. Comm., 83: 710-714, 1978

26. Woodcock, E.A., Funder, J.W., Johnston, C.I.: Decreased cardiac beta-adrenergic receptors in deoxycorticosterone-salt and renal hypertension rats, Circ. Res., 45: 560-565, 1979

27. Woodcock, E.A., Johnston, C.I.: Changes in tissue alpha- and beta-adrenergic receptors in renal hypertension in the rat, Hypertension 2: 156-161, 1980

28. Giachetti, A., Clark, T.L., Berti, F.: Subsensitivity of cardiac beta-adrenoceptors in renal hypertensive rats, J. Cardiovasc. Pharmacol., 1: 467-471, 1979

29. Limas, C.J.: Increased number of beta-adrenergic receptors in the hypertrophied myocardium, Biochem. Biophys. Acta, 588: 174-178, 1979

30. Chatelain, P., Robberecht, P., DeNeef, P., Camus, J.C., Heuse, D., Christophe, J.: Secretion and VIP-stimulated adenylate cyclase from rat heart. II: Impairment in spontaneous hypertension, Pfluegers Arch. 389: 29-35, 1980

31. Rodbell, M.: The role of hormone receptors and GTP-regulatory proteins in membrane transduction, Nature, 293: 17-22, 1980

32. Kumano, K., Upsher, M.E., Khairallah, P.: Beta-adrenergetic receptor response coupling in hypertrophied hearts, Hypertension 5 (suppl. I): I-174 - I-183, 1983

33. Goodyer, A.V.N., Goodkind, M.J., Landry, A.B.: Ventricular response to a pressure load. Left ventricular function curves in intact animals, Circ.Res. 10: 885-896, 1962

34. Pfeffer, M.A.. Pfeffer, J.M., Fishbein, M.C., Fletcher, P.J., Spardaro, J., Kloner, R.A., Braunwald, E.: Myocardial infarct size and ventricular function in rats, Circ. Res., 44: 503-512, 1979

35. Thoren, P. Noresson, E., Ricksten, S.E.: Cardiac reflexes in normotensive and spontaneously hypertensive rats, Am. J. Cardiol. 44: 884-888, 1979

36. Hallback, M., Isaksson, O. Noresson, E.: Consequences of myocardial structural adaptation on left ventricular compliance and the Frank-Starling relationship in spontaneously hypertensive rats, Acta Physiol. Scand., 94: 259-270, 1975

37. Pfeffer, J.M., Pfeffer, M.A., Braunwald, E.: Development of left ventricular dysfunction in the female spontaneously hypertensive rats, in: Perspectives in Cardiovascular Research, Myocardial Hypertrophy and Failure, ed. by Alpert, N.R., New York: Raven Press, 7, 73-84, 1983

38. Wicker, P., Tarazi, R.C.: Coronary blood flow in left ventricular hypertrophy: a review of experimental data, Eur. Heart J. 3: 111-118, 1982
39. Bache, R.J., Vrobel, T.R.: Effects of exercise on blood flow in the hypertrophied heart, Am. J. Cardiol. 44: 1029-1033, 1979
40. Wicker, P., Tarazi, R.C.: Coronary blood flow measurements with left arterial injection of microspheres in conscious rats, Cardiovasc. Res. 16: 580-586, 1982
41. Wicker, P., Tarazi, R.C.: Importance of injection site for coronary blood flow determinations by microspheres in rats, Am.J. Physiol., 242: H94-H97, 1982
42. Strauer, B.E.: Ventricular function and coronary hemodynamics in hypertensive heart disease, Am. J. Cardiol., 44: 999-1006, 1979
43. Pichard, A.D., Gorlin, R., Smith, H., Ambrose, J., Meller, J.: Coronary flow studies in patients with left ventricular hypertrophy of the hypertensive type, Am. J. Cardiol., 47: 547-554, 1981
44. Marcus, M.L., Mueller, T.M., Gascho, J.A., Kerber, R.E.: Effects on cardiac hypertrophy secondary to hypertension on the coronary circulation, Am. J. Cardiol. 44: 1023-1028, 1979
45. Wicker, P., Tarazi, R.C., Kobayashi, K.: Coronary blood flow with reversal of cardiac hypertrophy, Am. J. Cardiol., 51: 1744-1749, 1983
46. Tarazi, R.C., Sen, S., Fouad, F.J., Wicker, P.: Regression of myocardial hypertrophy: Conditions and sequelae of reversal in hypertensive heart disease, in: Perspectives in Cardiovascular Research, Myocardial Hypertrophy and Failure, ed. by Alpert, N.R., New York: Raven Press, 7, 637-652, 1983
47. Folkow, B.: Cardiovascular structural adaptation; its role in the initiation and maintenance of primary hypertension, Clin. Sci. Mol. Med., 55: 3s-22s, 1978

SUMMARY

The heart adapts itself to an alteration of the arterial system to match the change in the load. A quantitative description of both systems is required for studying the matching principle.

The pump function of the ventricle can be described by the relationship between mean ventricular pressure and mean output. This pump function graph is an inverse relationship, i.e. the output of the ventricle is higher when pressure is lower. The arterial system can be characterized by the relationship between mean aortic pressure and mean output at a given state of arteries and arterioles. This relationship is proportional, i.e. when the output of the ventricle is higher, pressure is higher. The combination of both relationships yields the work point.

The amount of work done by the ventricle on the arterial bed can be calculated from pressure and flow. At a given pump function, the amount of work done depends on the setting of the arterial load. Under control conditions, it can be demonstrated for left and right ventricle that the work point is at maximum work output.

When the oxygen consumption of the ventricle is measured, it can be shown that the left heart cannot combine maximum work output with minimum energy turnover or maximum efficiency.

It is concluded that:
1. *Matching between heart and arterial system implies that the ventricle works at maximum work output;*
2. *The work point for maximum work output is not the same as that for minimum energy turnover or maximum efficiency;*
3. *This could imply that demands of the body determine what output and pressure the heart has to generate, while the heart itself tries to execute the given task at as little cost as possible by operating at maximum work output.*

LEFT VENTRICULAR HYPERTROPHY, MATCHING BETWEEN HEART AND ARTERIAL SYSTEM

ELZINGA, G.

Free University, Laboratory for Physiology, Van der Boechorststraat 7, 1081 BT Amsterdam, The Netherlands

INTRODUCTION

The hemodynamic properties of heart and arterial system are adapted to each other. The well-known changes in cardiac dimensions occurring after a permanent change in arterial load demonstrate clearly the existence of matching. In general it may be assumed that the heart tries to adapt, as long as it can, to the requirements set by the vascular system. The vascular system in its turn is controlled by mechanisms outside the heart.

Although heart and arterial system appear to match hemodynamic properties, the precise matching principle is not known. A number of possibilities may be considered such as: (i) the heart tries to work at optimum efficiency, (ii) the heart tries to work at minimum energy turnover, (iii) the heart tries to work at optimum work output.

In order to learn what the matching principle is we need quantitative selective descriptions of the hemodynamic properties of heart and arterial system. This allows us to study changes of the two systems following an alteration of the hemodynamic situation.

CARDIAC PUMP FUNCTION

The ultimate task of the heart is to pump blood at a given pressure to the various organs of the body where it brings oxygen and substrates and removes waste products. A quantitative description of cardiac pump function can be obtained in analogy to ordinary fluid pumps (Elzinga and Westerhof, 1979). Pump function of such instruments is given by a graph relating the output capacity of the pump to the pressure head it has to overcome. An example of such a curve for a centrifugal pump is shown in figure 1 (head).

A pump function graph, or head capacity curve, can be obtained by measuring output at different pressures. During the determination of a given pump function graph, all control mechanisms of the pump function graphs will be obtained and the resulting graph will not describe one single functional state of the pump.

104

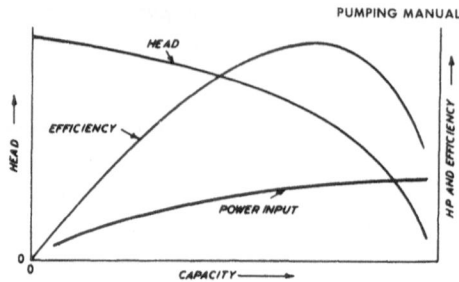

Figure 1: The specific characteristics of a centrifugal pump operated at constant speed. The head curve implies that (output) capacity of the pump increases when the (pressure) head decreases. Power input increases over that range and efficiency is optimum at some intermediate value.

The same approach can be used to quantify ventricular pump function of the heart. There are, however, two obvious differences as compared to the above example of the centrifugal pump: (i) the ventricle does have a valve which separates the ventricular cavity from the aorta. This implies that pressures in these two compartments are different when the valve is closed, which introduces the question what pressure to use for the pump function graph, (ii) the heart is an oscillatory pump, i.e. flow and pressure are not generated continuously, as is the case for the centrifugal pump, but at intervals. This raises the problem at what moments in time pressure and flow should be measured.

For various reasons (Elzinga and Westerhof, 1973; 1979) we choose to relate mean ventricular pressure with mean output. Such a choice ignores properties of the pump which determine oscillatory behavior, but stresses in particular the task of the heart to pump blood at a given pressure to the periphery.

As holds true for the centrifugal pump, ventricular pump function should be determined without changing cardiac control mechanisms. This means that during the pressure changes needed to obtain all points on the graph, heart rate, end-diastolic volume and inotropic state should remain constant. In our experiments we therefore used pressure changes for a single beat to avoid such effects. This requires an experimental technique which has not yet been accepted for studies in the closed chest situation.

A left ventricular pump function graph obtained from a cat heart by the method indicated above is shown in figure 2A. It shows that an inverse relationship exists between mean ventricular pressure and output reminiscent of the one shown for the centrifugal pump in figure 1 (head).

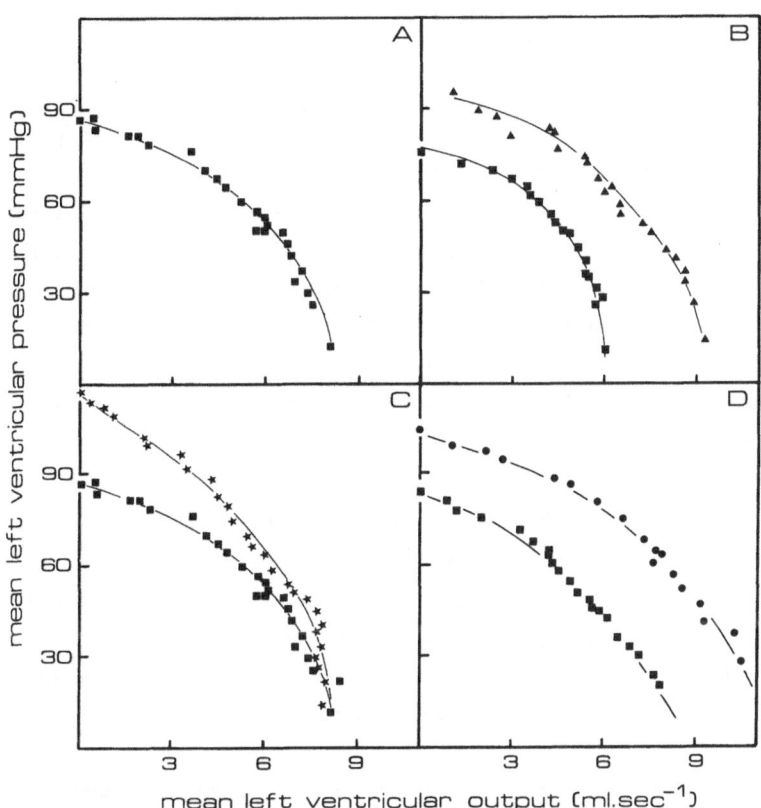

Figure 2: A. The left ventricular pump function graph is the inverse relationship between mean ventricular pressure and output obtained by varying the arterial load at a given functional state of the heart. B. Changes in end-diastolic volume shift the pump function graph in an almost parallel manner. C. An increase in inotropic state rotates the pump function graph around the intercept on the output axis. D. An increase in heart rate causes a parallel shift of the pump function graph, the magnitude of which is related to the frequency change.

Pump function of the left ventricle can change by changing cardiac control mechanisms: end-diastolic volume, inotropic state and heart rate (Elzinga and Westerhof, 1978, 1980). A selective increase in end-diastolic volume (figure 2B) and heart rate (figure 2D) move the pump function graph outwards in a parallel manner, while an increase in inotropic state rotates the graph around the intercept on the flow axis (figure 2C). The changes of ventricular pump function illustrate how important it is to keep control mechanisms constant during the determination of the pump function graph. They also demonstrate that the heart can adapt to changes in arterial load which is a crucial requirement for matching.

THE ARTERIAL SYSTEM

From the point of view of the left ventricle the hemodynamic properties of the arterial system are determined by the resistance, which mainly resides in the small blood vessels, the compliance which is located in the wall of the larger arteries, and the inductance which is determined by the mass of the ejected blood and the dimensions of the ascending aorta. All three components together determine the input impedance of the systemic arterial tree. The input impedance gives the amplitude ratio of, and the phase angle between, aortic pressure and flow as a function of frequency.

To obtain a quantitative description of the ventricular pump (see above), oscillatory phenomena were ignored. Since we want to describe interaction between ventricle and arterial system, the same will therefore be done for the latter. This simply means that the hemodynamic properties of the arterial system will be described by the ratio between mean aortic pressure and ventricular output, i.e. the peripheral resistance.

In contrast to the pump function graph of the ventricle, the pressure-flow relationship determining the peripheral resistance is not inverse. Because Ohms's law holds for the arterial system (McDonald, 1974), resistance is the slope of the straight line going through the origin of the mean pressure-mean flow relationship (figure 3). To measure the full line in the arterial system is not an easy task, because blood vessels tend to change their diameters when pressure alters and, according to Poisseuille's law (McDonald, 1974), this will dramatically affect the resistance. For such reasons pressure-flow relationships are often found which are not straight lines or/and do not go through the origin of the graph. However, as was the case for the ventricle, our interest is focussed on a description of the arterial system at a given state of the vascular bed.

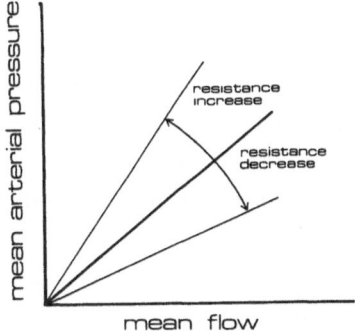

Figure 3: The peripheral resistance is the slope of the line between mean arterial pressure and mean flow. Rotation of the line signifies resistance changes.

Changes in peripheral resistance cause the line (figure 3) to rotate around the graph origin. This illustrates clearly that peripheral resistance should be determined at a fixed configuration of the arterial system. Moreover, it demonstrates that the arterial system can adapt its properties if necessary.

Comparison of the quantitative description of ventricular pump function (figure 2A) and that of the arterial system (figure 3) reveals that the same variable is plotted on the abscissa, but that the pressures on the ordinates have been measured in different cardiovascular compartments (ventricle and aorta). Since these pressures are not the same, the two relationships cannot without further consideration be plotted in the same graph, which, if possible, would simplify the comparison considerably.

We therefore studied (Van den Horn et al., in press) the relationship between mean ventricular and mean aortic pressure in open thorax cats under a wide range of hemodynamic conditions. Provided arterial compliance did not decrease below 25% of control, we found that in the cat:

$$\overline{P}_{ao} = 1.72 \ \overline{P}_{lv} \qquad (1)$$

where $\overline{P}_{ao}$ is mean aortic pressure and $\overline{P}_{lv}$ is mean ventricular pressure.

This finding allows us to combine the pump function graph with the peripheral resistance line in the same coordinate system as is shown in figure 4. The two relationships intersect at the point where the system works: the working point. Studying the position of the working point in the mean pressure-mean output plane, which is, in the intact animal, determined by the hemodynamic properties of heart and arterial system, may reveal some secrets of the nature of the matching principle.

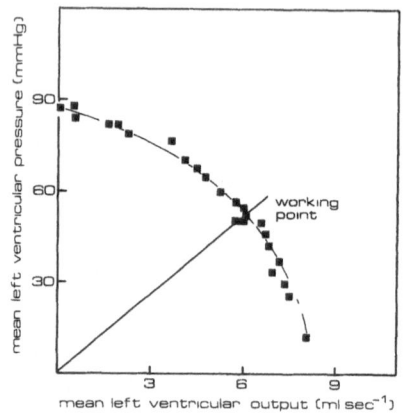

Figure 4: Because a simple relationship exists between mean ventricular and mean aortic pressure, the peripheral resistance line and the pump function graph can be plotted in the same coordinate system.

TRANSFER OF ENERGY FROM HEART TO ARTERIAL SYSTEM

Under normal conditions energy is liberated by the heart from the conversion of substrates into CO_2 and H_2O. Part of the liberated energy is used for contraction. When the left ventricle ejects blood into the ascending aorta at a given pressure, part of the energy used for contraction is converted into external work. That part of the liberated energy which is not converted into external work becomes heat in the myocardium (Ten Velden et al., 1982). The amount of energy transferred to the ascending aorta as work is converted into heat in the vascular system mainly at locations of resistance (see above).

Work output of the left ventricle is not constant but varies with the hemodynamic properties of heart and arterial system. Total external left ventricular work is calculated per unit time as:

$$W = \frac{1}{T} \int P_{(t)} \, F_{(t)} \, dt \qquad (2)$$

where W = work per unit time (power), T = the period of integration, P = pressure in aorta or ventricle and F = aortic blood flow. From this equation it can be learned that work output is zero when either pressure or flow is zero. These extreme situations, which will not occur in the in vivo situation, are found at the intercept of the pump function graph with both axes (figure 5A, B). At all other positions on the pump function graph a finite amount of work is done by the ventricle on the arterial system.

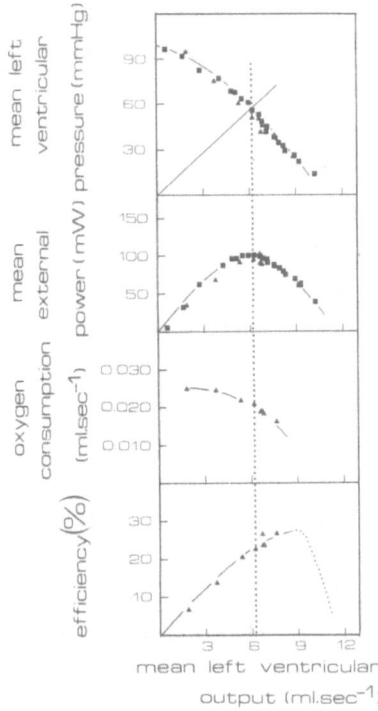

Figure 5: A. The left ventricular pump function graph. B. Work output of the left ventricle. C. Left ventricular oxygen consumption. D. The efficiency of the left ventricle. The comparison shows that optimum work output, minimum energy turnover (oxygen consumption), and optimum efficiency cannot occur at the same working point.

The total amount of energy liberated by the heart can be calculated from the amount of oxygen consumed times the caloric equivalent of the substrate burnt. The value of this product depends on the position of the working point. It is highest when the ventricle contracts isovolumically and lowest when it ejects at zero pressure (figure 5C). The absolute value of the amount of liberated energy is considerably higher than the amount of external work, which implies that most of the energy is lost as heat in the myocardium.

The percentage of liberated energy which is converted into work is called efficiency. If the amount of liberated energy would have been constant, independent of the load, optimum efficiency (figure 5D) would be found at the same working point as the optimum work output. However, this is not the case and optimum efficiency is found at higher outputs and therefore lower pressures.

Comparison of the energy turnover, external work output and efficiency when the working point travels over the pump function graph, indicates that the heart cannot operate simultaneously at the lower rate of energy turnover, maximum work output and maximum efficiency. To understand the matching principle, it is of interest to know at what point the heart wants to work in situ.

MATCHING OF HEART AND ARTERIAL SYSTEM

When in intact anesthetized cats the position of the working point is determined, it can be shown that it is found at optimum work output (Van den Horn et al., in press). A similar finding has been reported for conscious dogs, where pressures and flows were measured with implanted devices (Wilcken et al., 1968). These observations indicate that the heart is controlled to work at the optimum of the work output curve. Does a heart which has to deal with a permanent change in hemodynamic load, remain at this optimum?

Experiments to solve this question in the case of hypertrophy have not yet been performed. However, as is sometimes the case, nature gave us an experiment which can be used to provide an initial answer to the above query.

At birth the circulation of blood in the body changes dramatically and the hemodynamic load for left and right ventricle alters permanently. If the matching principle between heart and arterial system consists in the necessity to remain at the optimum of the work output curve, the working point of the right heart must be found at that very point too. For isolated cat hearts we could show (Elzinga et al., 1980) that work output of left and right heart are about five times different but that for each, when loaded with their respective arterial systems, maximum work output is found at the same cardiac output (figure 6). This implies that the two sides of the heart seem to operate at a similar working point, i.e. at optimum work output.

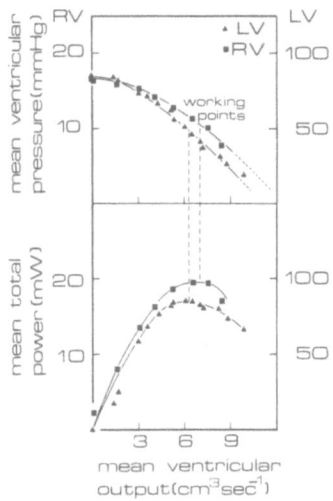

Figure 6: Pump function and work output graphs from right and left ventricle. Although the absolute magnitude of pressure and work differ by about a factor 5 (note different scales), optimum work output is found at the same cardiac output.

CONCLUSIONS

The suggestion that the heart tries to keep its working point at optimum work output raises questions about the mechanisms responsible for such a property. How does the heart sense that it operates at optimum work output? As far as we know, there are no work receptors in the heart. Moreover, we should realize that the rate of energy turnover is not a minimum at optimum work output (figure 5C). This means that the heart is not equipped with instruments needed for such a control mechanism. Therefore, the heart has to obtain information from another source.

The following sequence of events could serve as a working hypothesis for further tests: the tissues in the body require a certain amount of blood (chemoreceptors) at a given pressure (baroreceptors). The heart will try to generate that pressure and output at minimum cost, i.e. the required combination of output and pressure for as little energy turnover as possible. This working point is found at the optimum of the work output curve.

This hypothesis requires further experimental tests. In particular, it needs to be confirmed that a certain amount of work can be generated by the heart most economically at the maximum of the work output curve.

REFERENCES

Elzinga, G. and Westerhof, N.: Pressure and flow generated by the left ventricle against different impedances, <u>Circ. Res.</u>, 32:178-166, 1973

Elzinga, G. and Westerhof, N.: How to quantify pump function of the heart; the value of variables derived from measurements on isolated muscle, <u>Circ. Res.</u>, 44:303-308, 1979

Elzinga, G., Piene, H. and Jong, J.P. de: Left and right ventricular pump function and consequences of having two pumps in one heart; a study on the isolated cat heart, <u>Circ. Res.</u>, 46:564-574, 1980

Horn, G.J. van den, Westerhof, N. and Elzinga, G.: Interaction of heart and arterial system, <u>Ann. Biomed. Eng.</u> (in press)

McDonald, D.A.: <u>Blood flow in arteries</u>, Edw. Arnold, London, 1974

Velden, G.H.M. ten, Elzinga, G. and Westerhof, N.: Left ventricular energetics, <u>Circ. Res.</u>, 50:63-73, 1982

Wilcken, D.E.L., Charlier, A.A., Hoffman, J.I.E. and Guz, A.: Effects of alterations in aortic impedance on the performance of the ventricles, <u>Circ. Res.</u>, 14:283-293, 1964

SUMMARY

Until the recent past, cardiac function in hypertension has usually been assessed in terms of cardiac output or by analogy with other models of ventricular hypertrophy. Neither method was very satisfactory, but more direct studies of ventricular function were often impossible because of the ethical problems involved in the investigation of asymptomatic patients. The advent of non- or minimally invasive methods such as echocardiography and radionuclide first pass and gated blood pool techniques (99^m Tc) has allowed the integration of structural and functional aspects of ventricular hypertrophy and a better understanding of hypertensive heart disease. They have revealed an inverse relation between end-systolic stress and overall cardiac performance (measured as either LV %FS or V_{cf} (r = -0.76, p < 0.001). This approach has also helped distinguish afterload mismatch from myocardial depression. In addition, ventricular diastolic function was found to be altered in hypertension even before any clinical evidence of reduced systolic performance. Left ventricular filling rate was significantly reduced in hypertensive patients even though their cardiac output, ejection fraction and maximum rate of ejection were normal. This reduction in maximum LV filling rate correlated significantly with echocardiographically determined LV mass.

With therapy, regression of left ventricular hypertrophy occurred in some but not all patients. This change in left ventricular mass has not led in our experience to depression of cardiac performance. More studies, however, are needed to assess cardiac reserve in such cases.

ASSESSMENT OF THE FUNCTION OF THE HYPERTROPHIED HEART

FOUAD, F.M.

Research Division, Cleveland Clinic Foundation, Cleveland, Ohio

INTRODUCTION

A striking observation in most of the studies of cardiac structure and function in hypertension has been the dissociation between blood pressure levels and left ventricular mass. Berglund and co-workers[1] found a correlation of 0.26 between mean arterial pressure and echocardiographically determined left ventricular mass. In our laboratory, the correlation between left ventricular mass and systolic blood pressure was 0.46 (fig.1).

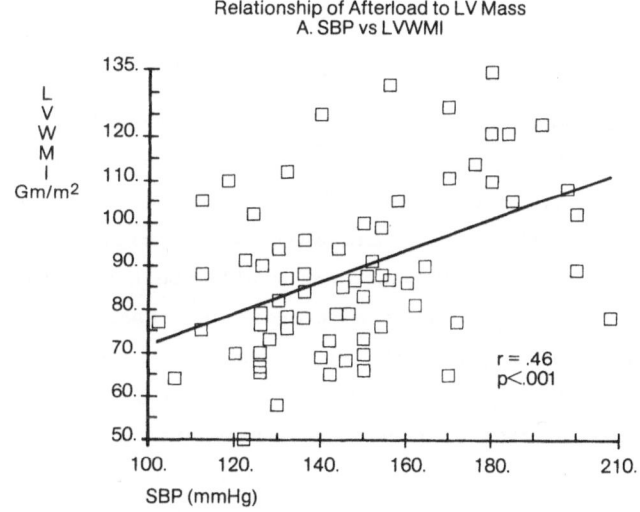

Figure 1. Correlation between systolic blood pressure (SBP) and left ventricular mass (LVM) in hypertensive patients. Although the correlation was significant, the r-value was only 0.46 and there was a marked dispersion of data points.

It is of interest that an even more striking dissociation between blood pressure and ventricular weight (or mass) was also observed during treatment both in clinical studies[2] and in animal experiments.[3] The reasons for this dissociation are many (table 1).

Table 1. Possible causes of dissociation between blood pressure and left ventricular mass.

1) HEMODYNAMIC CAUSES

    a) Inaccurate or approximate estimate of afterload

    b) Casual vs. continuous blood pressure recording

    c) Concomitant increase in volume load.

2) NEUROHUMORAL CAUSES

    a) Sympathetic stimulation

    b) Activation of the renin-angiotensin system

    c) Influence of other hormones (e.g. thyroxin, growth hormone)

3) ASSOCIATED CARDIAC DISEASE

4) AGING AND GENETIC FACTORS

In part, arterial pressure per se is not an accurate expression of afterload, since the latter also depends on left ventricular wall thickness and left ventricular cavity dimensions.[4] The relationship between calculated left ventricular wall stress and left ventricular mass, however, proved to be complex. On the one hand, one would expect that the greater the afterload, the more marked the hypertrophic response, but on the other hand, the greater thickening of the myocardium could help reduce wall stress.[5] In fact, an inverse correlation was reported between left ventricular peak systolic stress and left ventricular mass in hypertensive patients.

Among the other factors that can influence left ventricular mass and weight (table 1), circulating catecholamines have received the greatest attention. Clinical experience led Raab[7] to postulate that catecholamines play an important role in the evolution of hypertensive heart disease.[8]

Experimentally small doses of isoproterenol that did not produce myocardial necrosis, led to ventricular hypertrophy.[8,9] Moreover, Yamori and Tarazi[10] showed that alpha-blockade did not prevent the development of left ventricular hypertrophy secondary to norepinephrine infusions in rats, although it did blunt the rise in blood pressure; on the other hand, a beta-blocked parallel group had a higher blood pressure but a smaller left ventricular mass. Further, blood pressure control by antihypertensive drugs that produced reflex stimulation of adrenergic nervous system either failed to induce regression of LVH or resulted in a further increase of LVH in SHR.[11] Association of these vasodilators with beta-blocking[12] or sympatholytic[11] drugs, led to regression of hypertrophy even if blood pressure was not as well controlled.[12]

1) Left ventricular structural changes in hypertensive man

Studies of cardiac structure and function in clinical hypertension have lagged behind the rapid accumulation of knowledge in other forms of cardiac diseases,[13,14] mainly because of the invasiveness of the procedures needed and the asymptomatic nature of hypertension. These studies became possible with the introduction of non-invasive methods such as echocardiography and radionuclide techniques.

The following discussion is based on our experience with 73 hypertensive patients using M-mode echocardiography; the study has been reported in detail elsewhere.[15] Patients' ages ranged from 19 to 69 years (mean, 47.7 years); there were 40 men and 33 women; mean arterial pressure ranged from 77 to 159 mmHg [mean 112 mmHg $\pm$ 16 (SD)] and left ventricular wall mass corrected for body surface area (LVWMI) ranged from 50 to 135 g/m^2. There was no significant difference in average LV dimensions between the 37 untreated and the 36 treated patients in this series; so data from all patients were pooled together. The M-mode echocardiogram was recorded under two-dimensional echo monitoring to be sure of the position at which the M-mode tracing is recorded (at level of tip of mitral valve for LV measurements with the echo beam perpendicular to the long axis of the LV cavity). Left ventricular mass was calculated using the ellipsoid formula applied to both the inner and the outer volume of the left ventricle; the Teichholz correction factor was applied to the two volumes, each separately before subtraction.[15] The resulting volume (left ventricular wall volume) was multiplied by 1.05, the specific density of the myocardium.[16]

An important observation recently reported by Grossman et al.[17] and confirmed by others, has helped keep the study of hypertensive heart disease completely non-invasive. A high correlation between cuff blood pressure and left ventricular systolic pressure was repeatedly document-ed. We also found the same correlation in our laboratory in a separate group of patients with coronary artery disease.[18] Left ventricular wall stress was, therefore, calculated from cuff systolic blood pressure and echocardiographically recorded left ventricular dimensions (equation nos. 1 and 2).

$$ESS = \frac{.334 \times ESD \times SBP}{h_s \ (1 + h_s/ESD)} \tag{1}$$

$$PSS = \frac{.334 \times EDD \times SBP}{h_d \ (1 + h_d/EDD)} \tag{2}$$

Our hypertensive population showed a wide spectrum of structural cardiac findings: 42% had normal left ventricular dimensions, 22% had asymmetric septal hypertrophy, 20% had concentric left ventricular hypertrophy, and 16% had left ventricular dilatation in addition to hypertrophy. Another finding in hypertensive patients was the presence of left atrial enlarge-ment which was documented in 13 patients, with or without left ventric-ular abnormalities. In fact, five of them had completely normal left ventricles. Logan et al.[19] also reported the same observation in border-line hypertensives followed for a year. In this respect, electrocardio-graphic studies by Sodi Pallares[20] and by Tarazi et al.[21] had previously shown that isolated P wave abnormalities can sometimes be observed in hypertensive patients in the absence of any evidence of left ventricular hypertrophy. Presumably, these isolated left atrial abnormalities are related to abnormalities in left ventricular filling or compliance which may antedate any definite evidence of left ventricular hypertrophy. The evidence for this suggestion is further discussed later.

2) Left ventricular systolic function

Overall ventricular performance was evaluated in our patients (15) from the measurement of LV fractional shortening.[22] Since this index is load-dependent, it was assessed in relation to:

(a) an index of preload, derived from the left ventricular end-diastolic cavity dimension, (b) an index of afterload, the LV end-systolic stress, and (c) an index of contractility, the ratio of systolic blood pressure to end-systolic volume.[23] This latter index was based on the load independence of the relationship between LV end-systolic pressure and volume, E_{max}[24]; it was further simplified to avoid drug infusions during the study. The interaction between these three determinants of LV function was analyzed by a multivariant regression analysis.[25]

Left ventricular end-systolic stress correlated inversely with LV fractional shortening both in the hypertensive patients as well as in a parallel group of 20 normal volunteers (fig. 2).

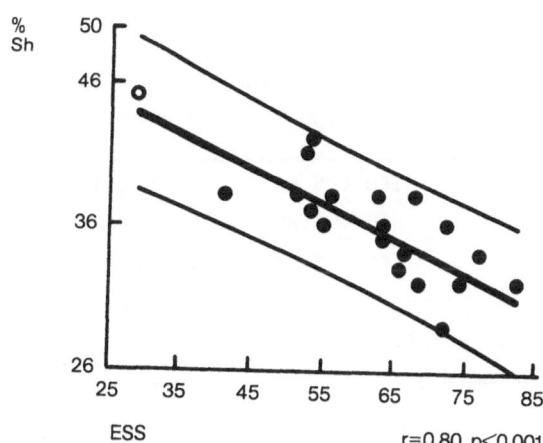

Figure 2. Inverse correlation between end-systolic stress (ESS) and left ventricular fractional shortening (% Sh) in 20 normal subjects.

A similar correlation was also reported in hypertensive patients by other centers.[6,26] In fact, the multivariate regression analysis confirmed that afterload was the major determinant of LV systolic function in hypertensive patients. Afterload became even more important and was the dominant factor in hypertensives with LV dilatation, whereas LV contractility was the major factor governing LV function in normal individuals and in patients with isolated septal hypertrophy (ASH). The mechanism(s) underlying the shift in factors controlling LV function are not completely clarified and the subject is further discussed in section 1, which deals with responsiveness of the hypertrophied heart to catecholamines and its dependence on the Frank-Starling mechanism.

3) Left ventricular diastolic function

Qualitative changes in left ventricular volume curve configuration (gated blood pool scanning) in hypertensive patients was described by Quereshi et al.[27] A significantly slower left ventricular peak filling rate in hypertensive patients compared to normotensive volunteers was then documented by Fouad et al.[28] In this latter study (radionuclide technique), the two groups of normotensives and hypertensives had similar heart rate, cardiac index, ejection fraction and peak LV ejection rate (table 2).

Table 2: LV ejection fraction and filling rates

	Normotensives (n=12)	Hypertensives (n=15)	P
SBP (mmHg)	109 + 3.90	160 + 5.81	< 0.001
DBP (mmHg)	70 + 1.35	99 + 2.80	< 0.001
HR (bpm)	62 + 2.50	65 + 3.18	ns
CI ($1/min/m^2$)	3.05 + 0.18	3.01 + 0.19	ns
EF	0.52 + 0.01	0.55 + 0.02	ns
Age (years)	21 - 66	20 - 63	

SBP = systolic blood pressure; DBP = diastolic blood pressure;
HR = heart rate; CI = cardiac index; EF = ejection fraction

Since LV pressure was not measured in these studies, this slower rate of filling could only be conceivably related to alterations in either LV compliance or LV relaxation. The fact that the major slowing occurred in early filling suggested, however, that this early alteration of LV function in hypertension was secondary to a slowed relaxation rate. Further studies were, therefore, developed to investigate this possibility (vide infra).

Whatever its mechanism, the slowed ventricular filling helped explain the frequent EKG and echocardiographic abnormalities of the left atrium in hypertension.[15,20,21] The occurrence of left atrial enlargement, even before unequivocal signs of LVH were seen, enhanced the clinical importance of this observation. Further, the presence of EKG-left atrial enlargement was associated with a greater incidence of atrial arrhythmias.[21]

4) Effect of therapy on left ventricular filling rate in hypertensive patients

The influence of therapy on left ventricular filling was studied in our laboratory in two groups of hypertensive patients using gated blood pool scanning (^{99m}Tc-HSA). To avoid the possible effects of structural changes, the duration of therapy was kept relatively short. The first group of 21 hypertensive patients was treated with beta-blockers, either with nadolol (non-cardioselective) or metoprolol (cardioselective). The differences in hemodynamic response (first pass technique) between the two treatment groups were not significant (figs. 3a and b). Therefore, data were pooled together and the results were analyzed according to blood pressure response only; nine patients (non-responders) had no significant change in blood pressure and 12 responders had a reduction in mean arterial pressure > 10 mmHg. Both non-responders and responders had similar reduction in heart rate and cardiac output during treatment. Both groups showed no significant change in ejection fraction or peak rate of left ventricular ejection. The two groups, however, had a different response of LV filling rate (figs. 4a and b); whereas responders increased the rate of filling, the non-responders showed a further slowing of filling rate compared to pretreatment values. A simple explanation would be that blood pressure reduction counterbalanced the effect of beta-

122

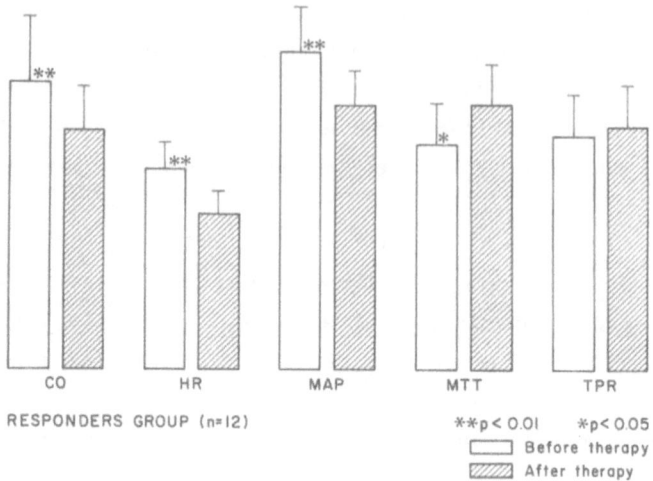

Figure 3a. Hemodynamic changes in association with blood pressure reduction in 12 patients treated with beta-blockers (either nadolol or metoprolol) for one month.

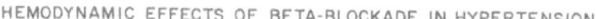
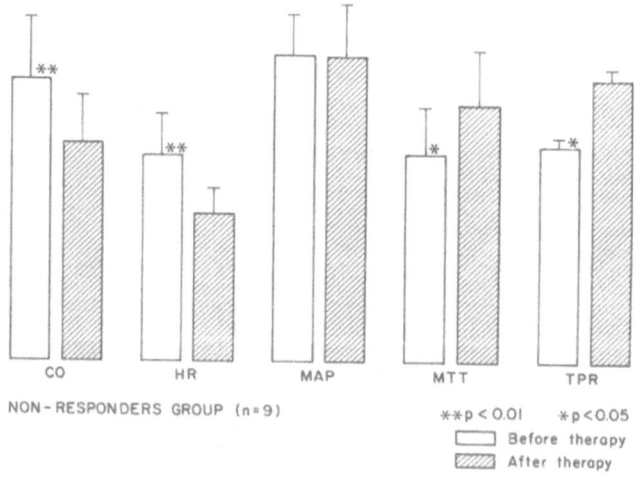

Figure 3b. Hemodynamic changes in nine patients, non-responders to beta-blockade therapy (either nadolol or metoprolol) for one month.

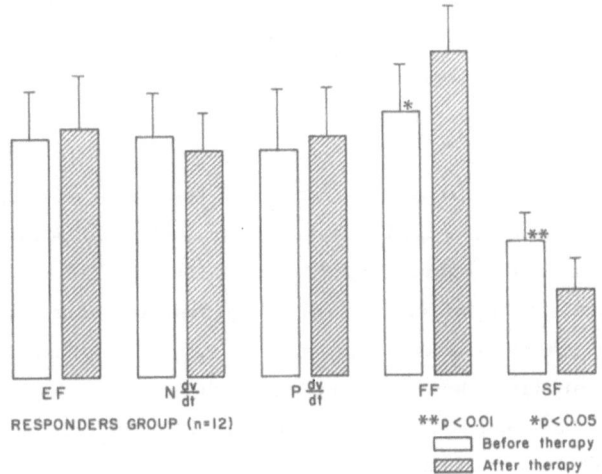

Figure 4a. Cardiac performance indices in association with beta-blockade therapy in 12 patients who showed blood pressure reduction (see figure 3a).

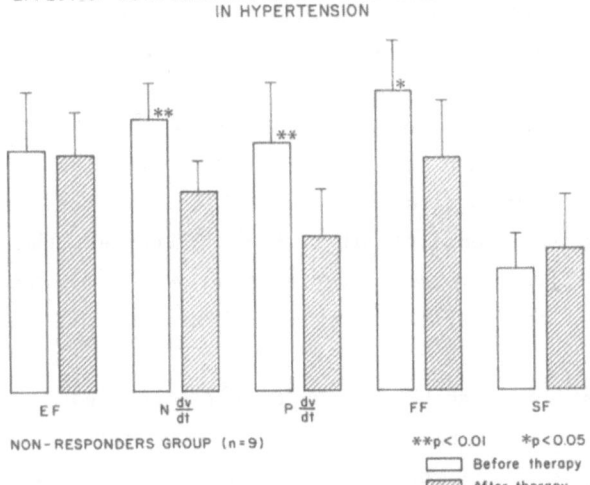

Figure 4b. Cardiac performance indices in association with beta-blockade therapy in nine patients who had no blood pressure change during treatment (see figure 3b).

blockade on the heart. In patients whose blood pressure did not change, the effect of adrenergic blockade was manifested by further slowing of relaxation. These observations were thus the clinical counterpart of the increase in relaxation produced by beta-stimulation in experimental studies.[29]

In the second study (11 patients) we utilized the calcium entry blocker, nitrendipine. Reduction of blood pressure was again associated with an increase in peak rate of ventricular filling (+dv/dt); it was difficult, however, to separate the effect of blood pressure reduction from the effect of calcium entry blockade per se because of the small number of patients. In both studies, however, the relatively early changes observed during treatment suggested that alterations in ventricular diastolic function could be due to functional factors such as level of arterial pressure or of adrenergic activity[30,31] and were not necessarily related to myocardial structural changes alone.

5) Regression of left ventricular hypertrophy

Reports from many centers over the past few years have unequivocally demonstrated that regression of LVH could be produced in hypertensive hearts, both in experimental models and in man.[6,32-36] The possible effects of that regression on cardiac function have not yet been, however, fully investigated. In our initial series of 11 patients treated with methyldopa, we did not observe significant changes in percent LV shortening in the four patients who showed a reduction in LV mass[33]; this was also the experience of others.[6,35,36] However, the interpretation of these results from group averages is difficult because of the concomitant changes in arterial pressure in different patients.

We extended our study to another group of patients treated with the new converting enzyme inhibitor, enalapril. This drug was chosen because it was shown to decrease total peripheral resistance without reflex stimulation of sympathetic nervous system, i.e., without change in heart rate or cardiac output.[37] Most patients responded to therapy and there was found, on the average, a reduction of left ventricular mass from 107 g/m^2 surface area to 94 g/m^2 ($p < 0.05$) during the seven months' follow-up (fig. 5). Blood pressure control might have played a role in the re-

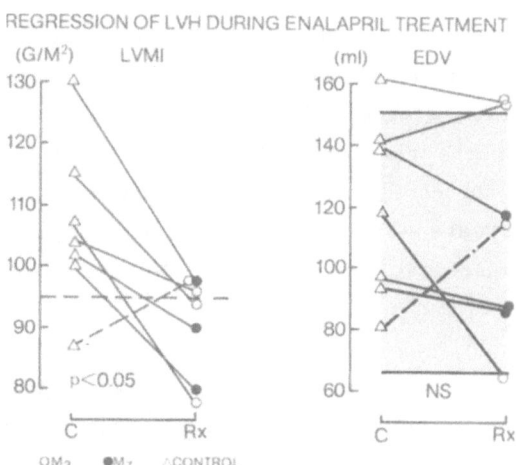

REGRESSION OF LVH DURING ENALAPRIL TREATMENT

Figure 5. Regression of left ventricular hypertrophy during enalapril
treatment. Left panel illustrates the change in left ventricular mass
(LVM); the dashed transverse line represents the upper limit of normal
LVM/m^2 BSA, in our laboratory. Right panel illustrates the corresponding
changes in end-diastolic volume (EDV).

gression of LVH in these patients, but other factors might also have been
involved, since there was no correlation between changes in pressure and
changes in LV mass. Indeed, angiotensin II was previously reported to
stimulate protein synthesis in the heart[38]; moreover, it is also known
to potentiate sympathetic activity both peripherally and centrally.[39,40]

Left ventricular performance during reduction of LV mass in patients
treated with enalapril was first evaluated by standard hemodynamic
indices:

(a) no changes were found in cardiac output, stroke volume, or pulmonary
circulation time; (b) ejection fraction (gated radionuclide technique)
did not change significantly. However, since these indices are load-dependent, we evaluated the relationship between LV stress and LV percent

shortening. This approach allowed us to take into account the concomitant changes in systolic blood pressure, LV wall thickness and internal diameter. Data were analyzed against our previous findings in 20 normal volunteers; these could serve as a point of reference for the study of changes in LV mass in hypertension, since the same relationship was also found in an independent study of untreated 37 hypertensive patients.[15] Data points from the hypertensive patients treated with enalapril fell within the 95% prediction limits of the normal regression line, both before treatment and at the time of maximum change of left ventricular mass. Thus, even when corrected for possible changes in afterload and with each patient evaluated individually, there was no evidence of altered cardiac performance, at least at rest, despite the reduction of left ventricular mass.

In conclusion, the heart in hypertension can show a wide variety of structural and functional changes. The alterations in function can affect not only systolic but also diastolic performance. Indeed, diastolic changes might occur much earlier than the reduction in systolic function. Both aspects can be influenced by treatment, either because of reduction in arterial pressure, of interference with neurohumoral factors, or secondary to regression of hypertrophy. The effect of the latter on LV function needs to be studied further with particular reference to pump function during physical exercise and stress.

REFERENCES

1. Hartford, M., Wikstrand, J., Wallentin, I., Lungman, S. Wilhelmsen, L. and Berglund, G.: Non-invasive signs of cardiac involvement in essential hypertension, Eur. Heart J., 3: 75-87, 1982.
2. Devereux, R., Savage, D.D., Sachs, I. and Laragh, J.H.: Effect of blood pressure control on left ventricular hypertrophy and function in hypertension, Circulation, 62 (suppl. II): III-36, 1980 (abstract).
3. Sen, S., Tarazi, R.C., Khairallah, P.A. and Bumpus, F.M.: Cardiac hypertrophy in spontaneously hypertensive rats, Circ. Res., 35: 775-781, 1974.
4. Quinones, M.A., Mokotoff, D.M., Nouri, S., Winters, W.L. and Miller, R.R.: Non-invasive quantification of left ventricular wall stress validation of method and application to assessment of chronic pressure overload, Am. J. Cardiol., 45: 782-790, 1980.
5. Grossman, W., Jones, D. and McLaurin, L.W.: Wall stress and patterns of hypertrophy in the human left ventricle, J. Clin. Invest., 56: 56-64, 1975.

6. Blackwood, R.A., Bloom, K.R. and Williams. C.M.: Aortic stenosis in children. Experience with echocardiographic procedure in severity, Circulation, 57: 263-268, 1978.
7. Raab, W.: Hormonal and Neurogenic Cardiovascular Disorders. Williams and Wilkins Co., Baltimore, 1953.
8. Alderman, E.L. and Harrison, D.C.: Myocardial hypertrophy resulting from low dosage isoproterenol administration in rats, Proc. of the Society for Experimental Biol. and Med., 136: 268-270, 1971.
9. Stanton, H.C., Brenner, G. and Maysfield, E.D.: Studies on isoproterenol-induced cardiomegaly in rats, Am. Heart J., 77: 72-8-, 1969.
10. Yamori, Y., Ooshima, A. and Tarazi, R.C.: Prevention of cardiovascular structural changes in norepinephrine-induced hypertension by alpha and beta blockers, Clin. Exp. Hypertension, 2: 347-357, 1980.
11. Sen, S., Tarazi, R.C. and Bumpus F.M.: Cardiac hypertrophy and antihypertensive therapy, Cardiovasc. Res., 11: 427-433, 1977.
12. Sen, S. and Tarazi, R.C.: Regression of myocardial hypertrophy and influence of adrenergic system, Am. J. Physiol., 13: H-97-H-101, 1983.
13. Tarazi, R.C. and Conway, J.: Hemodynamics of hypertension. In: Hypertension, 2nd edition (Genest, J., Kuchel, O., Hamet, P. and Cantin, M. eds), McGraw-Hill Book Co., New York, 1983 (in press).
14. Tarazi, R.C. and Dunbar, J.B.: Perspectives in Cardiovascular Research, vol. 8, Cardiac hypertrophy in hypertension. Raven Press, New York, pp. 349-352, 1983.
15. Abi-Samra, F., Fouad, F.M. and Tarazi, R.C.: Determinants of left ventricular hypertrophy and function in hypertensive patients. An echocardiographic study, Am. J. Med. (in press).
16. Troy, B.L., Pombo, J. and Rackley, C.E.: Measurement of left ventricular wall thickness and mass by echocardiography, Circulation, 45: 602-611, 1972.
17. Wilson, J.R., Reichek, N. and Hirshfeld, J.: Noninvasive assessment of load reduction in patients with asymptomatic aortic regurgitation, Am. J. Med., 68: 664-674, 1980.
18. El-Tobgi, S., Fouad, F.M., Kramer, J.R., Rincon, G., Sheldon, W.C. and Tarazi, R.C.: Left ventricular function in coronary artery disease. Evaluation of E_{max} and systolic P/Ve_s ratio, J. Am. Col. Cardiol. (in press).
19. Logan, A.G., Gilbert, B.W., Haynes, R.B., Milne, B.J., Flanagan, P.T.: Early effects of mild hypertension on the heart. A longitudinal study, Hypertension, 3 (suppl. II): II-187-II-190, 1981.
20. Sodi-Pallares, D. and Calder, R.M.: New Bases of Echocardiography. The C.V. Mosby Company, St. Louis, pp. 84 and 252, 1956.
21. Tarazi, R.C., Miller, A., Frohlich, E.D. and Dustan, H.P.: Electrocardiographic changes reflecting left atrial abnormality in hypertension, Circulation, 34: 818-822, 1966.
22. Feigenbaum, H.: Echocardiography, 2nd edition. Lea and Febiger, Philadelphia, 1976.
23. Nivatpumin, T., Katz, S. and Scheuer, J.: Peak left ventricular systolic pressure/end-systolic volume ratio: a sensitive detector of left ventricular disease, Am. J. Cardiol., 43: 969-974, 1979.
24. Suga, H., Sagawa, K. and Shoukas, A.A.: Load independence of the instantaneous pressure-volume ratio of the canine left ventricle and effects of epinephrine and heart rate on the ratio, Circ. Res., 32: 314-322, 1973.
25. Dixon, W.J. and Massay Jr, F.J.: Introduction to Statistical Analysis. McGraw-Hill Book Co., New York, p. 638, 1969.

26. Devereux, R.B., Savage, D.D., Sachs, I. and Laragh, J.H.: Relation of hemodynamic load to left ventricular hypertrophy and performance in hypertension, Am. J. Cardiol., 51: 171-176, 1983.

27. Quereshi, S., Wagner, H.N., Alderson, P.P., Housholder, D.F., Douglass, K.H., Lotter, M.G., Nickoloff, E.L., Tanabe, M. and Knowles, L.G.: Evaluation of left ventricular function in normal persons and patients with heart disease, J. Nucl. Med., 19: 135-141, 1978.

28. Fouad, F.M., Rarazi, R.C., Gallagher, J.H., MacIntyre, W.J. and Cook, S.A.: Abnormal left ventricular relaxation in hypertensive patients, Clin. Sci., 59: 411s-414s, 1980.

29. Morad, M. and Rolett, E.: Relaxing effects of catecholamines on mammalian heart, J. Physiol., 224: 537-558, 1972.

30. Brutsaert, D.L., Housmans, P.R. and Goethals, M.A.: Dual control of relaxation. Its role in the ventricular function in the mammalian heart, Circ. Res., 47: 637-652. 1980.

31. Paulus, W.J. and Brutsaert, D.L.: Relaxation abnormalities in cardiac hypertrophy, Eur. Heart J., 3 (suppl. A): 133-137, 1982.

32. Tarazi, R.C., Sen, S. and Fouad, F.M.: Regression of myocardial hypertrophy. In: Congestive Heart Failure: Current Research and Clinical Applications (Braunwald, E., Mock, M.B. and Watson, W., eds). Grune and Stratton, New York, pp. 151-163, 1982.

33. Fouad, F.M., Nakashima, Y., Tarazi, R.C. and Salcedo, E.: Reversal of left ventricular hypertrophy in hypertensive patients treated with methyldopa. Lack of association with blood pressure control, Am. J. Cardiol., 49: 795-801, 1982.

34. Nakashima, Y., Fouad, F.M., Tarazi, R.C. and Bravo, E.L.: Left ventricular function with reversal of left ventricular hypertrophy in hypertensive patients, Am. J. Col. Cardiol., 1: 599, 1983 (abstract).

35. Schlant, R.C., Felner, J.M., Blumenstein, B.A., Wollam, G.L., Hall, W.D., Shulman, N.B., Heymsfield, S.B., Gilbert, C.A. and Tuttle, E.P.: Echocardiographic documentation of regression of left ventricular hypertrophy in patients treated for essential hypertension, Eur. Heart J., 3 (suppl. A): 171-175, 1982.

36. Reichek, N., Franklin, B.B., Changler, T., Muhammad, A., Plappert, T. and St. John Sutton, M.: Reversal of left ventricular hypertrophy by antihypertensive therapy, Eur. Heart J., 3 (suppl. A): 165-169, 1982.

37. Fouad, F.M., Tarazi, R.C., Bravo, E.L. and Textor, S.C.: Hemodynamic and antihypertensive effects of the new oral angiotensin converting enzyme inhibitor MK-421 (enalapril), Hypertension (in press).

38. Khairallah, P.A. and Kanabus, J.: Angiotensin and myocardial protein synthesis. In: Perspectives in Cardiovascular Research, vol. 8, Cardiac hypertrophy in hypertension (Tarazi, R.C. and Dunbar, J.B., eds). Raven Press, New York, pp. 337-347, 1983.

39. Ferrario, C.M., Dickinson, C.J. and McCubbin, J.W.: Central vasomotor stimulation by angiotensin, Clin. Sci., 30: 239-245, 1970.

40. Antonaccio, M.J. and Kerwin, L.: Pre- and post-junctional inhibition of vascular sympathetic function by Captopril in SHR. Implications of vascular angiotensin II in hypertension and antihypertensive actions of Captopril, Hypertension, 3 (suppl. I): I-54-I-62, 1981.

THE CORONARY CIRCULATION IN THE HYPERTROPHIED HEART

SUMMARY

Vulnerability of subendocardial muscle to ischemia is enhanced by acquired hypertrophy. The basis of subendocardial ischemia is that an imbalance between myocardial oxygen supply and demand causes selective loss of coronary flow reserve in subendocardial vessels. This can be demonstrated in experiments in which left ventricular work and oxygen consumption are constant while coronary perfusion pressure is lowered in stages. At first, flow remains constant because vessels in all muscle layers dilate. There is, however, a progressive loss of coronary flow reserve, i.e. the extra flow that can be obtained at any pressure when the coronary vessels are maximally dilated. At some lower limit of pressure, total flow decreases due to a selective decrease in subendo-cardial blood flow. At this stage subendocardial vessels have lost their coronary flow reserve, while the remaining myocardial vessels still have some: thus any decrease in pressure below to critical pressure decreases subendocardial flow causing ischemia.

In acquired hypertrophy the total cross-sectional area of the vascular bed is not increased. Myocardial flow per gram of muscle is usually normal; total flow to the hypertrophied muscle is thus increased. The increased myocardial flow is achieved by increased vasodilation at rest. As a result, coronary flow reserve is reduced whenever there is hyper-trophy with normal perfusing pressures. Total blood flow is also in-creased in anemia or tachycardia, and the combination of these with hypertrophy is particularly deleterious. Another harmful combination is the polycythemia and hypoxemia of cyanotic heart disease. Increased viscosity decreases maximal coronary flow, and hypertrophy and hypoxemia raise resting myocardial flow; coronary flow reserve is thus drastically reduced. Similar effects occur when large coronary vessels are stenotic or when there is small-vessel disease of the coronary vascular system.

Two factors can prevent a decreased coronary flow reserve. In systemic hypertension the coronary perfusing pressure is high, so that there is a large coronary flow reserve. When ventricular hypertrophy begins in utero or in neonates, the total vascular bed seems to grow in parallel with the increase in muscle mass: coronary flow reserve is thus not compromised. The age at which vascular growth ceases, is unknown.

TOTAL AND TRANSMURAL PERFUSION OF THE HYPERTROPHIED HEART

HOFFMAN J.I.E., GRATTAN M.T., HANLEY F.L., MESSINA L.M.
Cardiovascular Research Institute and the Departments of Pediatrics
and Physiology, University of California, 1403 HSE San Francisco,
CA 94143, U.S.A.

INTRODUCTION

Ventricular hypertrophy in humans is associated with angina pectoris and electrocardiographic signs of subendocardial ischemia at rest or on exercise, even when there is no coronary stenosis; frequently it is accompanied by myocardial fibrosis that is often predominantly subendocardial. These changes are most prominent in left ventricular hypertrophy due to severe aortic stenosis[1-10] but have been described in aortic incompetence,[11] systemic hypertension,[12-15] and congestive cardiomyopathies.[16-18] They have been observed also in right ventricular hypertrophy due to pulmonic stenosis[19-21] or pulmonary hypertension.[22] Although there are many ways in which hypertrophy can damage the heart, current evidence suggests that the changes mentioned above are due primarily to the failure of myocardial blood flow to meet myocardial oxygen demands. Such failure could involve several mechanisms: inadequate growth of the extramural coronary arteries, increased diffusion distance from capillaries to the core of the myocardial cells, or impaired distribution of blood by the intramural coronary vessels to subendocardial muscle.

Despite a few contradictory reports, most studies have found that when ventricles hypertrophy the size of the extramural coronary arteries increases in proportion to the increase in heart weight,[23-27] so that the large arteries should offer no barrier to supplying blood to the increased muscle mass and thus are not involved in producing subendocardial ischemia. On the other hand, there is indeed an increased dif-

Supported by Program Project Grant HL-25847.

fusion distance that could lead to problems in supplying oxygen and substrates, even though capillaries are usually adequate in hypertrophy.[25,27-29] Tomanek et al.[30] have shown in the spontaneously hypertensive rat that capillary surface area did not increase in proportion to myocyte growth while hypertrophy was developing, but that during stable hypertrophy capillary growth restored capillary density and surface area to normal. The physiologic effects of an increased diffusion distance are uncertain because there can, for example, be compensatory changes in permeability,[31] and changes of diffusion distance appear to be uniform across the ventricular wall and so cannot explain the subendocardial localization of ischemia. This therefore leaves abnormal intramyocardial distribution of blood flow as the most likely cause of the ischemic subendocardial damage that occurs in hypertrophied ventricles.

BASIC PATHOPHYSIOLOGY

When pressure or volume loads cause ventricular hypertrophy, there is a period, often long, of stable hypertrophy[32,33] with no change of ventricular volume or muscle mass. At this stage, resting ventricular peak systolic wall stress is normal because the increased wall thickness compensates for the increased ventricular pressure or diameter.[34-38] Because wall stress is a major determinant of myocardial oxygen consumption,[38-41] the resting left ventricular oxygen consumption per unit muscle mass is usually normal;[38,42,43] thus the total resting left ventricular oxygen consumption is increased in proportion to the increased muscle mass. Because myocardial blood flow is regulated mainly by myocardial oxygen consumption, in stable left ventricular hypertrophy the resting myocardial blood flow per unit muscle mass is usually found to be normal,[42-51] although sometimes it has been found to be slightly below normal;[52-55] all studies, however, have found an increased total resting blood flow in the increased left ventricular muscle mass.

Except for patients who have severe aortic stenosis or coronary stenosis, hypertrophy does not usually cause ischemia at rest. There are, however, many perturbations that can cause ischemia either by altering myocardial oxygen demand or by interfering with myocardial blood supply. To understand the basis for these changes, consider figure 1, which represents myocardial pressure-flow relations during autoregulation and during maximal vasodilatation. To obtain these data, a cannula is placed in

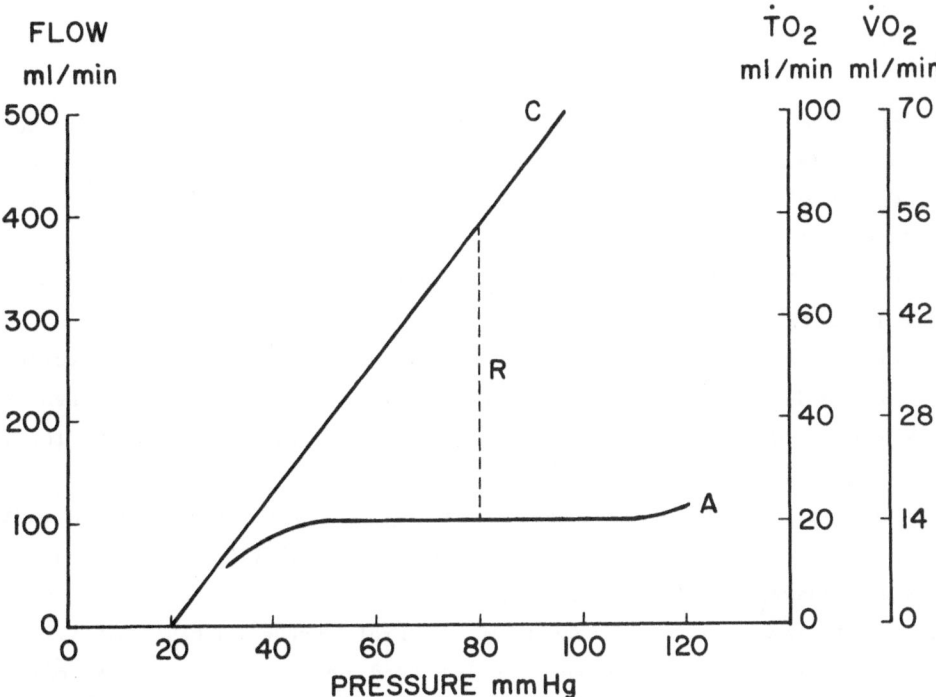

Figure 1. Coronary pressure-flow relations in a normal left ventricle during autoregulation (A) and maximal vasodilatation (C). The dashed vertical line indicates the coronary flow reserve at that perfusing pressure. Right-hand scales show the values of coronary oxygen transport ($\dot{T}O_2$) and myocardial oxygen consumption that correspond to the flows on the left-hand scale.

the left main coronary artery so that coronary perfusion pressure can be varied while left ventricular work remains constant. If coronary arterial pressures are raised or lowered from their initial resting level, coronary flow will change transiently and then return to or near to the control value; the resulting pressure-flow line during autoregulation (A) is horizontal or nearly horizontal over a wide range of pressures. Within this range, changes of coronary perfusing pressure are compensated for by changes in vascular conductance. Below some lower limit of perfusing pressure, however, coronary flow falls below the resting level because at these low pressures the vessels in the subendocardial muscle are maximally dilated and cannot compensate for further decreases in perfusion pressure.[56,57]

If pressure flow relations are determined after the coronary vessels have been dilated maximally with pharmacologic agents like adenosine, then a steep, almost straight line (C) is obtained; the points on this line indicate the maximal flow that can be achieved at each perfusion pressure. The vertical dashed line (R) between the other two lines represents the coronary flow reserve, that is, the increase in flow above the resting level that can be obtained at any given pressure when the vessels are maximally dilated. In normal hearts at normal perfusing pressures, maximal coronary flow is about four to five times the resting level.

On the right-hand side of figure 1 are two vertical scales, which indicate the values of myocardial oxygen transport ($\dot{T}O_2$) and myocardial oxygen consumption ($\dot{V}O_2$) that correspond to the flows on the left-hand scale. Transport is the product of arterial oxygen content (ml/dl) and coronary blood flow (ml/min), and is based on a normal arterial oxygen content of 20 ml/dl. The figures for myocardial oxygen consumption are based on a myocardial oxygen extraction of 70%.

Figure 2 is a similar diagram expanded to include a second autoregulation line A_2. This represents the effects of hypertrophy that doubles left ventricular mass. As a result, resting total myocardial oxygen consumption is doubled, and total autoregulated flow to the left ventricle (A_2) will be approximately double that of the normal ventricle (A_1). This increased autoregulated flow is achieved by vasodilatation. By contrast, many studies[38,43-46,49,55,58,59] have shown that the total coronary flow during maximal vasodilatation is similar in normal and hypertrophied ventricles, thereby indicating that the total cross-sectional area of the vascular bed is not much altered by hypertrophy. The coronary flow reserve is reduced, as indicated by the dotted line R_2.

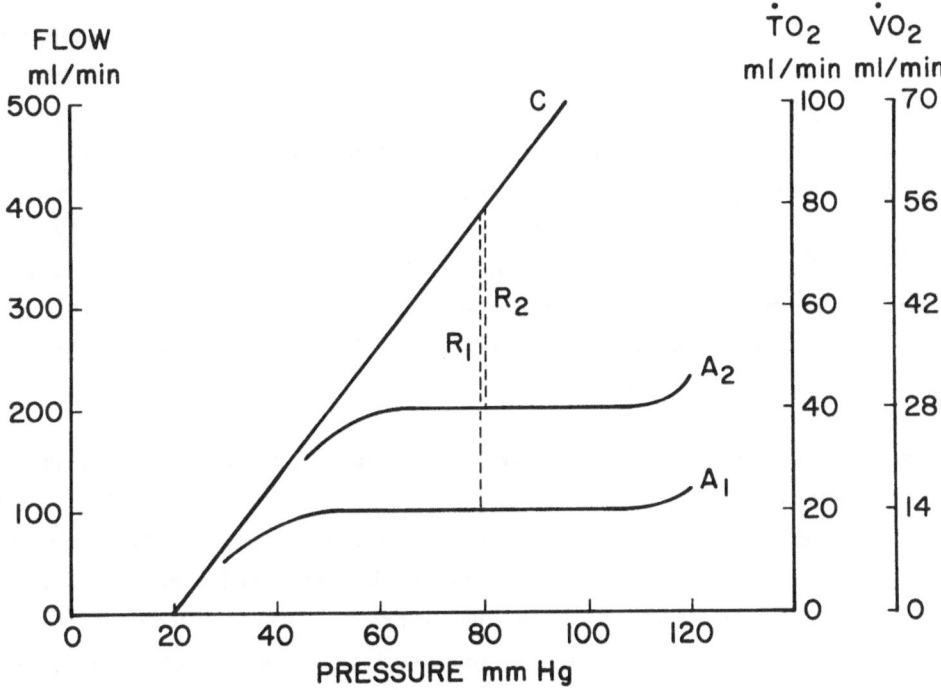

Figure 2. Coronary pressure-flow relations during maximal vasodilatation (C) and autoregulation in normal (A_1) and hypertrophied (A_2) left ventricles. The coronary flow reserve is shown by the vertical dashed lines: R_1 - normal ventricle, R_2 - hypertrophied ventricle. Right-hand scales as in figure 1.

The only group in whom coronary flow reserve may be normal are those who have systemic hypertension[38,60] (see below). It is important to use total ventricular flows in these assessments, because flows per unit mass can be misleading.[44,45] If, for example, a left ventricle increases in mass from 100 g to 200 g but maximal coronary flow is 400 ml/min at both weights (indicating no change in the conducting vessels), then maximal flow per unit mass will change from 5 ml/min per gram to 2 ml/min per gram and lead to the erroneous conclusion that minimal vascular resistance had doubled.*

Figure 2 shows also that coronary flow reserve is exhausted and subendocardial ischemia begins at higher perfusing pressures when there is hypertrophy than in the normal ventricle. With more hypertrophy than is indicated in this diagram, the coronary flow reserve at rest will be further reduced until even a slight increase in myocardial oxygen demand will produce an imbalance between myocardial oxygen supply and demand with resultant subendocardial ischemia. This type of hypertrophy in which perfusing pressures are normal occurs typically in valvar or subvalvar aortic stenosis, aortic or mitral incompetence, or cardiomyopathies.

EFFECTS OF DECREASED MYOCARDIAL OXYGEN TRANSPORT OR INCREASED MYOCARDIAL OXYGEN DEMAND

For a given degree of hypertrophy, the resting coronary flow can be elevated still further above normal either by decreased oxygen transport (anemia,[62-67] hypoxemia[67,68]) or by increased oxygen demand (thyrotoxicosis[69,70]). The new raised autoregulated resting flow is shown as A_3 in figure 3. This figure shows that the combination of these changes with hypertrophy causes a high resting coronary flow that barely supplies myocardial oxygen needs, and leaves little coronary flow reserve (R_3)** so that any further increase in myocardial oxygen demand will produce subendocardial ischemia at perfusing pressures that are normal or even above normal.

---

* To allow for variations in body weight among animals of the same species, one can calculate flows and resistances per kg of body weight.[45] Normally ventricular weight is proportional to body weight so that, provided there have not been acute changes in body weight, then the body weight can be used to normalize the expected flow and vascular resistance of the ventricle prior to hypertrophy.

** It is true that anemia decreases blood viscosity which increases normal maximal coronary flow, but this change is not enough to correct the decrease in coronary flow reserve.

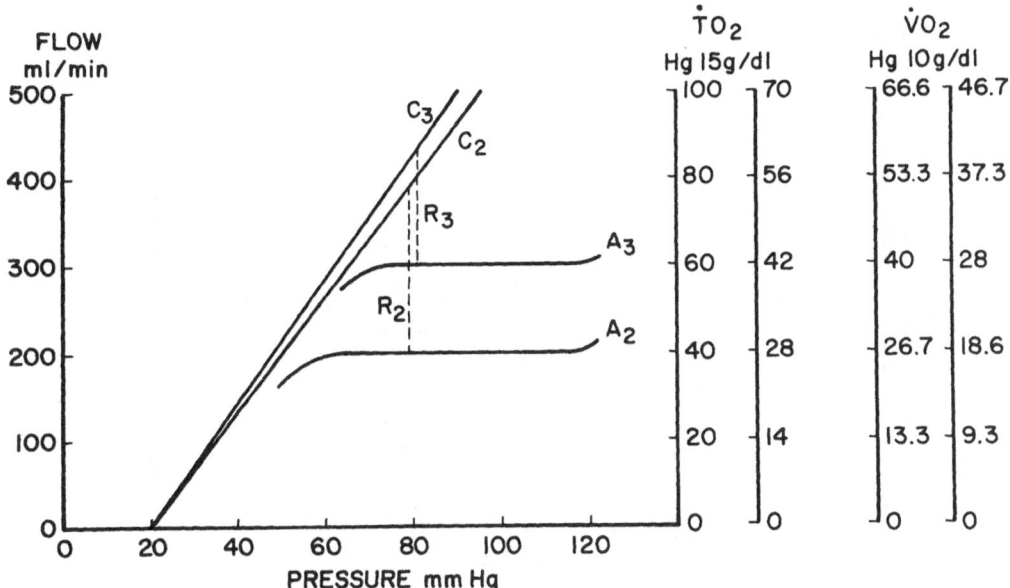

Figure 3. Coronary pressure-flow relations in a hypertrophied left ventricle when hemoglobin concentration is 15 g/dl (9.3 mmol/1) (A_2, C_2) and when hemoglobin concentration is 10 g/dl (6.2 mmol/1) (A_3, C_3). The coronary flow reserve is lower in anemia (R_3) than with a normal hemoglobin (R_2). A - autoregulation; C - maximal vasodilatation; R - coronary flow reserve. Right-hand scales show systemic oxygen transport ($\dot{T}O_2$) and myocardial oxygen consumption ($\dot{V}O_2$) for both hemoglobin concentrations.

Another harmful mechanism is shown in figure 4, where two autoregulation lines (A_1 - normal; A_2 - hypertrophy) are shown together with two maximal pressure-flow lines, C_1 and C_2. C_1 is the normal maximal pressure-flow line, and C_2 is a decreased maximal pressure-flow line, due either to a decreased cross-sectional area of the coronary vascular bed (fewer or narrower vessels[10,45,71]) or to an increased blood viscosity (polycythemia[64,66]) or an increased rigidity of red blood cells.[72] If these changes occur, then at any pressure the maximal coronary flow

138

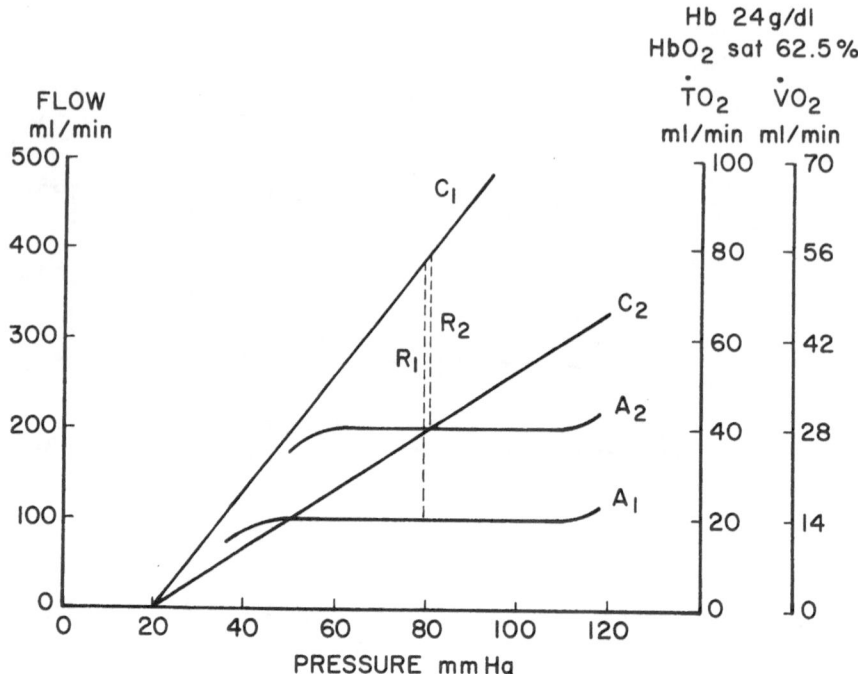

Figure 4. Coronary pressure-flow relations in a normal left ventricle (A_1, C_1, R_1) in a person with normal hemoglobin concentration and arterial oxygen saturation and in a hypertrophied left ventricle (A_2, C_2, R_2) in a patient with polycythemia and arterial hypoxemia. A - autoregulation; C - maximal vasodilatation; R - coronary flow reserve. Right-hand scales show systemic oxygen transport ($\dot{T}O_2$) and myocardial oxygen consumption ($\dot{V}O_2$) for the polycythemic patient.

will be reduced, causing a decrease in the corresponding coronary flow reserve. It probably is the disastrous combination of hypoxemia, polycythemia and hypertrophy that accounts for the diffuse subendocardial necrosis and fibrosis so common in children with cyanotic heart disease.[20]

TACHYCARDIA AND EXERCISE

Up to this point, we have described the effects of hypertrophy on only resting coronary flows, and now need to consider what happens to coronary flow when the hypertrophied left ventricle is stressed, for example, by tachycardia or exercise. Tachycardia per se has several effects. It increases contractility moderately, and this plus the increased number of beats per minute will increase myocardial oxygen consumption and blood flow per minute.[73-78] In addition, at high rates, two other mechanisms come into play. Because of a reduced filling time of the ventricles, cardiac output and blood pressure fall; this lowered aortic pressure decreases maximal coronary flow that can be attained when vessels are maximally dilated. Even more important is the relative decrease in diastolic time that occurs at high heart rates.[79] Because all subendocardial flow, and perhaps most myocardial flow, occurs during diastole, a decrease in diastolic time per minute reduces the maximal flow possible at any given perfusion pressure. Therefore even in the normal ventricle, tachycardia can cause subendocardial ischemia.[75,77,80] In the hypertrophied ventricle the risk of ischemia due to tachycardia is increased.[44,51]

The effects of exercise on coronary flow go beyond the effects attributed to the tachycardia. Further increases in myocardial oxygen consumption occur because the increased pressure and volume loads of exercise cause peak systolic wall stress to rise, and because contractility is increased.[77,80-87] In normal ventricles, maximal exercise does not appear to produce subendocardial ischemia.[81-88] With hypertrophy, exercise may cause modest reduction in subendocardial blood flow[50,87] although there may not be evidence of ischemia. However, it should be noted that in these experimental studies the hypertrophy was mild because ventricular mass was not even twice normal. In addition, the hypertrophy was induced by supravalvar aortic banding, so that the diastolic pressure in the coronary arteries was higher than normal. We would expect that, if there were a greater degree of hypertrophy, the loss of coronary flow reserve would be greater, and if the diastolic perfusing pressure is lower, as occurs in valvar or subvalvar aortic stenosis, then exercise is more likely to bring out ischemic changes.[89]

EFFECTS OF CHANGES IN VENTRICULAR VOLUME

An increase in ventricular volume will have different effects on the hypertrophied ventricle, depending on whether the volume increase has developed acutely or chronically. If hypertrophy is due to a volume load, as in valvar incompetence or complete heart block, then peak systolic wall stress remains normal,[34,35,37,38] and myocardial blood flow and oxygen consumption per unit muscle mass remain normal or are slightly increased.[59] Once again, total ventricular coronary flow is increased and coronary flow reserve is reduced. If there were acute or subacute ventricular dilatation, however, then peak systolic wall stress would rise[17,38] as would myocardial oxygen consumption per unit mass. This would decrease coronary flow reserve still more and increase the risk of subendocardial ischemia with any further increase in myocardial oxygen demand.

SYSTEMIC HYPERTENSION

One of the commonest causes of left ventricular hypertrophy is systemic hypertension which has some specific effects on coronary blood flow in the hypertrophied ventricle. Tarazi and his colleagues[61] have pointed out that in the hypertrophy which accompanies systemic hypertension, the increased muscle mass requires an increased resting coronary blood flow, as in other forms of hypertrophy; however, during maximal coronary vasodilatation the high perfusing pressure yields a normal coronary flow reserve (figure 5). They have observed in studies on spontaneously hy-

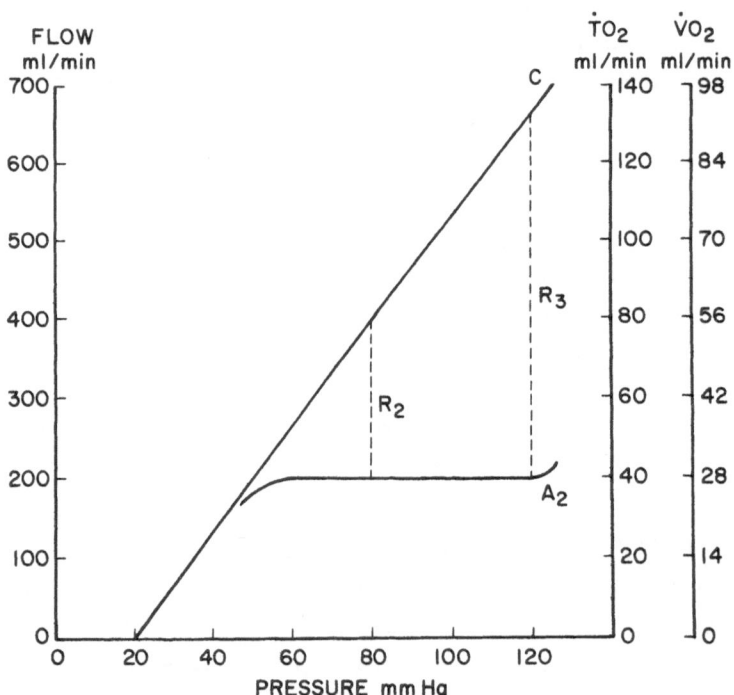

Figure 5. Coronary pressure-flow relations in a patient with systemic hypertension during autoregulation (A_2) and maximal vasodilatation (C). R_2 and R_3 are the coronary flow reserves at normal and high perfusing pressures respectively. Right-hand scales as in figure 1.

pertensive rats that a reduction in pressure without a corresponding
reduction in muscle mass will reduce coronary flow reserve; this would
occur when treatment lowers blood pressure but hypertrophy has not had
time to regress. That this is likely can be seen from figure 6, but it
is clear that, with the reduced myocardial oxygen need consequent on
lowered ventricular pressures, the relative flow reserve can actually be
increased.

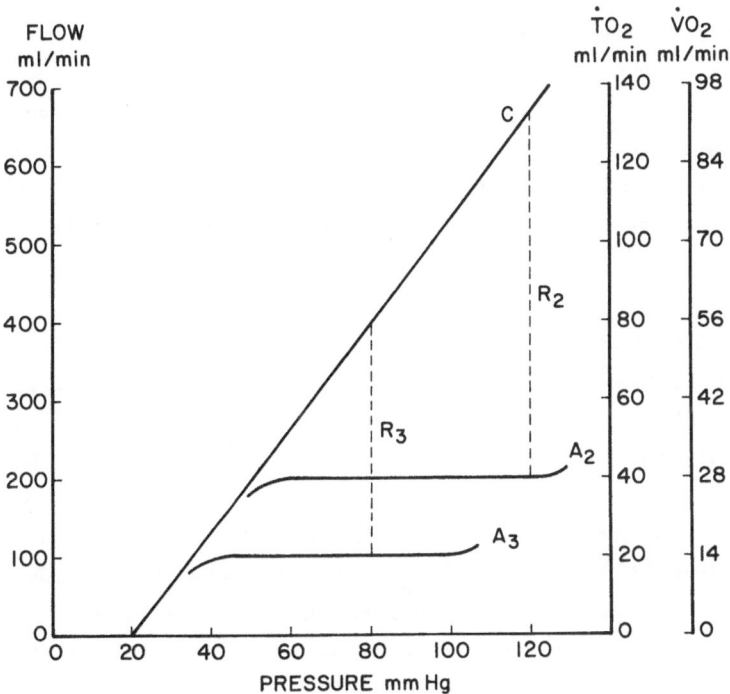

Figure 6. Coronary pressure-flow relations in a patient with systemic
hypertension and left ventricular hypertrophy. R_2 is the coronary flow
reserve before treatment, R_3 is the coronary flow reserve soon after
systemic pressure has been returned to normal by therapy. A_2 - autoregulation while hypertensive; A_3 - autoregulation while normotensive;
C - maximal vasodilatation. Right-hand scales as in figure 1.

For example, figure 6 shows that at a high perfusing pressure the coronary flow reserve (R_2) is 460 ml/min whereas at the low pressure the flow reserve (R_3) is 300 ml/min. However, at the higher perfusing pressure, the resting myocardial oxygen demand is twice what it will be at the lower perfusing pressure, so that when pressures are lowered the heart can safely attain four times the oxygen demand, whereas at the higher pressure it can only sustain a three and one-half fold increase.

These diagrams are only rough representations of actual data. What is important for any heart is the relationship between perfusing pressure, peak systolic wall stress, coronary blood flow and flow reserve, and myocardial oxygen consumption. Strauer[38] has made the important point that the relative coronary reserve (defined as the ratio of coronary vascular resistance in the resting state to that during maximal coronary vasodilatation) was inversely related to peak systolic wall stress in hypertensive patients; this wall stress in turn was a function of the left ventricular mass to volume ratio. Thus if the ventricle dilated, this would decrease and coronary vascular reserve would decrease.

RIGHT VENTRICULAR HYPERTROPHY

These principles that have been described for the left ventricle apply to the right ventricle as well. Stable right ventricular hypertrophy in adult dogs is manifested by a high wall mass to volume ratio[90] so that presumably peak systolic wall stress has been normalized. Furthermore, right ventricular hypertrophy produced by banding the main pulmonary artery in adult dogs[91,92] or ponies[93] or due to congenital pulmonic stenosis in dogs[21] increases resting flow to the right ventricle, decreases right ventricular coronary flow reserve, and usually leaves total right ventricular maximal pressure-flow relations unchanged; this demonstrates that, as in the left ventricle, the cross-sectional area of the right ventricular coronary vascular bed does not increase with hypertrophy. However, when right ventricular hypertrophy has been produced by banding the main pulmonary artery in fetal lambs,[94] newborn lambs,[95] or young calves[96] or by exposing young calves to simulated high altitude,[97] coronary flow reserve is not decreased, and the total right ventricular maximal conductance increases; this indicates growth of the coronary vascular bed in parallel with the increase in muscle mass.

The age at which the ability of coronary capillaries to proliferate is lost, is not known.

CORONARY STENOSIS

Finally, the association of significant coronary stenosis in a heart with hypertrophy will make it easier to produce subendocardial ischemia in the territory of the diseased artery, because the stenosis limits maximal flow to this territory and so further reduces its coronary flow reserve. This may be revealed by signs of ischemia when neither the degree of atheroma nor that of hypertrophy per se seems adequate to cause it.[3,6]

CONCLUSIONS

The framework presented above has been well substantiated by experiments in animals and confirmed to a large extent by observations in humans. At present, however, specific pressures and flows cannot be taken from these diagrams and applied to individual patients because of the many modifying variables that do not appear in the diagrams. For example, changes of contractility will affect myocardial oxygen consumption but to an extent not easy to predict. An increase in contractility per se will increase myocardial oxygen consumption[98-100] and so diminish coronary flow reserve; the increased contractility also tends, for independent reasons, to decrease the subendocardial to subepicardial flow ratio.[101] On the other hand, an increase in myocardial contractility may also decrease ventricular volume, thereby lowering peak systolic wall stress, and so limit the increase of myocardial oxygen consumption[100,102] that would otherwise occur. Other variables to be considered are the state of the intramural coronary arteries which have been observed to be abnormal in hypertrophy from certain causes.[103,104] Finally, the efficiency of myocardial oxygen utilization is not always constant; for example, experimentally induced pressure hypertrophy in animals has been shown to interfere with mitochondrial oxidation.[105]

What is clear is that ventricular hypertrophy occurring beyond infancy does not increase the cross-sectional area of the coronary vascular bed but does increase resting total ventricular oxygen consumption and resting total ventricular blood flow. To accomplish this increased flow the coronary vessels must dilate more than normal at rest, and therefore coronary flow reserve is reduced at any perfusing pressure. Any factors that increase resting flow still more (for example, anemia, hypoxemia, thyrotoxicosis, ventricular dilatation) will further decrease coronary flow reserve. Under these circumstances physiologic stimuli like exercise may exhaust coronary flow reserve and lead to subendocardial ischemia in the hypertrophied ventricle.

REFERENCES

1. Marquis, R.M. and Logan, A.: Congenital aortic stenosis and its surgical treatment, Br. Heart J., 17, 373-390, 1955
2. Moller, J.H., Nakeb, A. and Edwards, J.E.: Infarction of the papillary muscle and mitral insufficiency associated with congenital aortic stenosis, Circulation, 34, 87-91, 1966
3. Fallen, E.L., Elliott, W.C. and Gorlin, R.: Mechanisms of angina in aortic stenosis, Circulation, 36, 480-488, 1967
4. Maron, B.J. and Sissman, N.J.: The electrocardiogram in supravalvar aortic stenosis, Am. Heart J., 82, 300-306, 1971
5. Underhill, W.L., Tredway, J.B., D'Angelo, G.J. and Baay, J.E.M.: Familial supravalvar stenosis: comments on the mechanisms of angina pectoris, Am. J. Cardiol., 27, 560-565, 1971
6. Buckberg, G., Eber, L., Herman, M. and Gorlin, R.: Ischemia in aortic stenosis: hemodynamic prediction, Am. J. Cardiol., 35, 778-784, 1975
7. Trenouth, R.S., Phelps, N.C. and Neill, W.A.: Determinants of left ventricular hypertrophy and oxygen supply in chronic aortic valve disease, Circulation, 53, 644-650, 1976
8. Schwarz, F., Flameng, W., Schaper, J., Langebartels, F., Thormann, J., Hehrlein, F. and Schlepper, M.: Myocardial structure and function in patients with aortic valve disease and their relation to postoperative results, Am. J. Cardiol., 41, 661-669, 1978
9. Cheitlin, M.D., Robinowitz, M., McAllister, H., Hoffman, J.I.E., Bharati, S. and Lev, M.: The distribution of fibrosis in the left ventricle in congenital aortic stenosis and coarctation of the oarta, Circulation, 62, 823-830, 1980
10. Pyle, R.L., Lowensohn, H.S., Khouri, E.M., Gregg, D.E. and Patterson, D.F.: Left circumflex coronary artery hemodynamics in conscious dogs with congenital subaortic stenosis, Circ. Res., 33, 34-38, 1973
11. Harvey, W.P., Segal, J.P. and Hufnagel, C.A.: Unusual clinical features associated with severe aortic insufficiency, Ann. Intern. Med., 47, 27-38, 1957
12. Buchner, F.: Qualitative morphology of heart failure. Light and electron microscopic characteristics of acute and chronic heart failure, Methods Achiev. Exp. Pathol., 5, 60-120, 1971
13. Harris, C.N., Aronow, W.S., Parker, D.P. and Kaplan, M.A.: Treadmill stress in left ventricular hypertrophy, Chest, 63, 353-357, 1973

14. Hurst, J.W., Logue, R.B., Schlant, R.B. and Wenger, N.K.: The Heart, Arteries and Veins, New York, McGraw-Hill, fourth edition, 1556-1590, 1978

15. Opherk, D., Weihe, E., Zebe, H., Mall, G., Mehmel, H.C., Stockins, B., Ryan, U. and Kubler, W.: Reduced coronary reserve and ultrastructural changes of the myocardium in patients with angina pectoris, arterial hypertension and normal coronary arteries. In: The Heart in Hypertension, Strauer, B.E. (ed), Springer Verlag, Berlin, 208-220, 1981

16. Olsen, I.G.J.: Pathology of primary cardiomyopathies, Postgrad. Med. J., 48, 732-737, 1972

17. Dick, M., Unverferth, D.V. and Baba, N.: The pattern of myocardial degeneration in nonischemic congestive cardiomyopathy, Hum. Pathol., 13, 740-744, 1982

18. Unverferth, D.V., Magorien, R.D., Lewis, R.P. and Leier, C.V.: The role of subendocardial myocardial failure in patients with nonischemic congestive cardiomyopathy, Am. Heart J., 105, 176-179, 1983

19. Lasser, R.P. and Genkins, G.: Chest pain in patients with isolated pulmonic stenosis, Circulation, 15, 258-266, 1957

20. Franciosi, R. and Blanc, W.A.: Myocardial infarcts in infants and children I. A necropsy study in congenital heart disease, J. Pediat., 73, 309-319, 1968

21. Lowensohn, H.S., Khouri, E.M., Gregg, D.E., Pyle, R.L. and Patterson, R.E.: Phasic right coronary artery blood flow in conscious dogs with normal and elevated right ventricular pressures, Circ. Res., 39, 760-766, 1976

22. Sleeper, J.C., Organ, E.S. and McIntosh, H.D.: Primary pulmonary hypertension, Circulation, 26, 1358-1369, 1962

23. Harrison, C.V. and Wood, P.: Hypertensive and ischemic heart disease: A comparative clinical and pathological study, Br. Heart J., 11, 205-229, 1949

24. Overy, H.R., Vogel, J.H.K., Grover, R.F. and Blount, S.G. Jr.: Coronary vascular development in response to increased right ventricular pressure loads, Circ. Res., 18, 634-640, 1966

25. Arai, S., Machida, A. and Nakamura, T.: Myocardial structure and vascularization of hypertrophied hearts, Tohoku J. Exp. Med., 95, 35-54, 1968

26. Hutchins, G.M., Bulkley, B.H., Miner, M.M. and Boitnott, J.K.: Correlation of age and heart weight with tortuosity and caliber of normal human coronary arteries, Am. Heart J., 94, 196-202, 1977

27. Hort, W.: Microscopic pathology of heart muscle and of coronary arteries in arterial hypertension. In: The Heart in Hypertension, Strauer, B.E. (ed), Springer Verlag, Berlin, 183-191, 1981

28. Roberts, J.T. and Wearn, J.T.: Quantitative changes in the capillary-muscle relationship in human hearts during normal growth and hypertrophy, Am. Heart J., 21, 617-633, 1941

29. Linzbach, A.J.: Hypertrophy, hyperplasia and structural dilatation of the human heart, Adv. Cardiol., 18, 1-14, 1976

30. Tomanek, R.J., Searls, J.C. and Lachenbruch, P.A.: Quantitative changes in the capillary bed during developing, peak, and stabilized cardiac hypertrophy in the spontaneously hypertensive rat, Circ. Res., 51, 295-304, 1982

31. Laughlin, M.H. and Diana, J.N.: Myocardial transcapillary exchange in the hypertrophied heart of the dog, Am. J. Physiol., 229, 838-846, 1975

32. Meerson, F.Z.: The myocardium in hyperfunction, hypertrophy and heart failure, Circ. Res., 25 (suppl. II), 1-163, 1969

33. Burger, S.B. and Strauer, B.E.: Left ventricular hypertrophy in chronic pressure load due to spontaneous essential hypertension. I. Left ventricular function, left ventricular geometry, and wall stress. In: The Heart in Hypertension, Strauer, B.E. (ed), Springer Verlag, Berlin, 13-36, 1981

34. Hood, W.P., Rackley, C.E. and Rolett, E.L.: Wall stress in the normal and hypertrophied left ventricle, Am. J. Cardiol., 22, 550-558, 1968

35. Falsetti, H.L., Mates, R.E., Grant, C., Greene, D.G. and Bunnell, I.L.: Left ventricular wall stress calculated from one-plane cine-angiography, Circ. Res., 26, 71-83, 1970

36. Sasayama, S., Ross, J., Franklin, D., Bloor, C.M., Bishop, S. and Dilley, R.B.: Adaptations of the left ventricle to chronic pressure overload, Circ. Res., 38, 172-178, 1976

37. Grossman, W., Jones, D. and McLaurin, L.P.: Wall stress and patterns of hypertrophy in human left ventricle, J. Clin. Invest., 56, 56-64, 1975

38. Strauer, B.E.: Hypertensive Heart Disease, Springer Verlag, Berlin, 1980

39. Sarnoff, S.J., Braunwald, E., Welch, G.H. Jr., Case, R.B., Stainsby, W.N. and Macruz, R.: Hemodynamic determinants of oxygen consumption of the heart with special reference to tension time index, Am. J. Physiol., 192, 148-156, 1958

40. Monroe, R.G. and French, G.N.: Left ventricular pressure-volume relationships and myocardial oxygen consumption in isolated heart, Circ. Res., 9, 362-374, 1961

41. McDonald, R.H., Taylor, R.R. and Cingolani, H.E.: Measurement of myocardial developed tension and its relation to oxygen consumption, Am. J. Physiol., 211, 667-673, 1966

42. Malik, A.B., Abe, T., O'Kane, H. and Geha, A.S.: Cardiac function, coronary flow, and oxygen consumption in stable left ventricular hypertrophy, Am. J. Physiol., 225, 186-191, 1973

43. Marchetti, G.V., Merlo, L., Noseda, V. and Visioli, O.: Myocardial blood flow in experimental cardiac hypertrophy in dogs, Cardiovasc. Res., 7, 519-527, 1973

44. Mueller, T.M., Marcus, M.L., Kerber, R.E., Young, Y.A., Barnes, R.W. and Abboud, F.M.: Effect of renal hypertension and left ventricular hypertrophy on the coronary circulation in dogs, Circ. Res., 42, 543-549, 1978

45. O'Keefe, D.D., Hoffman, J.I.E., Cheitlin, R., O'Neill, M.J., Allard, J.R. and Shapkin, E.: Coronary blood flow in experimental canine left ventricular hypertrophy, Circ. Res., 43, 43-51, 1978

46. Holtz, J., Restorff, W. von, Bard, P. and Bassenge, E.: Transmural distribution of myocardial blood flow and coronary reserve in canine left ventricular hypertrophy, Basic Res. Cardiol., 72, 286-292, 1977

47. Rembert, J.C., Kleinman, L.H., Fedor, J.M., Wechsler, A.S. and Greenfield, J.C. Jr.: Myocardial blood flow distribution in concentric left ventricular hypertrophy, J. Clin. Invest., 62, 379-386, 1978

48. Bache, R.J. and Vrobel, T.R.: Effects of exercise on blood flow in the hypertrophied heart, Am. J. Cardiol., 44, 1029-1033, 1979
49. Mittmann, U., Brückner, U.B., Keller, H.E., Kohler, U., Vetter, H. and Waag, K.L.: Myocardial flow reserve in experimental cardiac hypertrophy, Basic Res. Cardiol., 75, 199-206, 1980
50. Bache, R.J., Vrobel, T.R., Ring, W.S., Emery, R.W. and Anderson, R.W.: Regional myocardial blood flow during exercise in dogs with chronic left ventricular hypertrophy, Circ. Res., 48, 76-87, 1981
51. Borkon, A.M., Jones, M., Bell, J.H. and Pierce, J.E.: Regional myocardial blood flow in left ventricular hypertrophy, J. Thorac. Cardiovasc. Surg., 84, 876-885, 1982
52. Weiss, M.B., Ellis, K., Sciacca, R.R., Johnson, L.L., Schmidt, D.H. and Cannon, P.J.: Myocardial blood flow in congestive and hypertrophic cardiomyopathy, Circulation, 54, 484-494, 1976
53. Johnson, L.L., Sciacca, R.R., Ellis, K., Weiss, M.B. and Cannon, P.J.: Reduced left ventricular myocardial blood flow per unit mass in aortic stenosis, Circulation, 57, 582-590, 1978
54. Nichols, A.B., Sciacca, R.R., Weiss, M.B., Blood, D.K., Brennan, D.L. and Cannon, P.J.: Effects of left ventricular hypertrophy on myocardial blood flow and ventricular performance in systemic hypertension, Circulation, 62, 329-340, 1980
55. Pichard, A.D., Gorlin, R., Smith, H., Ambrose, J. and Meller, J.: Coronary flow studies in patients with left ventricular hypertrophy of the hypertensive type, Am. J. Cardiol., 47, 547-554, 1981
56. Guyton, R.A., McClenathan, J.H., Newman, C.E. and Michaelis, L.L.: Significance of subendocardial S-T segment elevation caused by coronary stenosis in the dog, Am. J. Cardiol., 40, 373-380, 1977
57. Rouleau, J., Boerboom, L.E., Surjadhana, A. and Hoffman, J.I.E.: The role of autoregulation and tissue diastolic pressures in the transmural distribution of left ventricular blood flow in anesthetized dogs, Circ. Res., 45, 804-815, 1979
58. Wangler, R.D., Peters, K.G., Marcus, M.L. and Tomanek, R.J.: Effects of duration and severity of arterial hypertension and cardiac hypertrophy on coronary vasodilator reserve, Circ. Res., 51, 10-18, 1982
59. Gascho, J.A., Mueller, T.M., Eastham, C. and Marcus, M.L.: Effect of volume-overloading hypertrophy on the coronary circulation in awake dogs, Cardiovasc. Res., 16, 288-292, 1982
60. Marcus, M.L., Doty, D.B., Hiratzka, L.F., Wright, C.B. and Eastham, C.L.: Decreased coronary reserve. A mechanism for angina pectoris in patients with aortic stenosis and normal coronary arteries, New Engl. J. Med., 307, 1362-1366, 1982
61. Wicker, P. and Tarazi, R.C.: Coronary blood flow in left ventricular hypertrophy: a review of experimental data, Eur. Heart J., 3 (suppl. A), 111-118, 1982
62. Murray, J.F. and Rapaport, E.: Coronary blood flow and myocardial metabolism in acute experimental anaemia, Cardiovasc. Res., 6, 360-367, 1972
63. Restorff, W. von, Hofling, B., Holtz, J. and Bassenge, E.: Effect of increased blood fluidity through hemodilution on coronary circulation at rest and during exercise in dogs, Pfluegers Arch., 357, 15-24, 1975
64. Holtz, J., Bassenge, E. Restorff, W. von, and Mayer, E.: Transmural differences in myocardial blood flow and in coronary dilatory capacity in hemodiluted conscious dogs, Basic Res. Cardiol., 71, 36-46, 1976

65. Jan, K-M and Chien, S.: Effect of hematocrit variations on coronary hemodynamics and oxygen utilization, Am. J. Physiol., 233, H106-H113, 1977

66. Abendschein, D.R., Fewell, J.E., Carlson, C.J. and Rapaport, E.: Myocardial blood flow during acute isovolumic anemia and treadmill exercise in dogs, J. Appl. Physiol., 53, 203-206, 1982

67. Surjadhana, A., Rouleau, J., Boerboom, L.E. and Hoffman, J.I.E.: Myocardial blood flow and its distribution in anesthetized poly-cythemic dogs, Circ. Res., 43, 619-631, 1978

68. Heiss, H.W., Tupfer, M., Barmeyer, J., Wink, K., Huber, G. and Keul, J.: Studies in the regulation of myocardial blood flow in man II. Effects of acute arterial hypoxia, Clin. Cardiol., 1, 35-42, 1978

69. Strauer, B-E and Scherpe, A.: Experimental hyperthyroidism IV. Myocardial muscle mechanics and oxygen consumption in eu- and hyper-thyroidism, Basic Res. Cardiol., 70, 246-255, 1975

70. Talifah, K., Briden, K.L. and Weiss, H.R.: Thyroxine-induced hyper-trophy of the rabbit heart: effect of regional oxygen extraction, flow and oxygen consumption, Circ. Res., 52, 272-279, 1983

71. Strauer, B.E., Brune, I., Schenk, H., Knoll, D. and Perings, E.: Lupus cardiomyopathy; cardiac mechanics, hemodynamics and coronary blood flow in uncomplicated systemic lupus erythematosus, Am. Heart J., 92, 715-722, 1976

72. Dintenfass, L.: Rheology of Blood in Diagnostic and Preventive Medicine, Butterworths, London, 1976

73. Pitt, B. and Gregg, D.E.: Coronary hemodynamic effects of increasing ventricular rate in the unanesthetized dog, Circ. Res., 22, 753-761, 1968

74. Holmberg, S. and Varnauskas, E.: Coronary circulation during pacing-induced tachycardia, Acta Med. Scand., 190, 481-490, 1971

75. Buckberg, G.D., Fixler, D.E., Archie, J.P. and Hoffman, J.I.E.: Experimental subendocardial ischemia in dogs with normal coronary arteries, Circ. Res., 30, 67-81, 1972

76. Neill, W.A., Phelps, N.C., Oxendine, J.M., Mahler, D.J. and Sim, D.N.: Effect of heart rate on coronary blood flow distribution in dogs, Am. J. Cardiol., 32, 306-312, 1973

77. Buckberg, G.D., Fixler, D.E., Archie, J.P., Henney, R.P. and Hoffman, J.I.E.: Variable effects of heart rate on phasic and regional left ventricular muscle blood flow in anaesthetized dogs, Cardiovasc. Res., 9, 1-11, 1975

78. Ball, R.M., Bache, J., Cobb, F.R. and Greenfield, J.C. Jr.: Regional myocardial blood flow during graded treadmill exercise in the dog, J. Clin. Invest., 55, 43-49, 1975

79. Boudoulas, H., Rittgers, S.E., Lewis, R.P., Leier, C.V. and Weissler, A.M.: Changes in diastolic time with various pharmacologic agents. Implications for myocardial perfusion, Circulation, 60, 164-169, 1979

80. Domenech, R.J. and Goich, J.: Effect of heart rate on regional coronary blood flow, Cardiovasc. Res., 10, 224-231, 1976

81. Khouri, E.M., Gregg, D.E. and Rayford, C.R.: Effect of exercise on cardiac output, left coronary flow and myocardial metabolism in the unanesthetized dog, Circ. Res., 17, 427-437, 1965

82. Barnard, R.J., Duncan, H.W., Livesay, J.J. and Buckberg, G.D.: Coronary vasodilator reserve and flow distribution during near-maximal exercise in dogs, J. Appl. Physiol.: Respirat. Environ. Exercise Physiol., 43, 988-992, 1977

83. Holmberg, S., Serzysko, W. and Varnauskas, E.: Coronary circulation during heavy exercise in control subjects and patients with coronary heart disease, Acta Med. Scand., 190, 465-480, 1971

84. Kitamura, K., Jorgensen, C.R., Gobel, F.L., Tayler, H.L. and Wang, Y.: Hemodynamic correlates of myocardial oxygen consumption during upright exercise, J. Appl. Physiol., 32, 516-522, 1972

85. Heiss, H.W., Barmeyer, J., Wink, K., Hell, G., Cerny, E.J., Keel, J. and Reindell, H.: Studies on regulation of myocardial blood flow in man I. Training effects on blood flow and metabolism of healthy heart at rest and during standardized heavy exercise, Basic Res. Cardiol., 71, 658-675, 1976

86. Pannier, J.L. and Leusen, I.: Regional blood flow in response to exercise in conscious dogs, Eur. J. Appl. Physiol., 36, 255-265, 1977

87. Sanders, M., White, F.C., Peterson, T. and Bloor, C.M.: Effects of endurance exercise on coronary collateral blood flow in miniature swine, Am. J. Physiol.: Heart Circ. Physiol., 3, H614-H619, 1978

88. White, F.C., Sanders, M., Peterson, T. and Bloor, C.M.: Ischemic myocardial injury after exercise stress in the pressure overloaded heart, Am. J. Pathol., 97, 473-488, 1979

89. Halloran, K.H.: The telemetered exercise electrocardiogram in congenital aortic stenosis, Pediatrics, 47, 31-39, 1971

90. Laks, M.M., Morady, F., Garner, D. and Swan, H.J.C.: Relation of ventricular volume, compliance and mass in the normal and pulmonary arterial banded canine heart, Cardiovasc. Res., 6, 187-198, 1972

91. Murray, P.A. and Vatner, S.F.: Reduction of maximal coronary vasodilator capacity in conscious dogs with severe right ventricular hypertrophy, Circ. Res., 48, 27-33, 1981

92. Murray, P.A., Baig, H., Fishbein, M.C. and Vatner, S.F.: Effects of experimental right ventricular hypertrophy on myocardial blood flow in conscious dogs, J. Clin. Invest., 64, 421-427, 1979

93. Manohar, M., Bisgard, G.E., Bullard, V. and Rankin, J.H.G.: Blood flow in the hypertrophied right ventricular myocardium of unanesthetized ponies, Am. J. Physiol., 240, H881-H888, 1981

94. Vlahakes, G.J., Turley, K., Verrier, E.D. and Hoffman, J.I.E.: Greater maximal coronary flow in conscious lambs with experimental congenital right ventricular hypertrophy, Circulation, 62 (suppl. III), 111, 1980

95. Archie, J.P., Fixler, D.E., Ullyot, D.J., Buckberg, G.D. and Hoffman, J.I.E.: Regional myocardial blood flow in lambs with concentric right ventricular hypertrophy, Circ. Res., 34, 143-154, 1974

96. Manohar, M., Thurmon, J.C., Tranquilli, W.J., Devous, M.D. Sr., Theodorakis, M.C., Shawley, R.V., Feller, D.L. and Benson, J.G.: Regional myocardial blood flow and coronary vascular reserve in unanesthetized young calves with severe concentric right ventricular hypertrophy, Circ. Res., 48, 785-796, 1981

97. Manohar, M., Parks, C.M., Busch, M.A., Tranquilli, W.J., Bisgard, G.E., McPherron, T.A. and Theodorakis, M.C.: Regional myocardial blood flow and coronary vascular reserve in unanesthetized young calves exposed to a simulated altitude of 3500 m for 8-109 weeks, Circ. Res., 50, 714-726, 1982

98. Sonnenblick, E.H., Ross, J. Jr., Covell, J.W., Kaiser, G.A. and Braunwald, E.: Velocity of contraction as a determinant of myocardial oxygen consumption, Am. J. Physiol., 209, 919-927, 1965

99. Sonnenblick, E.H., Ross, J. jr. and Braunwald, E.: Oxygen consumption of the heart: Newer concepts of its multifactorial determination, Am. J. Cardiol., 22, 328-335, 1968

100. Graham, T.P. Jr., Covell, J.W., Sonnenblick, E.H., Ross, J. Jr. and Braunwald, E.: Control of myocardial oxygen consumption: relative influence of contractile state and tension development, J. Clin. Invest., 47, 375-385, 1968
101. Marzilli, M., Goldstein, S., Sabbah, H.N., Lee, T. and Stein, P.D.: Modulating effect of regional myocardial performance on local myocardial perfusion in the dog, Circ. Res., 45, 634-640, 1979
102. Krasnow, N., Rolett, E.L., Yurchak, P., Hood, W.B. Jr. and Gorlin, R.: Isoproterenol and cardiovascular performance, Am. J. Med., 37, 514-525, 1964
103. Naeye, R. and Liedtke: Consequences of intramyocardial arterial lesions in aortic valvular stenosis, Am. J. Pathol., 85, 569-580, 1976
104. Vlodaver, Z. and Neufeldt, H.N.: The coronary arteries in coarctation of the aorta, Circulation, 37, 449-454, 1968
105. Cooper, G.I.V., Satava, R.M. Jr., Harrison, C.E. and Coleman, H.N. III: Mechanism for the abnormal energetics of pressure-induced hypertrophy of cat myocardium, Circ. Res., 33, 213-223, 1973

152

SUMMARY

_Patients with long-standing valvular disease of the heart or with severe
hypertension may develop typical angina pectoris, although their coronary arteries are normal and fully patent. Peak flow calculated per unit
mass and the ratio of peak flow to normal resting flow, called coronary
vascular reserve, are reduced in LVH._

_To explain the reduction of coronary reserve, Wearn postulated that in
the process of hypertrophy only the diameter of the muscle fibers
increases, whereas the ratio of the number of capillaries to the number
of muscle fibers remains the same, i.e. close to one. A number of
studies are reviewed in which capillary surface area is measured in both
normal and hypertrophied hearts with histological or in vivo optical
techniques. The results are in keeping with Wearn's postulate; only in
old adult, spontaneously hypertensive rats is capillary surface area
higher than expected, suggesting some capillary growth. Measurement of
coronary pressure and flow in dogs with experimental LVH also demonstrated a reduction of specific vascular resistance as predicted by Wearn.
We measured specific vascular resistance in isolated beating rat hearts,
taken from normal and spontaneously hypertensive rats. Specific vascular
resistance was the same in both groups. Resistance values obtained in
the hypertrophied hearts, however, did not differ significantly from
those predicted by Wearn's hypothesis. We found that, due to formation
of edema, perfusion at high pressure increases vascular resistance if
the vascular bed is fully dilated. Edema formation probably adds to the
reduction of coronary reserve in LVH and hypertension when a vasodilating agent is given or when ischemia dilates the precapillary vessels._

_Reduction of vascular reserve has been demonstrated in patients with
LVH, but complete measurements of vascular resistance at different
pressures and of LV mass in patients are lacking. Data from one clinical
study were used to make an estimate of vascular resistance in relation
to LV mass in patients with valvular aortic stenosis. Assuming normal
flow per unit mass, we found vascular resistance to be increased to
values closely fitting the Wearn hypothesis. In clinical cases of
valvular aortic stenosis, hypertrophy is far more extensive than that
found in experimentally induced LVH in dogs or rats._

LEFT VENTRICULAR HYPERTROPHY AND MYOCARDIAL ISCHEMIA

SCHIPPERHEYN, J.J. and JONAS, J.

Departments of Cardiology and Thorax Surgery, Leiden University, Leiden, the Netherlands

INTRODUCTION

Myocardial ischemia is one of the major problems in patients with left ventricular hypertrophy. It is known that patients with long-standing valvular disease or with severe hypertension may suffer from anginal pain although their coronary arteries are normal and fully patent.[1-3] Some of the patients may have episodes of myocardial ischemia without typical anginal pain. Myocardial ischemia eventually causes patchwise necrosis[4] leading to arrhythmias and cardiac failure. Myocardial ischemia in patients with hypertrophy of the left ventricle and normal coronary arteries is believed to be caused by a relative underdevelopment of the capillary bed in the hypertrophied heart.[5] Measurements of coronary flow in patients with ventricular hypertrophy[6] and in animals with experimentally induced hypertrophy[7,8] indicate that the so-called coronary vascular reserve is diminished. Coronary vascular reserve is defined as the ratio of maximal to normal coronary flow. To measure maximal flow, full vasodilation must be induced either by infusion of a vasodilating agent into the coronary artery or, alternatively, by reduction of perfusion pressure. Sudden reduction of pressure to below a mean value of 40-50 mm Hg rapidly induces complete vasodilation. After total occlusion for at least 15 seconds, the vascular bed is completely dilated and coronary vascular reserve can be calculated from the ratio of peak flow after reperfusion to normal resting flow. In patients with ventricular hypertrophy post-occlusion reactive vasodilation is reduced or is absent.[6] To explain the reduction or loss of reactive hyperemia found in hypertrophied hearts, a complete pressure-flow relationship of the coronary system must be measured, not only under normal resting conditions but also after induction of full vasodilation. The mean pressure-mean flow relationship of the fully dilated vascular bed of the heart is a straight line with a small intercept P_0 at zero flow on the pressure axis. The slope of the pressure-flow line is the minimal vascular resistance: $(P-P_0)/Q$ for any value of P.

154

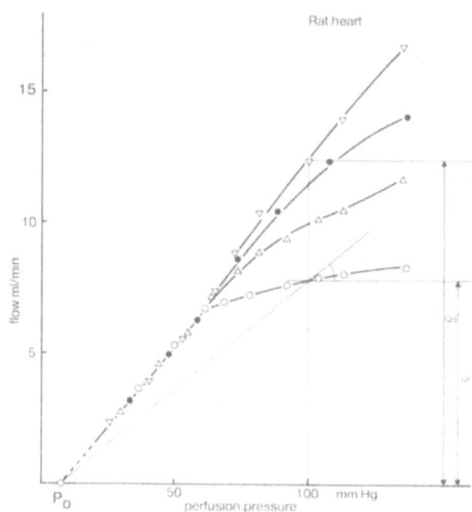

Figure 1. Pressure-flow relations in the isolated rat heart. Mean flow plotted versus mean perfusion pressure as measured in an isolated empty beating rat heart. The family of curves demonstrates the gradual loss of autoregulation during artificial perfusion. Open circles refer to measurements immediately after isolation. Upright triangles were obtained after ten minutes, closed circles after 30 minutes and downward pointing triangles after one hour of artificial perfusion. P_o is the extrapolated intercept on the abscissa, the so-called zero flow pressure. Q_d is the flow measured after full vasodilation and Q_n is flow under normal load conditions and normal autoregulation. The ratio Q_d/Q_n is used to define coronary vascular reserve. Vascular resistance is the slope of the line connecting P_o with any data point of a mean pressure-mean flow curve. After one hour the vascular bed is fully dilated, and the slope of the mean pressure-mean flow relation gives the minimal vascular resistance.

Figure 1 shows the results of a series of pressure-flow measurements in an isolated, empty, beating rat heart. The heart was taken from a 280-gram male Wistar rat, anesthetized with diethyl ether. Artificial perfusion was started within ten seconds after clamping and cannulation of the aorta. Perfusion pressure in the aorta was maintained by a roller pump. Pressure could be varied from 0 to 140 mm Hg; flow was measured with an electromagnetic flow meter. The perfusate was reconstituted blood made by adding 2% bovine serum albumin to a Krebs-Henseleit solution. Carefully washed bovine erythrocytes from blood freshly obtained from the slaughter house were added and the perfusate was equilibrated to a 5% CO_2, 95% O_2 gas mixture. The hemoglobin concentration was low, only 4.5 mmol/l. Open circles are the data points measured shortly after isolation.

Flow does not depend on perfusion pressure in isolated preparations, but only on oxygen demand of the tissue and oxygen content of the blood. In the empty beating rat heart, flow is not strictly independent of perfusion pressure, presumably because of an erectile mechanism that increases fiber length in the empty heart and thereby raises oxygen demand of the tissue.[9] In this experiment on rat heart, the curve above 50 mm Hg bends to the right, which means that resistance increases with pressure above this value. Coronary vascular resistance in this relatively flat portion of the curve above 50 mm Hg can be calculated from the slope of the line connecting data points with the zero flow point P_0. Resistance increases if perfusion pressure is raised. Below 50 mm Hg resistance is fixed at its minimal value. The critical pressure of 50 mm Hg is high in this experiment, because the hemoglobin concentration is low. The oxygen content of the blood is only about 50% of normal. Normally the critical perfusion pressure is about 30 mm Hg.

Coronary reserve at 100 mm Hg perfusion pressure is defined as the ratio of Q_d and Q_n. In this particular case, its value is only 1.6 because of the low concentration of hemoglobin we used. It would have been close to 3 if the heart had been perfused with normal blood.

Thus, coronary vascular reserve may be low because of anemia. In fact, patients with severe anemia may have practically no coronary vascular reserve and therefore suffer from angina although their coronary arteries are normal. Not only hemoglobin concentration has an effect on coronary reserve. From the curve given in figure 1 it is evident that coronary reserve increases steeply with perfusion pressure. This is largely due to the method we used to measure vascular resistance. In the normal beating heart with autoregulation, which maintains its own perfusion pressure and therefore requires more oxygen at high aortic pressures, the slope of the pressure-flow relation is only slightly less than the slope of the curve obtained after full vasodilation. As a result, the ratio of maximal to normal flow increases only slightly with blood pressure if measured in the intact organism, as Wicker and Tarazi have demonstrated.[10]

Artificial perfusion of isolated organs eventually damages autoregulation (figure 1). Gradually developing paresis of autoregulation rotates the flat portion of the pressure-flow curve until it corresponds to the straight line obtained after vasodilation. At the same time coronary vascular reserve diminishes. Loss of autoregulation, although it reduces vascular reserve, does not necessarily reduce oxygen supply to the myocardial tissue, and oxygen consumption remains the same. Maximal flow remains the same and loss of coronary reserve caused by paresis of autoregulation therefore does not restrict cardiac function nor does it cause ischemia.

If the larger coronary arteries are narrowed, coronary vascular reserve is of course also reduced. Coronary artery disease is probably the most important cause of reduced vascular reserve in clinical practice.

In hypertrophied hearts loss of coronary vascular reserve has been well documented, also in patients without significant coronary artery disease. Myocardial flow calculated per gram of tissue is normal in the hypertrophied heart[8,11] and these patients as a rule have normal hemoglobin concentrations. It is known that in hypertrophy wall stress and oxygen consumption per gram of cardiac tissue are usually normal[12], and since coronary flow is normal per gram of tissue, it looks as if autoregulation operates normally in the hypertrophied heart. Following exclusion of all other possible causes, only a rise of minimal vascular resistance remains as an explanation for the loss of coronary reserve.

CAPILLARY SURFACE AREA

It is close to 50 years ago that Wearn began to study capillary density in cardiac tissue using quantitative histological techniques.[13] He stated that the ratio of the number of capillaries to the number of muscle fibers remains close to one if hypertrophy develops. The number of muscle fibers did not seem to increase, only their size did and, as a result, the distance between adjacent capillaries increased and capillary density (number of capillaries per cross-sectional area) decreased. Later studies with similar methods by others, however, showed that the capillary to fiber ratio is not necessarily constant in hypertrophy and that it may increase slightly.[14,15] Henquell et al.[16] measuring intercapillary distances in beating rat heart after vasodilation also arrived at the conclusion that the number of capillaries may increase in hypertrophy, although the mean intercapillary distance as a rule increases. Their strongest evidence came from frequency distributions of intercapillary distances. These distributions kept the narrow flanks typical of the normal heart, while the frequency distribution of muscle fiber diameters had broad flanks in the hypertrophied heart. This implies that at least in the vicinity of extremely thick fibers capillaries must have increased in number.

Using delicate histological techniques, Tomanek et al.[15] demonstrated discrepancies in growth rate of muscle fibers and number of capillaries in hypertensive rats. In early cases they found the capillary surface area per gram of tissue reduced, but they demonstrated that capillary growth eventually catches up with increase in size of muscle fibers. In 15-month-old rats, intercapillary distance and capillary surface area per gram are again normal.

According tot Wearn's original idea of a constant ratio of number of fibers to number of capillaries, capillary surface area per gram will decrease with cardiac mass according to a power function, the square of the cubic root. If 1/CSA per gram (capillary surface area) is plotted against ventricular mass, the exponent of the power function fitting the data will be 0.66. For heart weights up to 300% of normal, this function can be closely approximated by a straight line (figure 2).

It is of interest to plot available data on intercapillary distances in hypertrophied hearts on a graph and to compare the data with a prediction based upon Wearn's statement. From histological studies by Rakusan[14], Henquell[16] and Tomanek[15] we calculated 1/CSA per gram, assuming, if not stated otherwise, that the capillary diameter was the same as that found by Tomanek. Tomanek's study provided us with four data points from

158

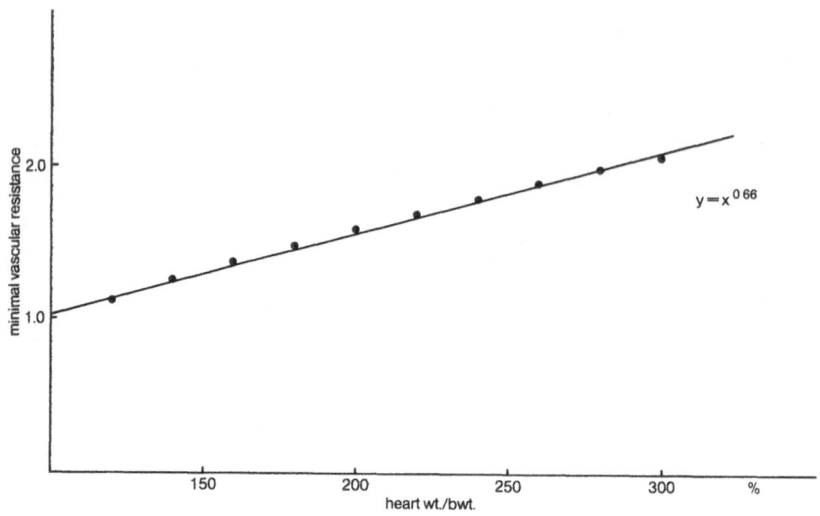

Figure 2. Theoretical relationship of minimal vascular resistance and relative heart weight. The theoretical relationship, according to Wearn's hypothesis, between minimal vascular resistance and heart/body weight ratio in hypertrophied hearts is a power function, the square of the cubic root. For a relative heart weight up to 300% of normal, the power function can be approximated by a linear function y = 0.50 x +0.53 (valid for 1 < x < 3).

rats of different age groups. The plot of the data (figure 3) shows that only Rakusan's values and those of Tomanek in 15-month-old rats differ significantly from the predicted values according to Wearn.

MINIMAL VASCULAR RESISTANCE IN ISOLATED HEARTS

In the fully dilated vascular bed, capillary vessels constitute the major part of the vascular resistance. In the hypertrophied heart, coronary arteries appear to grow in proportion to the flow demand[17], whereas capillary growth may be insufficient. Therefore, any reduction of capillary density in the hypertrophied heart can be expected to produce a rise in minimal vascular resistance calculated per gram of tissue mass. If so, vascular resistance measurements can be used to test Wearn's hypothesis.

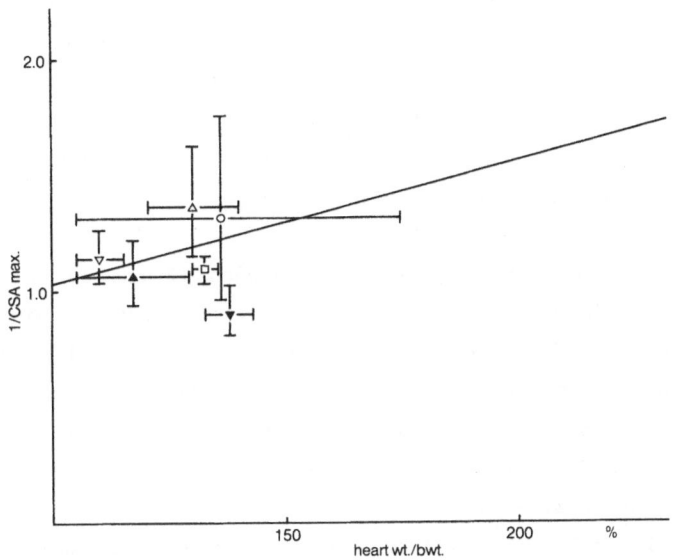

Figure 3. Capillary surface area in hypertrophic hearts. The reciprocal of the capillary surface area per gram as found by different authors in hypertrophic rat heart plotted versus relative heart weight. Henquell's data were measured in living hearts, all other data were obtained with histological techniques.

o	Henquell et al.[16]	6 normal	6 LVH	(salt-loaded after unilateral nephrectomy)
▽	Tomanek et al.[15]	5	6	(spontaneous hypertensive rat 1 mo)
▲	Tomanek et al.[15]	6	6	(spontaneous hypertensive rat 2.5 mo)
△	Tomanek et al.[15]	7	6	(spontaneous hypertensive rat 7 mo)
▼	Tomanek et al.[15]	5	7	(spontaneous hypertensive rat 15 mo)
□	Rakusan et al.[14]	18	10	(constriction of the descending aorta)

The straight line gives the theoretical relationship predicted by Wearn.

If Wearn's statement about the capillary to fiber ratio is correct, minimal vascular resistance can be expected to follow a power relation with an exponent of 0.66, when plotted against cardiac mass.

Data on minimal vascular resistance are not abundantly available in the literature. Especially data from clinical studies are scarce, because for obvious reasons only rough estimates of ventricular mass can be given. We measured minimal vascular resistance in spontaneously hypertensive rats, first to add a few data on resistance changes in hypertrophy to the available information and, secondly, to find out whether data obtained in isolated heart studies fit data obtained in studies in intact animals and in patients. This will be of importance in the assessment of the quality of our isolated heart preparations.

We used five spontaneously hypertensive rats between 12 and 14 months' old. Blood pressure in these rats was 152 mm Hg with a standard deviation of 5 mm Hg. Five normal Wistar rats of the same age were used as controls. Blood pressure in these rats is 112 mm Hg, standard deviation 5 mm Hg. The animals were anesthetized with diethyl ether; the hearts were exposed and taken out. Reperfusion started within ten seconds and the hearts did not stop or fibrillate. To perfuse the hearts reconstituted blood was used, as described above. Adenosine was added to the perfusate if needed to induce full vasodilation. But, if no drug was added, autoregulation disappeared spontaneously in these preparations as shown in figure 1. The absence of a typical post-occlusion hyperemic response was taken as proof of complete vasodilation.

Especially if the vascular bed was fully dilated, we found that high perfusion pressure is deleterious to the preparation. We therefore kept perfusion pressure as low as possible. We found in earlier experiments that a pressure only slightly above mean left ventricular pressure is high enough to prevent ischemia in the isolated heart. We did not measure intraventricular pressure in this study, but in view of our findings in earlier studies, we assumed it to be less than 20 mm Hg and we kept perfusion pressure at 30 mm Hg.

In the empty beating heart used for this study, end-diastolic pressure was 0, because the left atrium was left open. To measure coronary flow an electromagnetic flow-through probe was used, mounted 2 cm above the aortic valve. The probe was calibrated by collecting the blood pumped out of the right ventricle and by measuring its volume with a calibrated syringe. Pressure flow plots were obtained by changing perfusion pressure to values up to 130 mm Hg for short periods of time (15 seconds).

In the fully dilated vascular bed, perfusion pressure had a distinct effect on vascular resistance. This is demonstrated in figure 4, which gives pressure flow relations measured in the same heart kept at different perfusion pressures. In this experiment perfusion pressure was initially kept at 50 mm Hg. Upward and downward pointing triangles refer to data obtained at this pressure before and after a period of high pressure perfusion respectively. Circles refer to high pressure data obtained at 124 mm Hg. High pressure perfusion raised minimal vascular

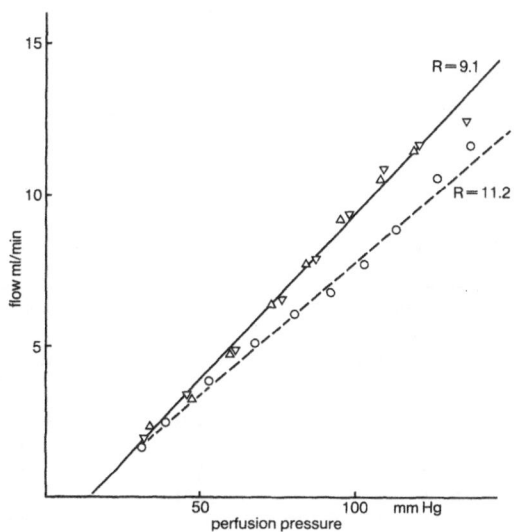

Figure 4. The effect of perfusion pressure on minimal vascular resistance. Mean pressure-mean flow plots obtained in an isolated rat heart kept at two different perfusion pressures. Upward and downward pointing triangles refer to data measured at a perfusion pressure of 50 mm Hg before and after a period of high perfusion pressure (124 mm Hg). To obtain data points, only short perturbations of perfusion pressure were induced in order to avoid pressure effects. Minimal resistance at low pressure was 9.1 mm Hg/ml per minute and at high pressure 11.2 mm Hg/ml per minute, which is 1.21 times higher. The pressure effect develops with a time constant of one minute, it is fully reversible and is related to the formation of edema.

resistance to 123% of its original value in this case. Perfusion pressure-induced changes are fully reversible and they develop rapidly with a time constant of less than one minute. To avoid pressure influences on vascular resistance we reduced exposure to high perfusion pressure as much as possible in the experiments.

Formation of edema seems the most likely explanation for the pressure-induced changes of resistance. Autoregulation, among other things, serves to keep the pressure drop across the capillaries constant and protects the capillary bed from arterial pressure overload. Paresis of autoregulation exposes the tissue to high pressure and causes edema formation.

Hearts including both ventricles and atria were weighed immediately after the experiment. Heart weight expressed as a percentage of body weight was significantly greater in the hypertensive rats, 121% of normal (table 1).

	normal Wistar rat		spontaneously hypertensive rat	
	heart wt/ body wt	minimal vascular resistance mm Hg/ml/min/g	heart wt/ body wt %	minimal vascular resistance mm Hg/ml/min/g
	0.396	8.86	0.458	8.07
	0.389	8.17	0.490	7.57
	0.379	8.58	0.447	9.50
	0.358	8.95	0.453	9.12
	0.400	8.24	0.480	8.60
mean	0.384	8.56	0.465	8.57
SD	0.017	0.35	0.018	0.78
percentage of normal			121%	100%
SD			10%	13.2%

Table 1. Heart weight/body weight ratios and minimal vascular resistance values as measured in five spontaneously hypertensive rats and in five normal Wistar rats. Isolated heart preparations perfused with reconstituted blood.

Data on vascular resistance in this small series of experiments did not show a significant difference between hypertensive rats and controls (figure 5).

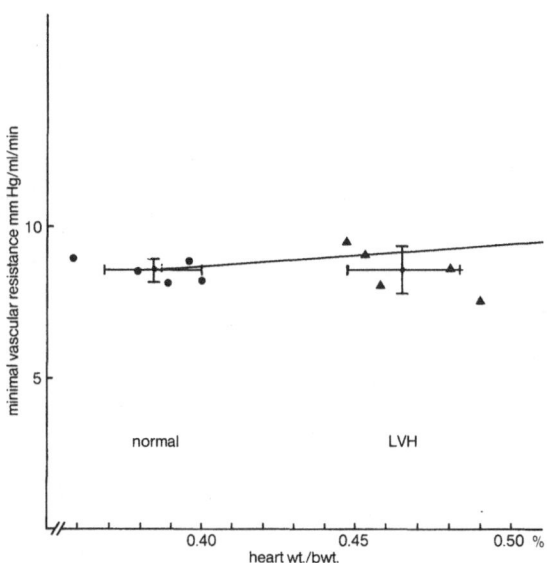

Figure 5. Minimal vascular resistance in hypertrophic rat heart. Minimal coronary vascular resistance values measured in isolated hypertrophic hearts of spontaneously hypertensive rats as compared to values obtained in hearts of normal Wistar rats. Artificial perfusion with reconstituted blood at a perfusion pressure of 50 mm Hg. The straight line is the linear approximation of the Wearn hypothesis as given in figure 2.

MINIMAL VASCULAR RESISTANCE IN THE INTACT ANIMAL

Several authors have published data on minimal vascular resistance measured in the exposed heart of an intact animal. O'Keefe et al.[7] measured vascular resistance in dogs with LVH induced by banding of the ascending aorta. Mueller et al.[8] did the same in dogs with renovascular hypertension. Interestingly, the latter measured it not only in the hypertensive state but also several days after reconstruction of the renal artery when blood pressure had returned to normal. O'Keefe's measurements were done only at normal coronary artery pressures.

Both authors find an increased minimal vascular resistance in the animals
with ventricular hypertrophy. The specific vascular resistance values
taken from their publications are plotted against heart weight normalized
for body weight (figure 6).

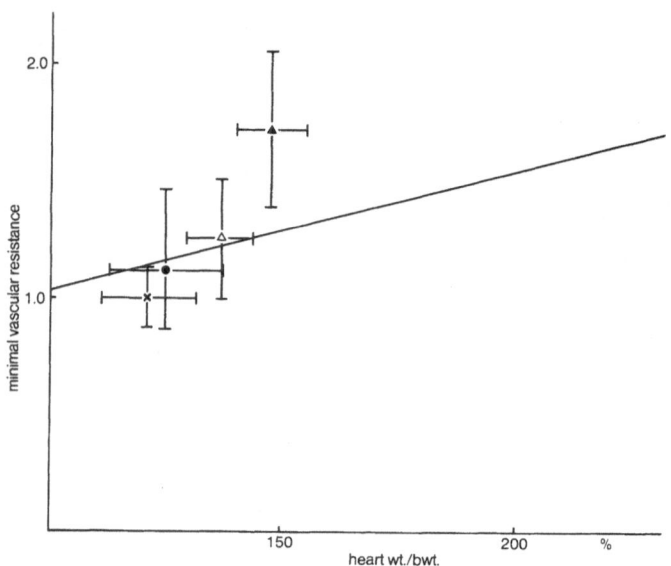

Figure 6. Minimal vascular resistance measured in intact dogs. Minimal
vascular resistance as measured by two different authors in the intact
dog is plotted against heart/body weight ratio. The straight line again
gives the predicted relation according to Wearn.
- O'Keefe et al.[7]   12 normal   9 LVH (constriction of the ascending
                                       aorta)
▲ Mueller et al.[8]   9 normal   11 LVH (unilateral renal artery con-
                                       striction and hypertensive)
△ Mueller et al.[8]   9 normal   6 LVH (after reconstruction of the
                                       renal artery and normotensive)
x author's data added for comparison, data obtained in isolated rat
   heart (figure 5).

Heart weight/body weight is expressed as a percentage of normal, and the
normal vascular resistance per gram measured by the authors in their
control experiments is taken as a unit of specific resistance. Our data
obtained in isolated rat hearts are added for comparison.

Surprisingly, vascular resistance measured in the hypertensive dog hearts is significantly higher than in the other hypertrophied hearts, and also significantly higher than predicted by the Wearn hypothesis.[13] Mean values of the other two sets of data measured in hypertrophied hearts at normal pressure lie close to the 0.66 power function. The variation of the data, however, is too large to allow for discrimination between Wearn's hypothesis and other models up to full compensatory growth of capillaries. We found a normal minimal resistance per gram in rats with hypertrophy, which is in keeping with Tomanek's histological data[15] in spontaneously hypertensive rats with long-standing hypertension.

It would be unlikely that the relatively high resistance found by Mueller et al.[8] in hypertensive dogs is caused only by a low capillary density, since, after return to normal pressure, resistance decreases considerably in only a few days. In view of our observations on the effect of high perfusion pressure on vascular resistance it seems likely that the high pressure measurements yielded higher resistance values because of edema formation induced by vasodilation.

Measurements of minimal vascular resistance can be used to estimate capillary density in the in situ heart as well as in the isolated preparation. Data on normal hearts measured under the same conditions should be available for comparison. Exposure to high perfusion pressure after vasodilation should be avoided, since it rapidly raises vascular resistance by formation of edema. Resistance measurement is not a sensitive method to detect minor changes of capillary density.

MINIMAL VASCULAR RESISTANCE IN CLINICAL PRACTICE

Reduction of coronary vascular reserve has been demonstrated beyond doubt in different types of ventricular hypertrophy in man. Most authors believe this to be caused by an underdevelopment of the capillary bed, similar to the pathologically low capillary density found in experimental hypertrophy in rats and dogs. Evidence from experimental work summarized above indicates that hypertrophy caused by hypertension or aortic valvular stenosis indeed raises vascular resistance to values closely predicted by Wearn.[13] Rats with hypertension for more than one year are an exception.[15] Other studies[16] give some evidence of growth of the number of capillaries around very thick muscle fibers, but the mean capillary surface area per gram is in close agreement with Wearn's constant ratio hypothesis.

The question can be raised whether hypertrophied hearts in man show the same changes of capillary density with respect to relative heart weight as those found in animals. Although coronary reserve is undoubtedly reduced in man with LVH, it may be that late capillary growth at least in part compensates for the hypertrophy of the muscle fibers, as in the adult hypertensive rat. If so, minimal vascular resistance would be lower than expected according to Wearn's power function. It may also be that secondary changes, such as myocardial fibrosis or infiltration of the myocardium, add to the vascular resistance and increase it to values above those predicted by the power function.

Only very few data on coronary resistance measurements and ventricular dimensions exist. Minimal vascular resistance can be estimated from the post-occlusion hyperemic response. Recently Marcus et al.[6] published flow measurements obtained in the intact coronary artery of the exposed heart prior to cardioplegia. The authors present data on 13 patients with aortic stenosis and eight controls, all with normal coronary arteries. Echocardiographic measures of the ventricles are given, from which ventricular mass can be roughly estimated. The mean value of vascular resistance plotted against ventricular mass is given in figure 7 together with data points taken from the publications summarized above. The single point at the extreme right of the figure is the one obtained in the human hearts. Standard deviations of the experimental data are already given in figures 3 and 6; the standard deviations of the data from Marcus' paper are undoubtedly very large, but the conversion of echocardiographic measures to ventricular mass makes it impossible to calculate their magnitude. This renders this plot of limited value, but the figure shows a few interesting things. First of all it is clear that the ventricular mass and the minimal vascular resistance in the human hearts far exceed any value measured in the experimental animals with induced hypertrophy. This should make us very careful in drawing any conclusion from the

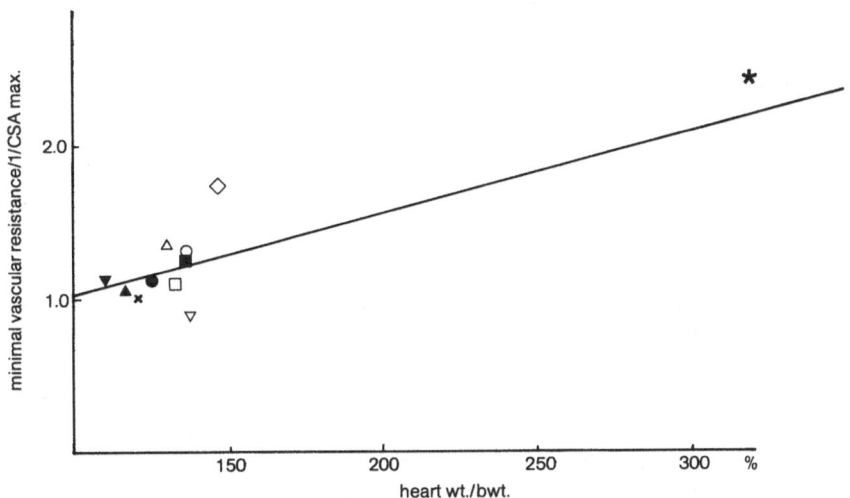

Figure 7. Capillary density or minimal vascular resistance in hyper-trophic heart. Data on the reciprocal of the capillary surface area combined with minimal vascular resistance measurements as given in figures 3 and 6. For comparison, estimates of the minimal vascular resistance measured in patients with aortic valve stenosis are added.

▼ Tomanek et al.[15]   1-mo-old SHR (spontaneously hypertensive rat)
▲ Tomanek et al.[15]   2.5-mo-old SHR
× author's data   adult SHR
● O'Keefe et al.[7]   dogs, after constriction of the ascending aorta
△ Tomanek et al.[15]   7-mo-old SHR
□ Rakusan et al.[14]   adult rat, after constriction of the descending
                          aorta
■ Mueller et al.[8]   dogs, normotensive after a period of renovascular
                          hypertension
○ Henquell et al.[16]   rats, salt-loaded after unilateral nephrectomy
▽ Tomanek et al.[15]   15-mo-old SHR
◇ Mueller et al.[8]   dogs, hypertensive after unilateral renal artery
                          constriction
* Marcus et al.[6]   men, severe aortic valvular stenosis

The data point calculated from the results obtained by Marcus et al. re-quired some additional assumptions. Coronary artery flow was assumed to be normal and autoregulation was assumed to be fully intact. Ventricular mass was estimated from echocardiographic data given by the authors. A standard deviation could not be calculated, but it is undoubtedly large. The standard deviations of the other data points are given in the previous figures.

168

animal studies. Another interesting point is that the data obtained in 13 patients with aortic stenosis are in close agreement with values predicted by Wearn's power function, which suggests that very little if any compensatory growth of capillaries occurs in man, at least in this type of hypertrophy, despite the fact that LVH occurring in man is far more extensive than that found in experimental situations.

REFERENCES

1. Fallen, E.L., Elliott, W.C. and Gorlin, R.: Mechanisms of angina in aortic stenosis, Circulation, 36, 480-488, 1967
2. Buckberg, G., Eber, L., Herman, M. and Gorlin, R.: Ischemia in aortic stenosis: hemodynamic prediction, Am. J. Cardiol., 35, 778-784, 1975
3. Opherk, D., Weihe, E., Zebe, H., Mall, G., Mehmel, H.C., Stockins, B., Ryan, U. and Kubler, W.: Reduced coronary reserve and ultra-structural changes of the myocardium in patients with angina pectoris, arterial hypertension and normal coronary arteries. In: The Heart in Hypertension, Strauer, B.E. (ed), Springer Verlag, Berlin, 208-220, 1981
4. Cheitlin, M.D., Robinowitz, M., McAllister, H., Hoffman, J.I.E., Bharati, S. and Lev, M.: The distribution of fibrosis in the left ventricle in congenital aortic stenosis and coarctation of the oarta, Circulation, 62, 823-830, 1980
5. Roberts, J.T. and Wearn, J.T.: Quantitative changes in the capillary-muscle relationship in human hearts during normal growth and hypertrophy, Am. Heart J., 21, 617-633, 1941
6. Marcus, M.L., Doty, D.B., Hiratzka, L.F., Wright, C.B., Eastham, C.L.: Decreased coronary reserve. A mechanism for angina pectoris in patients with aortic stenosis and normal coronary arteries, N. Engl. J. Med., 307, 1362-1367, 1982
7. O'Keefe, D.D., Hoffman, J.I.E., Cheitlin, R., O'Neill, M.J., Allard, J.R. and Shapkin, E.: Coronary blood flow in experimental canine left ventricular hypertrophy, Circ. Res., 43, 43-51, 1978
8. Mueller, T.M., Marcus, M.L., Kerber, R.E., Young, Y.A., Barnes, R.W. and Abboud, F.M.: Effect of renal hypertension and left ventricular hypertrophy on the coronary circulation in dogs, Circ. Res., 42, 543-549, 1978
9. Gregg, D.E.: Effect of coronary perfusion pressure or coronary flow on oxygen usage of the myocardium, Circ. Res., 13, 497-500, 1963
10. Wicker, P. and Tarazi, R.C.: Coronary blood flow in left ventricular hypertrophy: a review of experimental data, European Heart J., 3, suppl. A, 111-118, 1982
11. Malik, A.B., Abe, T., O'Kane, H. and Geha, A.S.: Cardiac function, coronary flow, and oxygen consumption in stable left ventricular hypertrophy, Am. J. Physiol., 225, 186-191, 1973
12. Marchetti, G.V., Merlo, L., Noseda, V. and Visioli, O.: Myocardial blood flow in experimental cardiac hypertrophy in dogs, Cardiovasc. Res., 7, 519-527, 1973
13. Shipley, R.A., Shipley, L.J., Wearn, J.T.: The capillary supply in normal and hypertrophied hearts of rabbits, J. Exp. Med., 65, 29-42, 1937

14. Rakusan, K., Poupa, O.: Differences in capillary supply of hypertrophic and hyperplastic hearts, Cardiologica, 49, 293-298, 1966
15. Tomanek, R.J., Searls, J.C., Lachenbruch, P.A.: Quantitative changes in the capillary bed during developing, peak, and stabilized cardiac hypertrophy in the spontaneously hypertensive rat, Circ. Res., 51, 295-304, 1982
16. Henquell, L., Odoroff, C.L., Honig, C.R.: Intercapillary distance and capillary reserve in hypertrophied rat hearts beating in situ, Circ. Res., 41, 400-408, 1977
17. Arai, S., Machida, A. and Nakamura, T.: Myocardial structure and vascularization of hypertrophied hearts, Tohoku J. Exp. Med., 95, 35-54, 1968

SUMMARY

The main determinants of coronary flow are coronary artery pressure and coronary vascular resistance. The extent of the latter depends on the contractile state of the blood vessel wall, and on the amount of compression of the vessels through intramyocardial-intravascular pressure differences.

In the autoregulated hypertrophied heart, under resting conditions the resistance vessels are more dilated at any given arterial pressure than in the normal heart, because the increased muscle mass requires a larger resting flow. As a result, vasodilatory reserve is diminished in the hypertrophied heart. If hypertrophy is caused by hypertension or supravalvular constriction of the aorta, loss of vascular reserve can in part be compensated by the high coronary perfusion pressure. This is because maximal flow increases more steeply with aortic pressure than resting flow, which increases as oxygen demand increases with aortic pressure. In aortic valvular stenosis, compression of the intramyocardial blood vessels may have additional unfavorable effects on coronary vascular reserve. Increased intramyocardial pressure not balanced by an increased perfusion pressure may be expected to increase minimal vascular resistance especially in the subendocardium and thereby reduce the flow reserve.

Coronary pressure and flow patterns can be analyzed by assuming a hemodynamic model of the coronary circulation comprising intramyocardial compliance, loaded by intramyocardial pressure, and inflow and outflow resistances. The model has been validated in open-chest experiments in which the coronary arterial inflow and coronary venous outflow are measured simultaneously. Variations of intramyocardial blood volume can be calculated from these measurements. From these studies it follows that the use of coronary vascular resistance values calculated from end-diastolic pressures and flows is questionable. It can be demonstrated that resistances calculated in this way partly depend upon the shape of the arterial pressure pulse.

The typical reversal of the coronary flow pattern found in severe aortic insufficiency is in keeping with the myocardial compression model. It can be predicted that systolic flow will exceed diastolic flow if the arterial pulse pressure becomes larger than half the intraventricular systolic-diastolic pressure difference. Low diastolic flow in aortic insufficiency does not imply that coronary vascular resistance is raised.

CORONARY FLOW MECHANICS OF THE HYPERTROPHIED HEART

SPAAN, J.A.E., BRUINSMA, P., LAIRD, J.D.

Department of Physiology and Physiological Physics, Leiden University, Wassenaarseweg 62, 2333 AL Leiden, the Netherlands

INTRODUCTION

Cardiac contraction impedes coronary flow. This can be shown directly in the experimental situation in which a large coronary artery is cannulated and the coronary bed is fully dilated. Mean coronary flow will then increase after cardiac arrest although coronary artery pressure remains constant.[1,2] Cardiac contraction reduces coronary reserve not only in normal but also in hypertrophied hearts.

Coronary arterial flow in a beating heart is pulsatile even when arterial pressure is constant. The phasic coronary flow pattern results from the interplay between arterial pressure pattern and the systolic compression of intramyocardial blood vessels. In particular the coronary arterial pressure pattern in hypertrophied hearts may differ from that in normal hearts. The magnitude of coronary flow variations, being partly determined by the coronary vascular resistance, is larger in the hypertrophied heart compared to the normal. This is because vascular resistance at rest is lower in the hypertrophied heart.

Diastolic coronary flow is partly determined by the amount of blood expelled from intramyocardial blood vessels during systole.[3,4] The interaction between systole and diastole complicates the prediction of the effect of compression on net myocardial perfusion. Analyzing diastolic and systolic coronary arterial flow independently is not always justified. In this chapter we shall first analyze the interwovenness of determinants of coronary arterial systolic and diastolic flow. Thereafter we shall attempt to analyze the consequences of the compression of intramyocardial blood vessels for the perfusion of the hypertrophied heart.

This study was supported in part by the foundation for fundamental medical research, FUNGO, and the Dutch Heart Foundation.

PHASIC CORONARY FLOW

Cardiac contraction exerts an influence on blood in the coronary vascular bed which is similar to the pumping action of the myocardium on ventricular blood mass. In systole, pressure is exerted on blood within the intramyocardial vessels. As a result, blood is squeezed out of the intramyocardial blood compartment. In diastole, the similarity holds as well: the volumes expelled in systole are replaced in diastole. Hence the term "intramyocardial pump action" of the heart on the coronary blood flow is fully justified.

The differences between cardiac pump action and intramyocardial pump action relate to ejection fraction and the presence or absence of valves. The aortic valve offers minimal resistance to left ventricular outflow and an ejection fraction of 80% can be attained. The intramyocardial blood compartment is distributed over many tiny vessels offering high resistance to flow. Because of this, the amount of blood ejected from this compartment during systole is of the order of a few percent of its volume. Due to the absence of valves in the coronary circulation, the intramyocardial pump action results only in pulsatility of coronary arterial and venous flow and does not contribute to a net forward flow.

The intramyocardial pump model

A model for this pump is depicted in figure 1. The compliance of all intramyocardial blood vessels has been lumped into one overall intramyocardial compliance, C_{im} The compliance C_{im} is simulated by the spring. Extravascular compression (P_{im}) forces blood out of the intramyocardial vessels and increases blood pressure within the vessels, which leads to reduction of arterial inflow and enhances venous outflow. In diastole, the opposite occurs. The mean intramyocardial blood pressure is represented by P_{ib}. R_{in} and R_{out} are overall resistances representing the intramyocardial resistances to the squeezing out of blood.

By analyzing systolic-diastolic coronary arterial flow differences caused by intramyocardial pressure variations, Spaan et al.[4] found the following correlation: R_{in} = 0.63 x (R_{in} + R_{out}) - 12.9 (mmHg.s/ml). In the experi-

Intramyocardial pump model

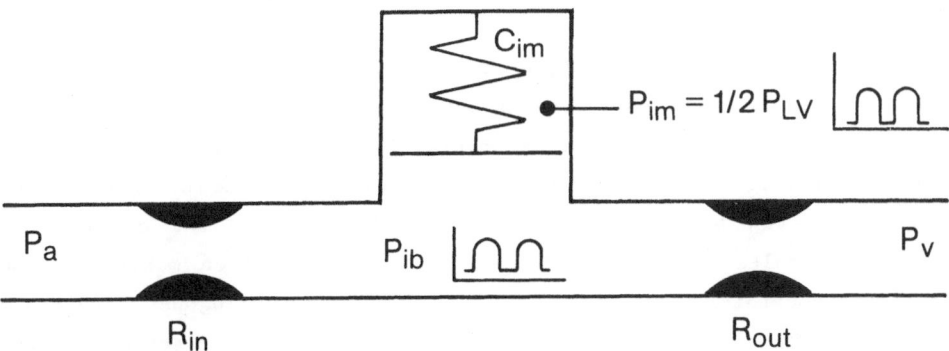

Figure 1. Hydraulic analog of the coronary circulation. Compliance of all intramyocardial blood vessels is lumped into one overall intramyocardial compliance, C_{im}, represented by a spring. Intramyocardial blood pressure varies periodically since C_{im} is loaded by intramyocardial pressure P_{im}. R_{in} and R_{out} represent resistances impeding the squeezing out of blood through the arteriolar and venous side of the coronary circulation respectively. P_a and P_v represent arterial and venous pressure respectively.

ments total coronary resistance was varied by changing perfusion pressure, heart rate and left ventricular pressure. The overall resistance R_{in} + R_{out} was calculated by assuming an outflow pressure of 14 mmHg, which was the mean peripheral coronary artery pressure measured 15 s after interruption of coronary flow. Intramyocardial systolic-diastolic blood pressure variations due to cardiac contraction were 53.1 $\pm$ 7 (SD) mmHg, while systolic-diastolic ventricular pressure variations were 100 $\pm$ 10 (SD) mmHg. The correlation between R_{in} + R_{out} was determined in the autoregulating coronary bed. As a result, the simulations will have reference only to this situation. In the simulations, the resistances are calculated from arterial pressure assuming an autoregulated flow per 100 grams of 1 ml/s. The extravascular pressure is approximated by a square wave in order to facilitate the recognition of charging and discharging effects within the simulated curves. Systolic P_{im} = 50 mmHg and diastolic P_{im} = 5 mmHg. As explained above, this means that ventricular systolic pressure is 100 mmHg and diastolic pressure is 10 mmHg. Compliance is taken to be 0.07 ml/mmHg as was estimated for a ventricle of 100 g.[4]

174

Simulations applying to the steady beating heart and transients after
cardiac arrest are shown in figure 6 and are discussed below.

INTRAMYOCARDIAL COMPLIANCE LOADED BY VENTRICULAR CONTRACTION
Extravascular compression decreases intramyocardial blood volume. Because
of the compliance of the intramyocardial blood compartment, this volume
will be restored after release of compression. Volume changes of any
compartment can be quantified only when both inflow and outflow are
measured simultaneously. Below, we shall discuss three manifestations
of intramyocardial compliance as studied by measuring both coronary
arterial inflow and coronary venous outflow. All three observations can
be understood with the aid of the intramyocardial pump model given in
figure 1.

Phasic coronary arterial flow and coronary venous flow
The effect of contraction on coronary arterial and venous flow is shown
in figure 2. The measurements have been obtained in an experiment on an
open-chest anesthetized dog. Both left main coronary artery and the great
cardiac vein were cannulated in that experiment. The artery was perfused
via a perfusion system that maintained coronary arterial pressure.[4]

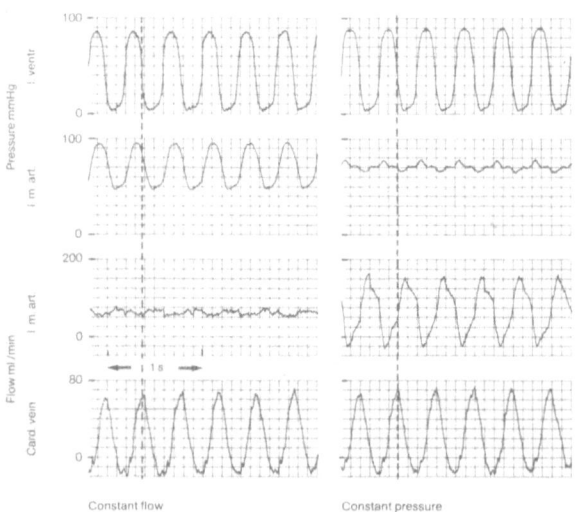

Figure 2. Comparison between constant pressure perfusion and constant
flow perfusion. Note that the venous outflow pattern is independent of
the arterial inflow pattern.

The flow from the great cardiac vein was drained into a pressure-controlled container. Results of constant flow perfusion and constant pressure perfusion are shown in figure 2. Systolic compression of intramyocardial blood vessels reduces inflow and enhances outflow.[5] Note that systolic arterial flow became negative although perfusion pressure was as high as 70 mmHg. During constant flow perfusion, coronary arterial pressure became pulsatile. The pulse of the coronary arterial pressure during constant flow perfusion results from compression of intramyocardial vessels througout the wall. Compression effects are stronger in the subendocardium than in the subepicardium. The pressure pulse during constant flow perfusion equals the intramyocardial blood pressure variation, which causes pulsatile flow during constant pressure perfusion. Note that the venous outflow pattern is almost identical for both perfusion methods. Apparently, the transients in venous flow are independent of the wave form of arterial flow.

Venous outflow during arterial occlusion

The results shown in figure 3 have been obtained in a study on a goat with the same experimental procedure as described above. The coronary venous pressure was measured with a 0.1-mm catheter in an epicardial vein. After sudden arterial occlusion, venous flow decayed to zero. During the occlusion, the epicardial venous pressure was kept constant by adjusting the venous reservoir pressure. The venous outflow during the decay of coronary arterial pressure results from the discharge of intramyocardial compliance. The mean coronary arterial pressure after occlusion was extrapolated to obtain $P_{ib,o}$, which is an estimate of mean intramyocardial blood pressure before occlusion. Typical of this kind of experiment is the delay of recovery of venous outflow after resumption of arterial flow. This cannot be accounted for by a single compliant compartment as shown in figure 1. In engineering terms, these are the characteristics of a higher-order system. This means that one should consider a number of intramyocardial pumps in series rather than single ones.

Venous outflow during cardiac arrest

The effect of intramyocardial compliance on venous outflow following cardiac arrest, is shown in figure 4. The experiment was performed in a goat with the same experimental set-up as used to obtain the results of figures 2 and 3. Coronary arterial pressure was kept constant.

Coronary venous outflow dropped to almost zero at cardiac arrest, although coronary inflow continued. This can only mean that intramyocardial blood volume increased in this period. Venous outflow reached a maximum after 3.2 ± 0.54 (mean $\pm$ 1 SD) seconds (four animals, 10 long diastoles). We have calculated the increase of intramyocardial blood volume from the arterial and venous flow curves. Before we subtracted venous from arterial flow, the former was multiplied by the ratio of arterial to venous flow after the first four seconds of diastole. Thereafter the ratio remained constant.

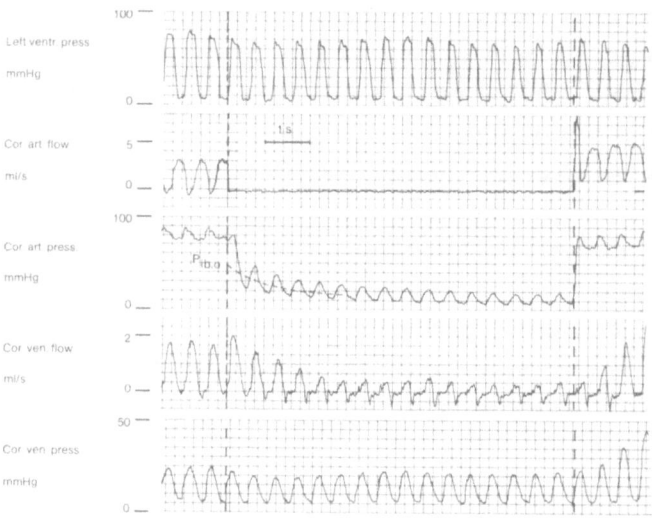

Figure 3. Venous outflow during arterial occlusion.
Coronary venous pressure was measured with a 0.1-mm catheter within a large epicardial vein. Note the concomitant fall of mean arterial pressure (-----) and coronary venous outflow. $P_{ib,o}$ = estimated mean intramyocardial blood pressure in the beating heart.

The result given in figure 4 is a change of intramyocardial blood volume of about 2 ml/100 g LV. Intramyocardial blood volume constitutes up to 15% of tissue weight.[6] Thus during cardiac arrest, intramyocardial blood volume increased by about 13% of its end-systolic volume.

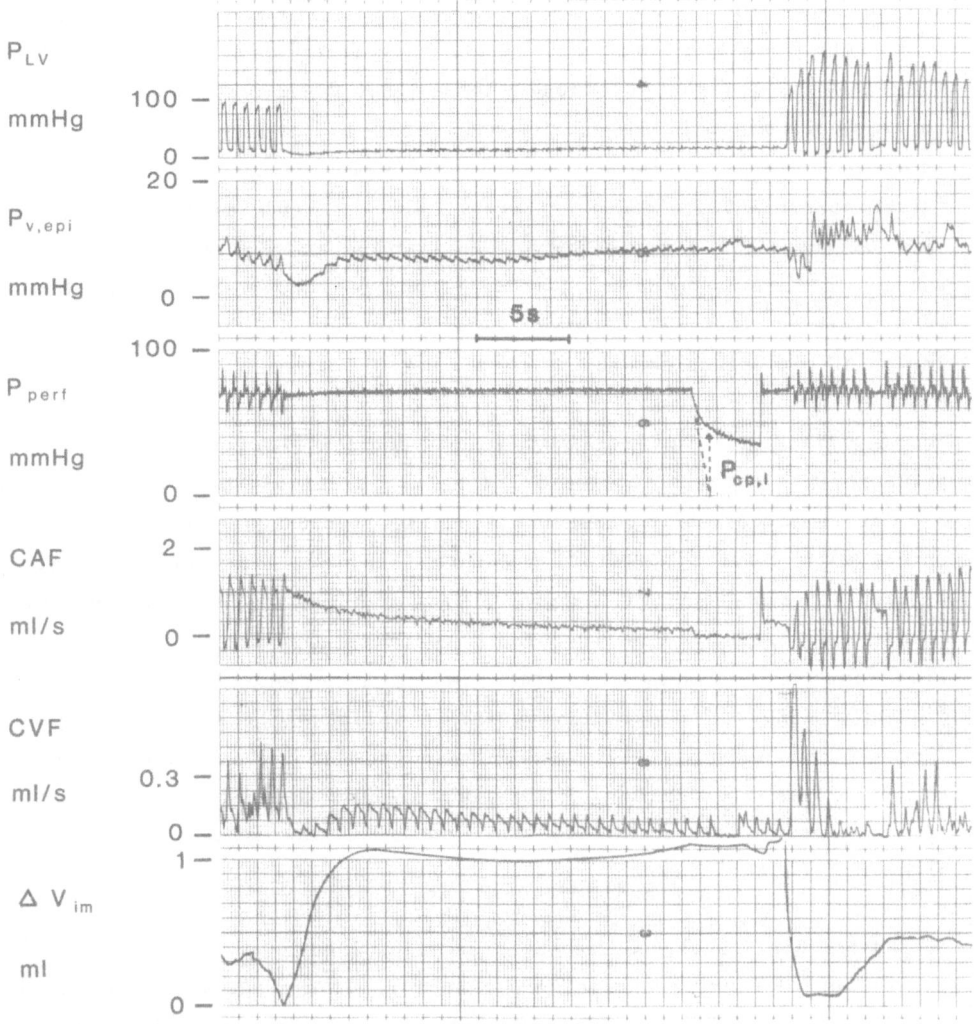

Figure 4. Arterial and venous flow during a long diastole at constant perfusion pressure. P_{LV} = left ventricular pressure, $P_{v,epi}$ = epicardial venous pressure, P_{perf} = perfusion pressure measured at the tip of a Gregg cannula, CAF = coronary arterial flow, CVF = coronary venous flow, ΔV_{im} = calculated intramyocardial volume change. Note the drop in CVF and $P_{v,epi}$ with the onset of the long diastole. This indicates that blood is withheld, or even sucked back into the intramyocardial veins in the early part of cardiac arrest. Left ventricular weight was 65 g.

CORONARY ARTERIAL PRESSURE-FLOW RELATIONS AND CORONARY RESISTANCE

The presence of a relatively large intramyocardial compliance causes independence of the transients of coronary arterial and coronary venous flow (see also figure 6 below). In the intramyocardial pump model all intramyocardial compliances are considered to be lumped together. The intramyocardial compliance is in reality distributed over the whole intramyocardial vasculature. Moreover, its magnitude will depend on the type of vessel, _e.g._ arterioles, capillaries, or venules. As a result, shapes of flow patterns will be different in the various types of vessels. This in fact was observed by Tillmans et al.[7] in the microcirculation of the dog epicardium.

The equilibration time for both venous outflow and coronary peripheral pressure with arterial occlusion is in the order of three seconds (fig. 3). The same equilibrium time was found for venous outflow after cardiac arrest with constant arterial pressure (fig. 4). The equilibrium times reflect time constants of charging and discharging of the intramyocardial compliance. Pressure-flow relations are often obtained by varying arterial flow and pressure at a rate faster than, or comparable to, the discharge rate of the intramyocardial compliance. If so, the pressure-flow relation will be determined only in part by the coronary resistance at the arterial side (R_{in} of the model), and in addition by the downstream pressure determined by the charge of the intramyocardial compliance.

Intramyocardial compliance and pressure-flow lines

The effect of intramyocardial compliance is clearly demonstrated in the example of diastolic pressure-flow relationships as given in figure 5. The curves in figure 5 are calculated by means of the intramyocardial pump model. The arterial pressure before the intervention was taken to be constant at 90 mmHg. For the sake of argument, we shall assume that the values of resistances do not change as a result of autoregulation. The change of coronary inflow following a rapid change in arterial pressure during diastole can be represented by any curve parallel to and in between the bold lines in figure 5.

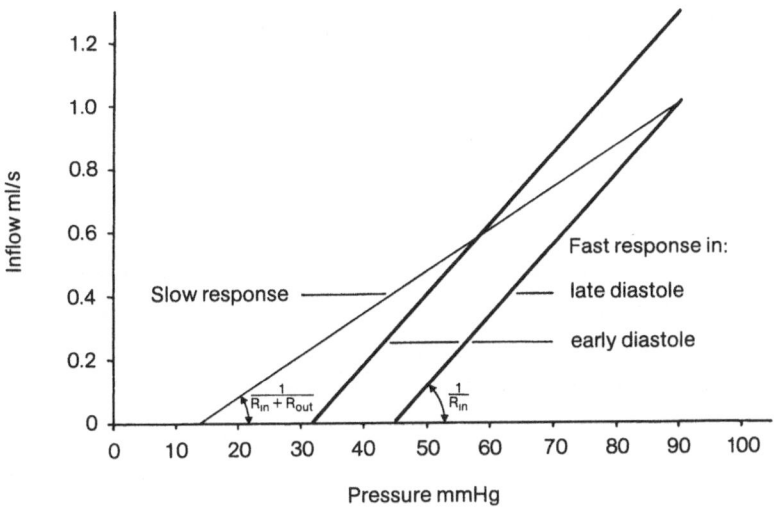

Figure 5. Predictions of arterial pressure flow relations in the auto-regulated heart by the intramyocardial pump model. Heavy lines represent relationships in the case in which coronary flow is not allowed to stabilize for a period several times that of the characteristic time constant of the intramyocardial compliance. The late diastolic line is shifted to the right because the intramyocardial compliance is charged before the pressure change. The thin line is the relationship if stabilization is allowed.

The inverse of the tangent of such a diastolic pressure-flow relation equals R_{in}. The pressure intercept equals the intramyocardial blood pressure at the moment of pressure change. If the pressure is varied at the onset of diastole, the pressure intercept is low because intramyocardial blood pressure is low as a result of the release of extravascular pressure. This is shown in figure 5 by the heavy line on the left. However, if pressure changes after the intramyocardial compliance is charged (e.g fig. 6), the intercept will be higher. This is shown by the heavy line on the right. Note that under this condition initial coronary flow equals mean coronary flow in the beating heart. When the intramyocardial compliance is allowed to equilibrate after a pressure change to a new steady pressure level, one will find the slow response line of figure 5. This slow response line is identical to the mean flow-mean pressure curve in the beating heart if coronary resistance would not be influenced by autoregulation. Obviously, the late diastolic pressure-flow line will only be parallel to the early diastolic pressure-flow line if autoregulation does not change R_{in}. Figure 5 shows that due to compliance of

180

intramyocardial vessels, pressure-flow lines in the coronary circulation
are not unique, but strongly depend on the way they are obtained. Note
that the actual value of intramyocardial compliance is not critical to
the above analysis.

Intramyocardial compliance and long diastoles

The theoretical pressure-flow lines of figure 5 are relevant to experimental curves obtained by perfusion of the coronary artery at constant
pressure.[8,9] Let us now consider the diastolic pressure-flow relation as
a result of an exponential arterial pressure decay.[10] The simulation of
a cardiac arrest after a period of steady beating is shown in figure 6.

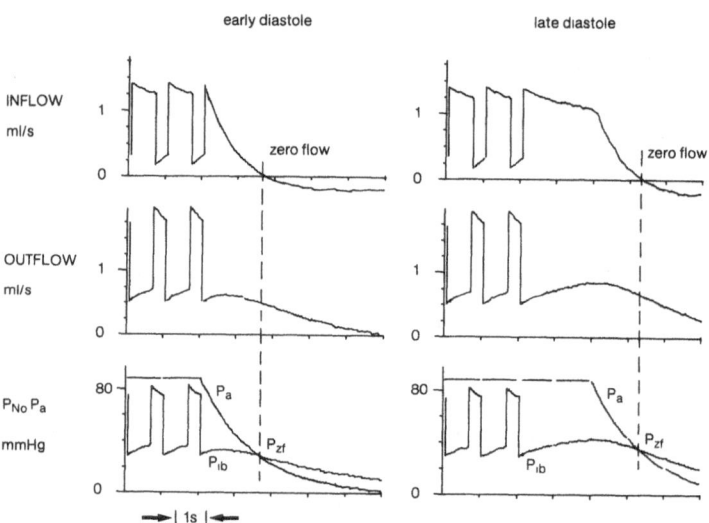

Figure 6. Simulation of arterial inflow, venous outflow, arterial pressure (P_a) and intramyocardial blood pressure (P_{ib}) of the coronary
circulation. In the left-hand panel P_a decays exponentially from the
onset of cardiac arrest. Inflow decreases immediately but outflow and
P_{ib} increase first. Inflow becomes zero when arterial pressure equals
intramyocardial blood pressure at the value P_{zf}. With later diastolic
arterial pressure decay, P_{zf} is higher because the intramyocardial
compliance has been charged in the period before pressure decay. Note the
similarity of the simulated and the measured venous outflow curve just
after cardiac arrest in figure 4.

The periodic diastolic charging and systolic discharging of the intramyocardial blood compartment is shown by the wave form of the resulting intramyocardial blood pressure. As is clear from figure 6, the model predicts phasic variations of intramyocardial blood pressure, arterial inflow and venous outflow. As explained above, systole and diastole are just too short to allow for steady coronary inflow.

Arresting of the heart was simulated by fixing intramyocardial pressure at its diastolic level of 5 mmHg. Two cases were simulated. In the left-hand panels arterial pressure fell exponentially starting immediately after cardiac arrest. In the right-hand panels the drop in arterial pressure was delayed by two seconds.

Because of the intramyocardial compliance, intramyocardial blood pressure does not follow the time course of arterial pressure. In the early period of a long diastole, intramyocardial compliance is still being charged. This is the case even when the drop in arterial pressure starts immediately after cardiac arrest. Coronary inflow is zero when arterial pressure equals intramyocardial blood pressure. Arterial pressure at zero flow is called P_{zf}. When arterial pressure decay is delayed, P_{zf} is higher because the intramyocardial compliance charges up to a higher pressure during the early period of constant arterial pressure.

In figure 7, theoretical values of P_{zf} are compared with experimental values as presented by Dole and Bishop[9] and Klocke et al.[11] The experimental dependence of P_{zf} on pre-arrest perfusion pressure[9] agrees well with the model. Dole and Bishop determined P_{zf} at about 1.5 to 2 seconds after cardiac arrest, Klocke et al.[11] did this at the onset of cardiac arrest. The higher P_{zf} values found by Dole and Bishop[9] can be accounted for by the differences in charging of the intramyocardial compliance.

End-diastolic coronary resistance
The end-diastolic coronary resistance of the normal beating heart has been defined as the ratio between arterial-venous pressure difference and coronary flow at the end of diastole.[12] It is assumed that all transients in the coronary flow signal due to inertia and/or compliance are

damped out at the end of diastole. As is clear from the analysis above, this is not the case. Therefore, one has to be cautious with the interpretation of intervention-effect relations based on the analysis of end-diastolic resistance values.

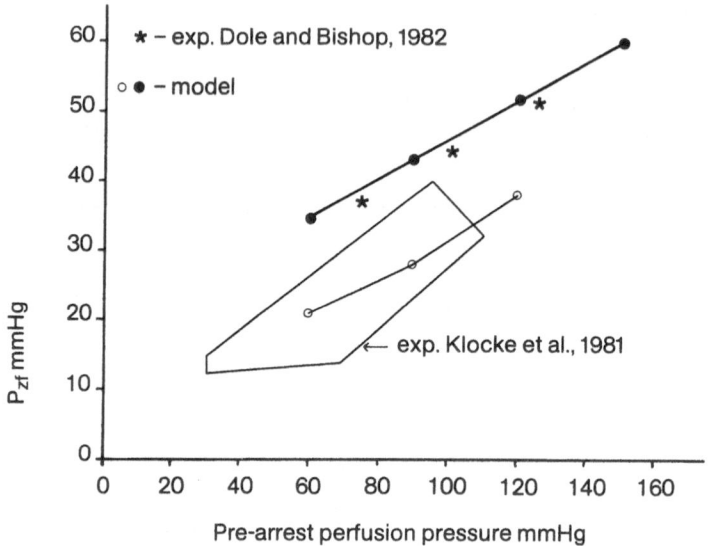

Figure 7. Comparison of P_{zf} predictions by the intramyocardial pump model and experimental results. The data of Dole and Bishop[9] are obtained with late diastolic pressure decays. The encircled area represents the results of Klocke et al.[11] obtained in the autoregulated heart with early diastolic pressure decay. The theoretical values are the results of simulations of the constant pressure technique (fast response), (●)P_{zf} two seconds after and (o)P_{zf} at cardiac arrest.

To illustrate this point, let us consider the effect of a drug that decreases systemic peripheral resistance. Assume that this drug does not influence heart rate nor coronary resistance. A decreased peripheral resistance will result in a larger fall of aortic pressure during diastole. Coronary diastolic flow will follow aortic pressure according to the early diastole-fast response curve of figure 5. As a result, one would probably conclude that end-diastolic coronary resistance has increased. Apparently, the shape of the aortic pressure pattern in itself has influenced the value obtained for the end-diastolic resistance. One has to remember this point especially in studies on the hypertrophied heart. Hypertrophy is mostly secondary to an abnormality in the circulation strongly influencing the coronary perfusion pressure pattern.

PHASIC CORONARY FLOW IN HYPERTROPHIED HEARTS

Hypertrophy usually results from chronic hypertension, valvular aortic stenosis, supravalvular aortic stenosis, or aortic insufficiency. All these abnormalies influence the phasic coronary flow pattern. Most alterations in the flow patterns can be explained on the basis of changes in both intramyocardial extravascular compression and coronary arterial pressure. The magnitude of coronary flow variations is also determined by the coronary resistance vessels. Before discussing the coronary flow patterns related to different forms of hypertrophy, we shall discuss in general terms the contribution of extravascular compression and coronary resistance to the shape of the phasic coronary flow pattern.

Extravascular compression and hypertrophy

Phasic coronary flow is caused by phasic coronary arterial pressure on the one hand and the squeezing out of blood by compression of intramyocardial vessels on the other hand. One usually considers intramyocardial tissue pressure to be the major source of compression of blood vessels. Tissue pressure is in fact the pressure of the extravascular fluid.[13,14]

Tissue pressure in the heart muscle cannot be measured directly without distortion of the tissue, influencing the pressure measurement. This problem has recently been discussed in a review by Feigl.[15] There is more or less a consensus about the distribution of systolic-diastolic tissue pressure variations. In the subendocardium these variations equal the ventricular pressure variations in magnitude and they gradually disappear towards the sub-epicardium. The gradient of tissue pressure across the wall will be smaller when the wall is thicker. However, the overall effect of vascular compression on coronary flow will be relatively independent of wall thickness.

Other factors may contribute to the squeezing out of blood. Geometrical changes in the myocardial wall may also contribute to the squeezing effect. Contraction of muscle fibers may well have a direct mechanical effect on the vessel walls. For example, the walls of microvessels are coupled to the myocytes by connective tissue.[16,17] Fiber shortening is quite homogeneous across the wall[14], and consequently the contribution of direct mechanical effects to the squeezing effect on blood vessels will be uniform across the myocardial wall. Therefore, the direct contribution of fiber shortening to vascular compression can also be expected to be independent of wall thickness.

Since wall thickness is unlikely to be important for the height of the overall intramyocardial pressure, we extrapolated the findings from the normal heart to the non-ischemic hypertrophied heart. In the analysis of phasic flow in normal hearts of the anesthetized dog the squeezing pressure was found to be 53.1 ± 7.02 (SD) mmHg, while systolic left ventricular pressure equaled 100 ± 10 (SD) mmHg. This fact demonstrates the dominating role of tissue pressure in vascular compression of intramyocardial vessels.

Effect of decreased coronary resistance in hypertrophied hearts

As discussed above, the resistance to the squeezing out of blood by vascular compression at the arterial side of the coronary circulation (R_{in} of the model) correlates fairly well with total coronary resistance ($R_{in} + R_{out}$ of the model).

Due to autoregulation, the coronary resistance vessels of hypertrophied hearts have a lower resistance as compared to normal hearts under similar hemodynamic conditions. This lower resistance results in a decreased coronary vasodilatory reserve (Hoffman et al., chapter 9 of this book). As a result, the coronary flow variations during the cardiac cycle will be larger in hypertrophied hearts than in normal hearts under equal conditions of coronary arterial and ventricular pressures.

Hypertension and supravalvular aortic constriction

In hypertension and supravalvular aortic constriction, intramyocardial pressure variations are larger than normal, which will lead to larger coronary flow variations. However, especially in the case of supravalvular aortic constriction, the coronary arterial pressure variations will increase as well.[18,19] As a result, the net effect of the increased systolic ventricular pressure on phasic coronary flow pattern will be small. The increased work of the heart will result in metabolic vasodilation and thus in larger coronary flow variations. However, increased coronary arterial pressure will lead to vasoconstriction due to autoregulation, which will reduce flow variations.[20,21]

Two studies[20,21] have shown a marked decrease in the difference between mean systolic and mean diastolic flow in hypertrophied hearts after weeks of aortic banding. This would mean that the factors causing a reduction of pulsatility probably dominate in these cases.

Valvular aortic stenosis

A valvular aortic stenosis increases intramyocardial pressure and work of the heart but has little effect on coronary arterial pressure. Hence, only those factors which increase systolic-diastolic coronary flow differences are intensified. Indeed, a strong reduction of coronary systolic inflow compared to diastolic inflow has been measured in dogs with congenital subvalvular stenosis.[19,22]

Aortic insufficiency

The most marked change in perfusion condition of the heart with an incompetent aortic valve is found in the shape of the coronary arterial pressure pulse. The large systolic-diastolic pressure difference reduces the systolic-diastolic coronary flow difference. Experimental studies have shown that diastolic flow can become systolic flow and may even become negative.[23-26]

The reduction of systolic-diastolic flow differences with increasing arterial pressure pulse is in agreement with the measurements given in figure 2. Reversal of the coronary flow pattern so that systolic flow exceeds diastolic flow, is caused by the increase of the arterial pressure pulse when it exceeds the pulse of the intramyocardial pressure in size. However, as long as mean coronary arterial pressure remains within the autoregulatory range, mean coronary flow will be independent of the pressure wave form.[4]

The extreme of aortic insufficiency is the situation in which the coronary arterial pressure equals ventricular pressure during the whole cardiac cycle. Evidently, the perfusion condition of the heart with complete aortic insufficiency can only be obtained with the aid of an extracorporeal circuit and a cannulated coronary artery, as has been done by Downey and Kirk.[27]

We simulated this extreme form of aortic insufficiency and used ventricular pressure as coronary arterial pressure. Two intramyocardial pump units of the type shown in figure 1 were arranged in parallel. One simulated the subendocardium, and intramyocardial pressure was set equal to ventricular pressure and arterial pressure; the second simulated the subepicardium where intramyocardial pressure was taken as zero. The overall resistance was assumed to be equal for both layers.

Results of the simulation are shown in figure 8. In the left-hand panel the assumed ventricular pressure curve is shown. For the sake of simplicity, the pressure was assumed to be a square wave. Systole and diastole were assumed to have the same duration, which holds true for a heart rate of around 120 beats/min. In the middle panel the simulated endocardial inflow is shown at the top and epicardial inflow at the bottom. As one may expect, arterial inflow is quite steady in the endocardial model. Inflow in the epicardial model is phasic and out of phase with arterial pressure. This is the result of systolic charging of intramyocardial compliant vessels in the epicardium. In diastole, the intramyocardial compliance discharges, resulting in this particular case in a negative diastolic flow. Note that, because of the equal overall resistances in both layers, mean flow through the layers is equal.

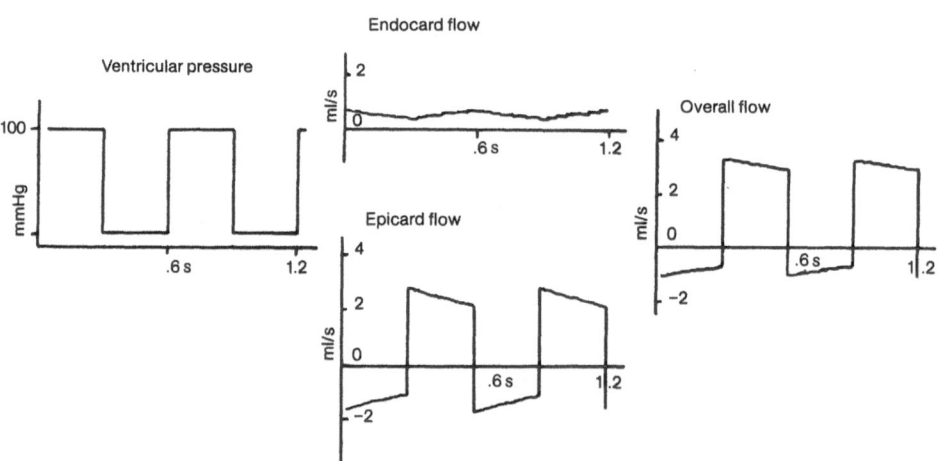

Figure 8. Simulation of coronary arterial flow pattern with complete aortic valve incompetence. Left panel is the assumed left ventricular pressure curve which equals the coronary pressure curve. The panels in the middle show simulated endocardial flow (top) and epicardial flow (bottom). Note that epicardial flow is out of phase with coronary pressure. The panel at the right shows simulated overall coronary flow.

The total coronary inflow is the sum of the inflow into both layers, as is shown in the right-hand panel. The total coronary inflow remains pulsatile but, because of the steady endocardial component, the ratio between peak flow and mean flow is smaller than in the case of epicardial inflow alone. The simulated total coronary inflow will be identical if one divided the myocardium into more layers and assumed intramyocardial pressure to vary linearly with distance through the myocardial wall.

Obviously, our model is too simple. Still, it may explain the reversal of coronary flow pattern with aortic insufficiency as a result of systolic charging of compliant intramyocardial vessels in those parts of the heart where arterial pressure exceeds extravascular pressure. As we shall discuss in the next section, extravascular pressure adds to coronary resistance. As a result, mean endocardial flow will be lower than mean epicardial flow, and the amplitude of the overall coronary flow pulse will appear to be larger with respect to mean flow. Moreover, the summation of endocardial flow and epicardial flow will show a lower overall diastolic flow due to the increased endocardial resistance.

One may summarize the arguments presented above as follows. Reversal of the coronary flow pattern in aortic insufficiency occurs if the diastolic-systolic coronary arterial pressure difference exceeds the magnitude of the overall intramyocardial pump pressure pulse. The intramyocardial pressure pulse is about half the systolic-diastolic ventricular pressure difference. This is in agreement with the coronary flow recordings presented by Menno and Schenk,[26] Downey and Kirk[27] and Folts and Rowe.[23]

CORONARY RESERVE IN HYPERTROPHIED HEARTS

Mechanism of flow impediment

Cardiac contraction impedes coronary flow. This has been convincingly demonstrated by the increase of net coronary flow after cardiac arrest at constant mean coronary arterial pressure.[1,2] The impediment is larger in the subendocardium than in the subepicardium. Microsphere studies on which this conclusion can be based, have recently been reviewed by Feigl.[15] The fully dilated coronary bed of the arrested heart has an endo/epi ratioof perfusion flows of 1.4-1.6, indicating a low resistance in the endocardium when extravascular compression is absent. The endo/epi ratio of perfusion flows decreases with increasing heart rate and becomes 0.4 in hearts paced at 250 beats/min.

The models commonly used to explain the influence of extravascular compression are the so-called extravascular resistance model and the waterfall model. In the first model, it is assumed that an extra resistance is added to the microcirculation during systole. The second model is based on the hydrodynamics of the collapsible tube. It is assumed that microvessels collapse locally and that the pressure needed to squeeze blood through the collapsed region equals the extravascular pressure. Since this pressure is high in systole, flow in the endocardium will occur only in diastole. However, neither model takes the compliance of the intramural vessels into account.

The resistance of a vessel is determined by its diameter. Because of the distensibility of vessels, their diameter and, therefore, the resistance will depend on the difference between extravascular pressure and intraluminal pressure. However, time is needed to decrease vessel diameter by extravascular compression because blood has to be squeezed out of the vessels. Because of the compliant nature of the vessels, this volume is restored in diastole. Thus, intramyocardial blood volume and resistance vary around a mean value during the cardiac cycle and mean coronary resistance will depend on mean extravascular pressure, while the magnitude of resistance variation will be determined by the rate at which blood within the vessels can be displaced.

All three models mentioned above predict a low arteriolar inflow into the endocardium during systole. The intramyocardial pump model even predicts endocardial arteriolar back flow during systole when perfusion pressure is constant, whereas diastolic arteriolar flow is expected to be increased. The crux that discriminates the intramyocardial pump model from the other two models is the interdependence of systolic and diastolic events.

This conclusion forces one to be careful in interpreting results obtained from experiments with separate systolic and diastolic interventions. For example, Hess and Bache[28] perfused the heart only during systole and found an endo/epi ratio of 0.36. When coronary flow was limited to a similar period during diastole, the transmural microsphere distribution was normal. However, when the artery was occluded in systole, the mean arterial pressure distal to the occluder must have been lower than when the flow was restricted during diastole. One has to attribute the difference in microsphere distribution at least in part to the difference in mean coronary arterial pressure.

Extravascular compression and coronary reserve in hypertrophied hearts
As has been discussed in this book by Hoffman, the relation between maximal coronary flow and coronary perfusion pressure does not change very much during the process of hypertrophy. Since oxygen consumption depends on ventricular mass, resting flow will increase with muscle growth. This reduces vasodilatory reserve in the hypertrophied heart. High extravascular pressure reduces vasodilatory reserve even further, especially in subendocardial regions.

As has been discussed above, it is not likely that increased ventricular wall thickness in itself will change the distribution of relative extravascular pressure across the wall. The magnitude of extravascular pressure in the endocardium does relate to ventricular pressure. The impediment to coronary flow produced by extravascular compression depends on the difference between the pressure inside and that outside the vessels. Consequently, if coronary pressure is increased simultaneously with left ventricular pressure, the increase in the extravascular contribution to coronary resistance will be neutralized at least partly. Obviously, this will not be the case in valvular aortic stenosis.

The interplay of the several factors determining coronary vasodilatory reserve is summarized schematically in figure 9. Pressure-flow relations for the maximally dilated coronary bed are shown in this figure. The relation is shifted to the right in the beating heart. The two horizontal lines represent the autoregulated flows of the endocardium before and after hypertrophy. The filled circles in the figure represent the condition before hypertrophy developed. The arrows show the changes one may expect as a result of three different kinds of hypertrophy. Hypertension hypertrophy is relatively harmless in this model, as relative coronary vasodilatory reserve remains unaltered. In both aortic insufficiency and valvular aortic stenosis, coronary vasodilatory reserve decreases due to increased flow. However, in aortic stenosis, coronary reserve decreases even more because of uncompensated extravascular compression. Note that an increased heart rate will decrease coronary reserve in all cases.

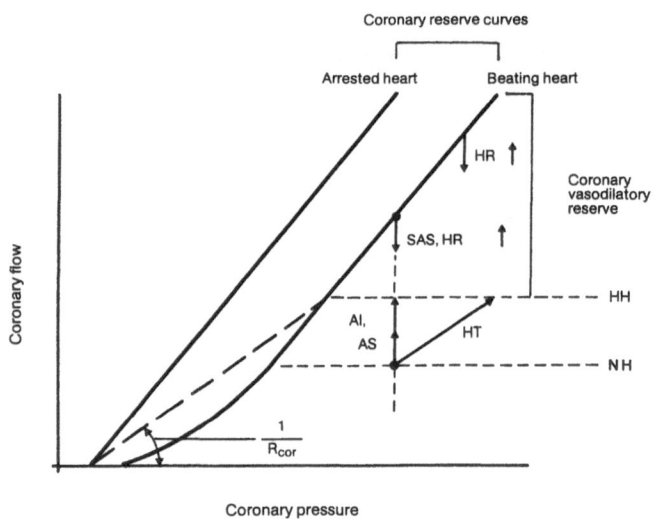

Figure 9. Schematic review of factors reducing coronary vasodilatory reserve within the endocardium. NH = normal heart, HH = hypertrophied heart, HR = heart rate, AI = aortic insufficiency, AS = aortic stenosis, HT = hypertension, hypertrophy. The horizontal broken lines indicate the increase of flow with hypertrophy. The conditions before hypertrophy are indicated by the filled circles. In the beating heart the coronary reserve is lower than in the arrested heart because extravascular compression increases coronary resistance. With aortic stenosis one may expect a further decrease of coronary reserve. Increasing HR reduces coronary reserve in all circumstances. Note that the coronary reserve curves may be explained by decreasing resistance at increasing coronary pressure.

CONCLUSIONS

In this chapter we analyzed the mechanics of the coronary flow based on compression of distensible intramyocardial blood vessels. Experiments with non-hypertrophied hearts showed the presence of intramyocardial compliance. The model used to analyze the consequences of intramyocardial compliance clearly illustrates the interwovenness of the determinants of systolic and diastolic flow, for both the endocardium and epicardium.

End-diastolic coronary resistance does not represent the resistance of the coronary bed free of systolic compression effects. This conclusion may be important, for example for pharmacologic studies. One may conclude that a drug dilates the coronary vessels while in fact the decrease in end coronary resistance is due to a change in coronary pressure pattern.

The interwovenness of systole and diastole may also have consequences for therapy. According to the intramyocardial pump model, an increase in diastolic coronary pressure results in an improvement of net coronary perfusion only if mean coronary pressure increases as well. At the moment, there is no evidence necessitating us to describe the mechanics of coronary flow in hypertrophied hearts as fundamentally different from those in normal hearts. However, only few studies are addressed to this specific question. It is not unlikely that other yet unknown determinants of coronary flow are of specific importance for the hypertrophied heart.

REFERENCES

1. Downey, J.M. and Kirk, E.S.: Inhibition of coronary blood flow by a vascular waterfall mechanism, Circ. Res., 36: 753-760, 1975
2. Sabiston, D.C. and Gregg, D.E.: Effect of cardiac contraction on coronary blood flow, Circ. Res., 15: 14-20, 1957
3. Porter, W.T.: The influence of the heart-beat on the flow through the walls of the heart, Am. J. Physiol., 1: 145-163, 1898
4. Spaan, J.A.E., Breuls, P.N. and Laird, J.D.: Diastolic-systolic coronary flow differences are caused by intramyocardial pump action in the anesthetized dog, Circ. Res., 49: 584-593, 1981a
5. Wiggers, C.J.: The interplay of coronary vascular resistance and myocardial compression in regulating coronary flow, Circ. Res., 2: 271-279, 1954
6. O'Keefe, D.D., Hoffman, J.I.E., Cheitlin, R., O'Neill, M.J., Allard, J.R. and Shapkin, E.: Coronary blood flow in experimental canine left ventricular hypertrophy, Circ. Res., 43: 43-51, 1978
7. Tillmans, H., Ikeda, S., Hansen, H., Sarma, J.S.M., Fauvel, J.M. and Bing, R.J.: Microcirculation in the ventricle of the dog and turtle, Circ. Res., 34: 561-569, 1974
8. Dole, W.P. and Bishop, V.S.: Regulation of coronary blood flow during individual diastoles in the dog, Circ. Res., 50: 377-385, 1982a
9. Dole, W.P. and Bishop, V.S.: Influence of autoregulation and capacitance on diastolic coronary artery pressure-flow relationships in the dog, Circ. Res., 51: 262-270, 1982b
10. Bellamy, R.F.: Diastolic coronary artery pressure-flow relations in the dog, Circ. Res., 43: 92-101, 1978
11. Klocke, F.J., Weinstein, I.R., Klocke, J.F., Ellis, A.K., Kraus, D.R., Mates, R.E., Canty, J.M., Anbar, R.D., Romanowski, R.R., Wallmeyer, K.W. and Echt, M.P.: Zero flow pressures and pressure-flow relationships during single long diastoles in the canine coronary bed before and during maximal vasodilation, J. Clin. Invest., 68: 970-980, 1981
12. Gregg, D.E. and Green, H.D.: Registration and interpretation of normal phasic inflow into a left coronary artery by an improved differential manometric method, Am. J. Physiol., 130: 114-125, 1940
13. Arts, T.: A mathematical model of the dynamics of the left ventricle and the coronary circulation, Ph.D. Thesis, State University of Limburg, Maastricht, the Netherlands, 1978
14. Arts, T., Veenstra, P.C. and Reneman, R.S.: Epicardial deformation and left ventricular wall mechanics during ejection in the dog, Am. J. Physiol., 243: H379-390, 1982
15. Feigl, E.O.: Coronary physiology, Physiol. Reviews, 63: 1-205, 1983
16. Borg, T.K. and Caulfield, J.B.: The collagen matrix of the heart, Federation Proc., 40: 2037-2041, 1981
17. Caulfield, J.B. and Borg, T.K.: The collagen network of the heart, Laboratory Investigation, 40: 364-372, 1979

18. Malik, A.B., Abe, T., O'Kane, H. and Geha, A.S.: Cardiac function, coronary flow, and oxygen consumption in stable left ventricular hypertrophy, Am. J. Physiol., 225: 186-191, 1973
19. Rembert, J.C., Kleinman, L.H., Fedor, J.M., Wechsler, A.S. and Greenfield Jr., J.C.: Myocardial blood flow distribution in concentric left ventricular hypertrophy, J. Clin. Invest., 62: 379-386, 1978
20. Laird, J.D., Breuls, P.N., Meer, P. van der, and Spaan, J.A.E.: Can a single vasodilator be responsible for both coronary autoregulation and metabolic vasodilation?, Basic Res. Cardiol., 76: 354-358, 1981
21. Spaan, J.A.E., Breuls, P.N. and Laird, J.D.: Forward coronary flow normally seen in systole is the result of both a forward and a concealed back flow, Basic Res. Cardiol., 76: 582-586, 1981b
22. Pyle, R.L., Lowensohn, H.S., Khouri, E.M., Gregg, D.E. and Patterson, D.F.: Left circumflex coronary artery hemodynamics in conscious dogs with congenital subaortic stenosis, Circ. Res., 33: 34-38, 1973
23. Folts, J.D. and Rowe, G.G.: Coronary and hemodynamic effects of temporary acute aortic insufficiency in intact anesthetized dogs, Circ. Res., 35: 238-246, 1974.
24. Green, H.D.: The coronary blood flow in aortic stenosis, in aortic insufficiency and in arterio-venous fistula, Am. J. Physiol., 115: 94-103, 1936
25. Karp, R.B. and Roe, B.B.: Effect of aortic insufficiency on phasic flow patterns in the coronary artery, Annals of Surgery, 164: 959-966, 1966
26. Menno, A.D., and Schenk, W.G.: Dynamics of coronary arterial flow: flow alterations resulting from certain surgical procedures and drugs of surgical importance, Surgery, 50: 82-90. 1961
27. Downey, J.M. and Kirk, E.S.: Distribution of the coronary blood flow across the canine heart wall during systole, Circ. Res., 34: 251-257, 1974
28. Hess, D.S. and Bache, R.J.: Transmural distribution of myocardial blood flow during systole in the awake dog, Circ. Res., 38: 5-15, 1976

SECTION 5

DIAGNOSTIC DEVELOPMENT IN DETECTION OF LEFT VENTRICULAR HYPERTROPHY

SUMMARY

The assumptions underlying the classical approach to the electrocardiographic diagnosis of LVH is that the hypertrophied ventricle generates increased electrical forces. Various sets of criteria based on voltage measurements have thus been proposed. A review of the literature indicates however that the classical Sokolow and Lyon criteria, the more elaborate Romhilt-Estes point score system and, even, various discriminant functions based on VCG measurements, all remain rather disappointing and often reveal a poor sensitivity with an acceptable specificity. Interestingly, for equivalent LV mass, the voltage criteria seem to be more sensitive in the presence of aortic regurgitation than stenosis. Application of the solid-angle theory of electrocardiography provides an explanation for these inconsistencies. It shows that a critical geometric relationship resulting from the interplay of wall thickness and chamber dilation is needed for LVH to appear on the surface electrocardiogram. The characteristics of intraventricular conduction may also be of paramount importance and electrocardiographic patterns of LVH may, for example, be transient and accompany paroxysmal intraventricular conduction disorders.

In the presence of cardiovascular disease (arterial hypertension or coronary artery disease), as well as in apparently healthy individuals, electrical LVH should always be considered a sign of guarded prognosis.

ELECTROCARDIOGRAPHIC ASPECTS OF LEFT VENTRICULAR HYPERTROPHY

KULBERTUS H.E.

Associate Professor of Medicine, Chief, Section of Cardiology,
University Hospital, University of Liege School of Medicine,
Liege, Belgium.

CORRELATION BETWEEN LEFT VENTRICULAR MASS AND SURFACE ELECTROCARDIO-
GRAM VOLTAGES

The classical approach to the electrocardiographic diagnosis of left
ventricular hypertrophy (LVH) has often been based on a simplistic
concept according to which "the bigger the muscle walls, the larger the
voltages recorded at the thoracic surface".

Recently, echocardiographic measurements of left ventricular wall thickness and internal dimensions as well as derived estimates of left ventricular mass (LV mass) were shown to correspond closely with measurements obtained by left ventriculography or post-mortem examination.[1,2,3]
Correlations between echocardiographic LV mass and electrocardiogram were
thus made possible; they have yielded interesting, albeit surprising,
results.

The conclusion derived from these studies is that the correlation between
LV mass and electrocardiographic voltage measurements is altogether
deceiving. This is illustrated by the results obtained by Reichek and
Devereux[4] in a non-selected clinical series of 100 consecutive subjects
in whom echocardiograms and electrocardiograms were performed (table).
The findings of Dunn et al.[5] and Ditchie et al.[6] are similar and gave
correlation values of the same order of magnitude.

The nature of the underlying disease also influences the correlation.
For example, in the patients with aortic stenosis studied by Ditchie et
al.[6], the precordial voltage S_{V1} or $V2$ + R_{V5} or $V6$ demonstrated a weak
correlation with LV mass (r = 0.58, p < 0.05); the R-wave amplitude in
aVL showed the highest correlation value (r = 0.77; p < 0.001). In
contrast, no correlation between LV mass and electrocardiographic
parameters were seen in normal subjects or patients with mitral or aortic
regurgitation.

Table 1. Quantitative relationship of ECG voltage to left ventricular mass

Authors	Correlation	r
Reichek, N. and Devereux, R.B.[4]	S_{V1} vs LVM	0.60
	R_{aVL} vs LVM	0.63
	Sokolow-Lyon voltage vs LVM	0.45
(Echo)	R_{V5} vs LVM	0.11
	R_{V6} vs LVM	0.18
Dunn, R.A. et al.[5] (ventriculography)	$S_{V1} + R_{V5 \text{ or } V6}$ vs LVM	0.61
Ditchey, R.V. et al.	$S_{V1 \text{ or } V2} + R_{V5 \text{ or } V6}$ vs LVM	0.59
(Echo)	R_{aVL} vs LVM	0.64

LVM = left ventricular mass

These differences may be due to geometric factors which will be discussed in the following paragraph.

DETERMINANTS OF THE ELECTROCARDIOGRAPHIC PATTERN OF LVH

The relatively weak correlations which exist between the electrocardiographic signs of LVH and the angiographical or echocardiographical measurements of left ventricular mass lead to the postulation that the latter is probably not the only determinant of electrocardiographic LVH and that additional geometric factors must be involved.

In a very interesting study, Antman, Green and Grossman[7] have demonstrated that it is the relative interplay between wall thickness and chamber dilatation which determines whether LVH will be recorded on the surface electrocardiogram. They studied a group of 93 patients who had undergone left ventriculography. Among other things, they measured the left ventricular wall thickness (h) and the semi-minor radius of the left ventricle (R). By plotting left ventricular wall thickness on the vertical axis against semi-minor radius on the horizontal axis, they observed that the hyperbolic function described by h.R = 2.6 best discriminates the patients with electrocardiographic evidence of left ventricular hypertrophy (h.R values greater than 2.6) from those without LVH (h.R values lower than 2.6). Patients with h.R close to 2.6 had borderline voltages (fig. 1).

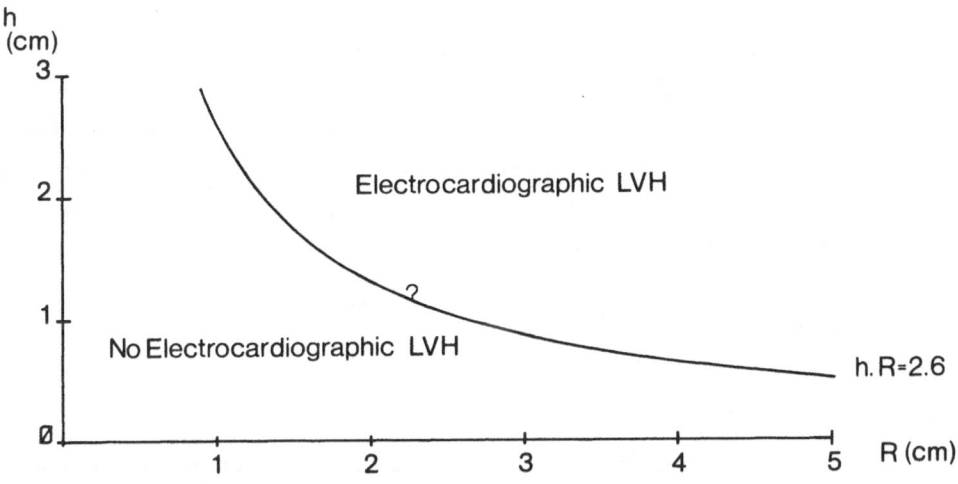

Figure 1. LV wall thickness (h) plotted against semi-radius of the left ventricle (R). The hyperbolic function h x R = 2.6 best separates patients with electrocardiographic LVH from those without LVH. (Redrawn from Antman et al.[7])

This explains why some individuals with markedly dilated ventricles and only slightly thickened left ventricular wall (cardiomyopathy) may have electrocardiographic LVH whereas, in haemodynamic situations of pressure overload where the volume chamber remains rather small, marked thickening of the left ventricular free wall is required for the electrocardiographic evidence of LVH to appear. The latter thus almost always results from a combination of thickened free wall and dilated chamber. This observation is not yet fully understood.

Some authors have pointed to the fact that a dilated ventricle carries the heart closer to the electrodes and, thereby, increases QRS voltages by a proximity effect.[8] Brody[9] has also suggested that a dilated chamber, because of the increase of intracavity blood, augments radially directed dipoles. Antman et al.[7] add another hypothesis: they believe that their findings can be explained by the solid angle theory of electrocardiography. Bayley[10] has shown that the electrical potential at a given point P in a conducting medium surrounding a closed surface double-layer dipole source is directly related to the dipole moment of each element of the surface and to the solid angle, Ω, subtended by the boundaries of the surface at a point P. The solid angle is defined as the area of spherical surface cut off a unit sphere inscribed about P. For a region in the heart with different transmembrane voltages, Vm_1 and Vm_2, the electrical potential ($\mathcal{E}$) recorded at a point P of the body surface is given by the following equation:

$$\mathcal{E} = \frac{K \cdot \Delta Vm \cdot \Omega}{4\pi}$$

where

Ω = the solid angle subtended by the surface described by the limits of the region to be analysed (fig. 2);

$\Delta Vm = Vm_2 - Vm_1;$

and K = a constant related to the differences in conductivity and inhomogeneities within cardiac muscle.

This theory might explain the varying behaviour of QRS voltages in different conditions involving increased left ventricular mass.[11] For example, in volume overload, total LV mass is increased largely through chamber dilatation: the solid angle subtended at the recording site is

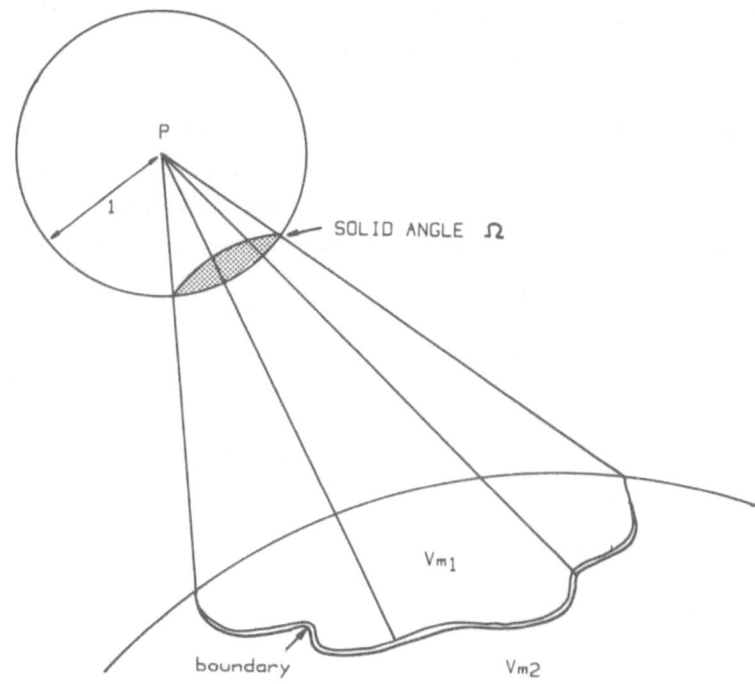

Figure 2. Description of the solid angle theory (redrawn from Antman et al.[7]). At point P, the electrical potential (ξ) is defined by

$$\xi = \frac{K \cdot \Delta Vm \times \Omega}{4\pi}$$

thus markedly increased and electrocardiographic LVH develops easily. In contrast, in pressure overload, LV mass increases through wall thickening; the solid angle subtended is not markedly enlarged unless chamber dilatation simultaneously occurs. Electrocardiographic LVH is therefore less frequent in this condition.[11] An illustration of this concept is found in the clinical observation that for a similar degree of increase of LV mass, the voltage criteria for LVH are more frequently fulfilled in aortic regurgitation (which induces LV enlargement) than in aortic stenosis (which does not).[4]

The views held by Antman et al. are in good agreement with those of Rudy et al.[12] who, using a mathematical model, hypothetized that chamber dilatation plays a greater role than wall thickening in augmenting surface potentials.

202

Intraventricular conduction undoubtedly also plays a role, at least in some cases of electrocardiographic LVH. As early as 1952, Segers et al.[13] described what they called the "acute development of the electrocardiographic pattern of left ventricular preponderance". It is only since Rosenbaum et al.[14] introduced the concept of the left hemiblocks that this phenomenon could be related to the transient appearance of a conduction disorder. An example of this phenomenon is illustrated in figure 3.

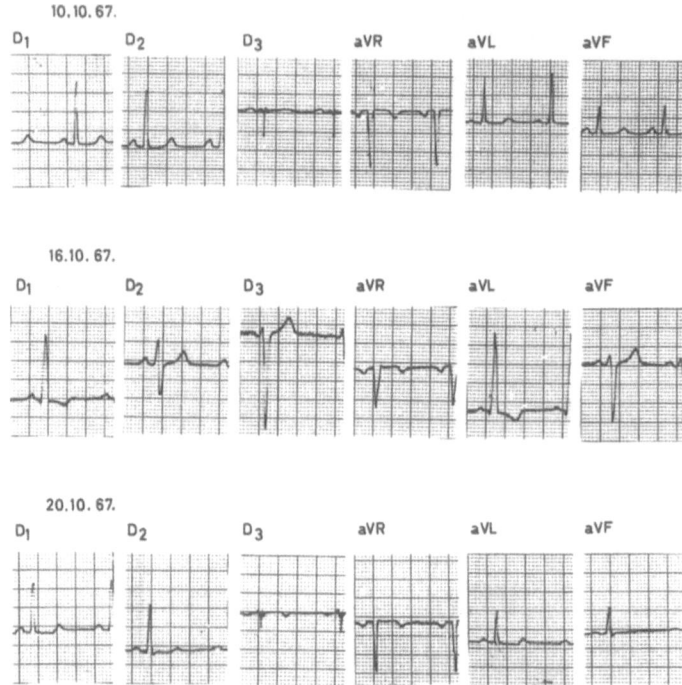

Figure 3. Serial electrocardiographic tracings of a 63-year-old subject with aortic stenosis and intermittent LAHB. Note in B the "acute development of the electrocardiographic pattern of left ventricular preponderance" appearing concomitantly with left anterior hemiblock.

These are the tracings of a 63-year-old man with senile aortic valve disease and transient left anterior hemiblock. Every time he presented with transient left anterior hemiblock, he showed increased voltage of R_I, S_{III} and R_{aVL} and inversion of the T wave in leads I and aVL, thus realizing the pattern of LVH with strain. The precise role played by minor intraventricular conduction alterations in the development of the electrocardiographic pattern of LVH remains to be further investigated.

PERFORMANCE OF SURFACE ELECTROCARDIOGRAM IN THE DIAGNOSIS OF LVH

The principles discussed in the preceding paragraph readily explain why the electrocardiographic diagnosis of LVH remains a very difficult task.

The most widely used criteria for LVH recognition are those of Sokolow and Lyon (S_{V1} + R_{V5} or R_{V6} > 3.5 mV). According to various investigations[4,5, 14-21], they show a sensitivity of 20 to 52% and a specificity of 84 to 100%.

The more elaborate point scoring system proposed by Romhilt and Estes[15] which takes into account parameters other than QRS voltages, is also somewhat disappointing. In their training group, i.e. the group used to develop the diagnostic criteria, Romhilt and Estes[15] observed a sensitivity of 62.2% and a specificity of 96.7%. However, a more recent study by Geva et al. (1979)[17] evaluated the Romhilt and Estes scoring system in a control group. This study was performed in chronic hypertensive subjects with echocardiographically recognized LVH. In this group, the sensitivity of the Romhilt and Estes scoring system was 42% and its specificity was 100%.

Another scoring technique described by MacFarlane et al.[20] utilizes various parameters (not all based on voltage) from the three orthogonal lead systems. It provides some limited improvement (sensitivity 65%; specificity 91%). More complex (multiple dipole electrocardiograms) and analytic (likelihood ratio) methods may offer an increased, although imperfect, accuracy in left ventricular mass prediction and in separation of individual patients into normal and abnormal categories.[5] The practical applicability of these techniques is, however, clearly limited.

At the present time, one must admit that the surface electrocardiogram remains a rather unsatisfactory tool for the recognition of left ventricular hypertrophy. In general, the existing voltage criteria are specific rather than sensitive. One should none the less realize that, when the prevalence of true left ventricular hypertrophy is less than 10%, the electrocardiogram yields more false positive than true positive results.[4] It is also interesting to note that non-voltage markers of LVH give diagnostic accuracy comparable to voltage criteria. They include ST-T changes, left atrial abnormality, QRS prolongation and intrinsic delay.[4] They might help the clinician in some individual cases. However, M-mode echocardiographic left ventricular mass determination is clearly superior to the electrocardiogram for the clinical diagnosis of LVH.

PROGNOSTIC SIGNIFICANCE OF ELECTROCARDIOGRAPHIC PATTERN OF LVH

The electrocardiographic pattern of LVH observed in apparently healthy individuals or in subjects with heart disease always carries useful prognostic information.

The Manitoba study[22] investigated a cohort of 3,983 apparently healthy men with a mean age of 30.8 years at entry who were regularly followed up for 30 years. During the observational period, 70 cases of sudden death were noted. 12.9% of these subjects who died suddenly had voltage criteria for left ventricular hypertrophy. The relative risk of sudden death (i.e. sudden death incidence in those with the electrocardiographic abnormality divided by the incidence in those without the abnormality) was 3.06. The risk clearly increased when the voltage criteria for LVH were found in association with ST segment or T wave abnormalities.

Hamby et al.[23] investigated the significance of LVH in the presence of ischaemic heart disease. Their study group with LVH consisted of 57 patients who were matched with age and sex controls. All patients were evaluated because of angina pectoris and none had a history or electrocardiographic evidence of prior myocardial infarction. The duration of symptoms was similar in both groups. Hypertension (75% vs 30%), congestive heart failure (25% vs 0%) and chest X-ray cardiomegaly (49% vs 4%) were more frequent among patients with LVH. The latter also demonstrated greater left ventricular dysfunction evidenced by a higher LVEDP (20 ± 8 vs 12 ± 9 mm Hg), a larger LVEDV (80 ± 28 vs 66 ± 22 ml/m^2) and a lower ejection fraction (0.55 ± 20 vs 0.64 ± 0.17). No significant group differences were seen in terms of severity of coronary artery disease. However, main left coronary artery stenosis was significantly more frequent in subjects with LVH and no hypertension (29% vs 7%, p < 0.05). Studies in the rat[24] have indicated that ligation of the LAD artery can result in hypertrophy of the left ventricle. It is possible that reparative processes following hypoxic necrosis may result in compensatory hypertrophy in the remaining myocardium. This, added to some chamber dilatation due to ischaemic dysfunction, will produce electrical LVH. Finally, the poor outcome of patients with arterial hypertension complicated by electrocardiographic evidence of LVH has been well documented in the Framingham study.[25]

CONCLUSION

This short review indicates that the various factors required to allow the development of the electrocardiographic pattern of LVH are very complex and that the electrocardiogram will therefore probably always remain a bad tool to make this diagnosis. Undoubtedly, echocardiography is much more reliable.

The electrocardiographic pattern of LVH results from the interplay of an increase in left ventricular mass and a dilatation of the ventricular cavity. Theoretically, electrocardiographic LVH may be absent in patients with obvious thickening of the left ventricular wall, and may, on the other hand, be present when the heart is grossly enlarged even if the ventricular wall remains relatively thin. In spite of these limitations, electrocardiographic LVH remains a very useful clinical sign: it carries a guarded prognosis both in patients with overt cardiac disease and in apparently healthy individuals.

REFERENCES

1. Feigenbaum, H., Popp, R.L., Chip, J.N. and Haine, C.L.: Left ventricular wall thickness measured by ultrasound, Arch. Intern. Med., 121, 391, 1968.
2. Murray, J.A., Hohn, W.E. and Reid, J.M.: Echocardiographic determination of left ventricular dimensions, volumes and performance. Am. J. Cardiol., 30, 252, 1972.
3. Troy, B.L., Pombo, J. and Rackley, C.E.: Measurements of left ventricular wall thickness and mass by echocardiography. Circulation, 45, 602, 1972.
4. Reichek, N. and Devereux, R.B.: Left ventricular hypertrophy: relationship of anatomic, echocardiographic and electrocardiographic finding, Circulation, 63, 1391, 1981.

5. Dunn, R.A., Pipberger, H.V., Holt, J.H. Jr., Barnard, A.C.L. and Pipberger, H.A.: Performance of conventional, orthogonal and multiple dipole electrocardiogram in estimating left ventricular muscle mass, Circulation, 60, 350, 1979.

6. Ditchey, R.V., Schuler, G. and Peterson, K.L.: Reliability of echo-cardiographic and electrocardiographic parameters in assessing serial changes in left ventricular mass, The Amer. J. of Medicine, 70, 1042, 1981.

7. Antman, F.M., Green, L.H. and Grossman, W.: Physiologic determinants of the electrocardiographic determinants of left ventricular hyper-trophy, Circulation, 60, 386, 1979.

8. Witham, A.C.: A system of vectorcardiographic interpretation, Year Book, Chicago, Medical Publishers, 116, 1976.

9. Brody, D.A.: Theoretical analysis of intracavitary blood mass in-fluence on the heart-lead relationship, Circulation Research, 4, 731, 1956.

10. Bayley, R.H.: Biophysical principles of electrocardiography, New York, Hoeber, 19, 1958.

11. Holland, R.P. and Arnsdorf, M.F.: Solid angle theory and the electro-cardiogram: physiologic and quantitative interpretations, Prog. Cardiov. Diseases, 19, 431, 1977.

12. Rudy, Y., Plonsey, R. and Liebman, J.: The effects of inhomogeneities and geometry of the electrocardiogram, Circulation, 56, suppl. III, III-17, 1977.

13. Segers, M., Regnier, M. and Delatte, E.: L'installation brusque de l'image électrocardiographique de prépondérance, Acta Cardiol., 7, 63, 1952.

14. Sokolow, M. and Lyon, T.P.: The ventricular complex in left ventric-ular hypertrophy as obtained by unipolar precordial and limb leads, Amer. Heart J., 38, 273, 1949.

15. Romhilt, D.W. and Estes, E.H. Jr.: A point score system for the ECG diagnosis of left ventricular hypertrophy, Amer. Heart J., 75, 752, 1968.

16. Romhilt, D.W., Bove, K.E., Norris, R.J., Conyers, E., Conradi, S. and Rowlands. D.T.: A critical appraisal of the electrocardiographic criteria for the diagnosis of left ventricular hypertrophy, Circula-tion, 40, 185, 1969.

17. Geva, B., Elkayam, U., Frishman, W., Terdiman, R. and Laniado, S.: Determination of left ventricular wall thickening in patients with chronic systemic hypertension, Chest, 76, 557, 1979.

18. Holt, J.H. Jr., Barnard, A.C.L. and Kramer, J.O. Jr.: Quantitative electrocardiography using a multiple dipole method. In: Abel, H., Ed., Advances in Cardiology, Basel, vol. 16, 117, 1976.

19. Liu, C.K. and De Cristofaro, D.: Sensitivity and specificity of electrocardiographic evaluation of LVH in 364 unselected autopsy cases, Am. Heart J., 76, 596, 1968.

20. Allenstein, B.J. and Mori, H.: Evaluation of electrocardiographic diagnosis of ventricular hypertrophy based on autopsy comparison, Circulation, 21, 401, 1960.

21. MacFarlane, P.W., Chen, C.Y., Boyce, B. and Fraser, R.S.: Scoring technique for diagnosis of ventricular hypertrophy from three orthog-onal lead electrocardiograms, Br. Heart J., 45, 402, 1981.

22. Rabkin, S.W., Mathewson, F.A.L. and Tate, R.B.: The electrocardio-gram in apparently healthy men and the risk of sudden death, Br. Heart J., 47, 546, 1982.

23. Hamby, R.I., Prakash, M.N., Wyne, U.A. and Hoffman, I.: Electrocar-
    diographic left ventricular hypertrophy and coronary artery disease:
    clinical haemodynamic and angiographic correlates, Am. Heart J., 100,
    794, 1980.
24. Norman, T.D. and Coers, C.R.: Cardiac hypertrophy after coronary
    ligation in rats, Arch. Pathol., 69, 181, 1960.
25. Kannel, W.B., Gordon, T. and Offut, D.: Left ventricular hypertrophy
    by electrocardiogram, Ann. Int. Medicine, 71, 89, 1969.

SUMMARY

Radionuclide studies of cardiovascular performance require only minute amounts of intravenously injected radioactive tracers, which do not perturb cardiovascular dynamics. Both equilibrium gated cardiac blood pool scanning and first pass radionuclide angiography (RNA) provide indices of global and regional left and right ventricular performance. Based upon the fact that at equilibrium ventricular counts are proportional to volume ejection fraction (LVEF), end-systolic volume (ESV), end-diastolic volume (EDV), mean ejection rate, peak left ventricular filling rate (PFR) and time to peak filling rate (TPFR) can be measured. These indices can be obtained both at rest and during exercise. Assessment of systolic and diastolic function by either scanning technique provides useful information in the evaluation of patients with left ventricular hypertrophy due to hypertension, valvular heart disease or cardiomyopathy, e.g. in determining whether abnormal systolic function or abnormal compliance is the predominant cause of heart failure. This will immensely aid in decisions regarding pharmacological and surgical therapy. Exercise RNA in patients with chronic aortic regurgitation (AI) may unmask ventricular dysfunction. Symptomatic patients with AI all have an abnormally low LVEF (< 0.55) during supine exercise. Sixteen of 22 asymptomatic patients with AI, however, had an abnormal EF during exercise only (Borer). Behavior of EDV and ESV at rest and during exercise appears to provide additional information about LV functional reserve in symptomatic patients with AI. In patients with hypertrophic cardiomyopathy, RNA demonstrates normal or supranormal systolic LV function, but 70% of the patients have a depressed PFR (< 2.5 EDV/s) or TPFR of > 180 ms. With verapamil diastolic dysfunction is seen in only 30% of the patients with this disorder. Tl-201 imaging is of additional use in assessment of hypertrophy. An increase in RV mass is observed in patients with pulmonary hypertension, whereas septal to free wall thickening is observed in patients with IHSS. Although one cannot measure wall thickness or cardiac mass directly and accurately, RNA allows detection of functional disturbances with a high degree of sensitivity. The recent development of nuclear magnetic resonance (NMR) techniques offers a powerful completely non-invasive method to study functional and structural properties of the heart. It is likely that NMR will become the most sensitive approach to quantitate LVH and RVH in the future.

RADIOISOTOPE STUDIES IN PATIENTS WITH LEFT VENTRICULAR HYPERTROPHY

BELLER, G.A.

Head, Division of Cardiology, Professor of Medicine, University of Virginia Medical Center, Charlottesville, VA 22908, U.S.A.

INTRODUCTION

Radionuclide studies of cardiovascular performance provide important physiologic insights into both right and left ventricular function in humans in a non-invasive manner. These techniques merely require the intravenous injection of small amounts of radioactive tracers such as technetium-99 m and thallium-201, which do not perturb hemodynamics or other aspects of cardiac function. Both equilibrium gated cardiac blood pool scanning and first-pass radionuclide angiography provide indices of global and regional left and right ventricular performance at rest and during exercise stress. Determination of relative left ventricular (LV) and right ventricular (RV) volumes can be made since the blood radio-activity in the ventricular chambers is proportional to blood volume. One can derive a volume curve (figure 1) by quantitating the radioactive emissions, after background correction, during the cardiac cycle. When this procedure is employed with the aid of a computer, a series of cardiac blood pool images are constructed during systole and diastole which can be displayed in rapid sequence, that is, in an endless-loop flicker-free movie format. This "radionuclide cineangiogram" provides qualitative information regarding spatial and temporal variation of the cardiac chambers. The ejection fraction of either the left or the right ventricle is measured by subtracting end-systolic counts within the chamber from end-diastolic counts and dividing by end-diastolic counts (figure 2).

In addition to measuring left ventricular ejection fraction (LVEF), end-systolic volume (ESV), end-diastolic volume (EDV), mean ejection rate, peak left ventricular filling rate and time-to-peak filling rate can be calculated. These measurements can be made utilizing either the first-pass or equilibrium gated approach to radionuclide angiography. LV volumes can be measured using a modification of the single plane area method.[1] Johnson et al.[1] found an excellent correlation between the

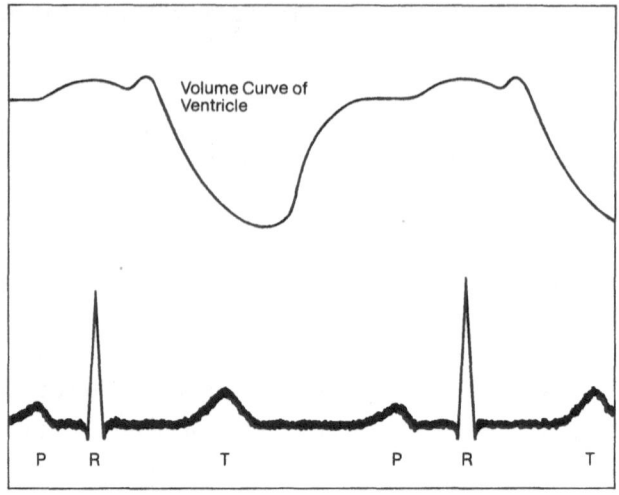

Relation of volume to EKG events. From Strauss, Zaret, et al.

Figure 1. Volume curve of the left ventricle showing the relation of changes in cardiac volume with the electrocardiogram. A similar volume curve can be computer-derived from a radionuclide angiogram by calculating LV cavity radioactivity over the time during the cardiac cycle and summing data from 100-200 beats in the equilibrium gated method.

LVEDV measured by contrast angiography at catheterization and the LVEDV measured by first-pass radionuclide angiography with an r-value of 0.89 and a standard error of the estimate of 14.5 ml. When the LVESV was plotted in a similar manner, an excellent correlation with an r-value of 0.93 was found between catheterization and radionuclide techniques. The left ventricular EDV and ESV can also be measured by radionuclide angiography employing non-geometric methods in which radioactive counts in the LV chamber are converted to milliliters after attenuation correction.

Both the LV and RV ejection fraction can be assessed during supine or upright bicycle exercise. In normal individuals, the LVEF should increase by at least 5% as long as the resting LVEF is below 75% (figure 3). Some patients with a very high resting LVEF will not show a significant increase with exercise. A decrease in LVEF or RVEF during exercise suggests the presence of underlying myocardial dysfunction with a diminution in cardiac reserve. Patients with coronary artery disease or valvular heart disease may demonstrate normal ventricular function at rest reflected by a normal LVEF or RVEF, but exhibit an abnormal response

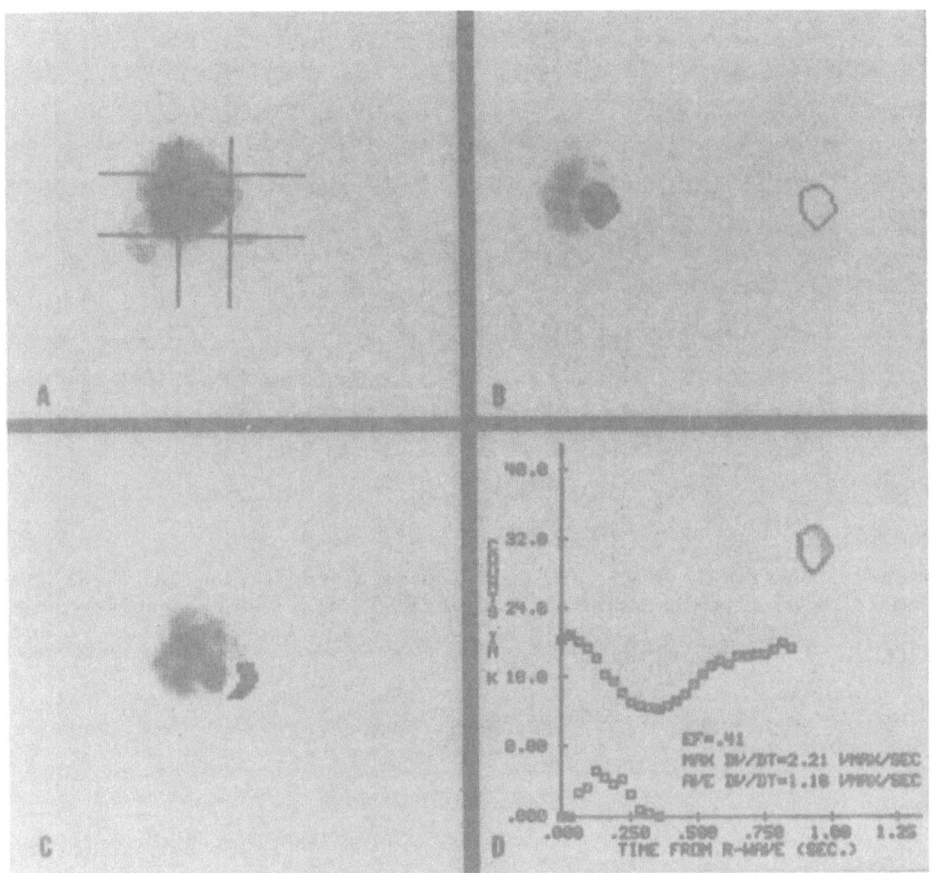

Figure 2. <u>Upper left panel</u>: A box is placed around the left ventricular cavity. <u>Upper right panel</u>: The outline of the left ventricular cavity is shown. <u>Lower left panel</u>: The region from which the background activity is measured is shown as a crescent-shaped region adjacent to the LV free wall. <u>Lower right panel</u>: LV time-activity curve from which the left ventricular ejection fraction is calculated by first subtracting end-systolic from end-diastolic counts and dividing by end-diastolic counts. In this example the LVEF is 41%.

to exercise stress. In patients with coronary artery disease a wall motion abnormality may appear during exercise if ischemia was induced.

Finally, indices of LV diastolic filling can be computed from the high-temporal resolution time-activity curve generated from the LV during gated equilibrium blood pool scintigraphy[2] (figure 4). The diastolic

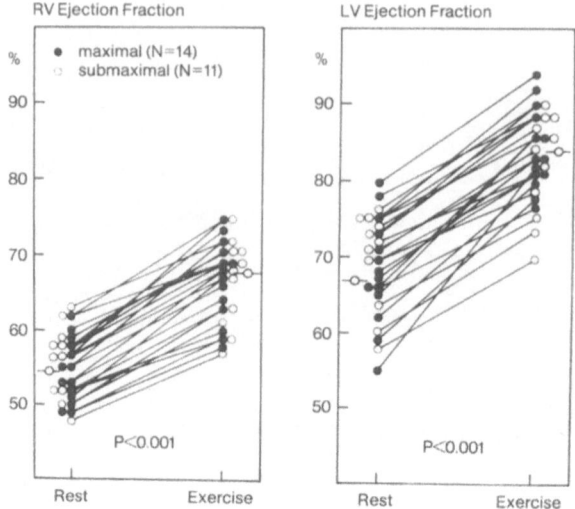

Figure 3. Changes in right and left ventricular ejection fractions from rest to submaximal exercise (open circles) or maximal exercise (solid circles). The normal response is for the ejection fraction of both ventricles to increase during exercise.

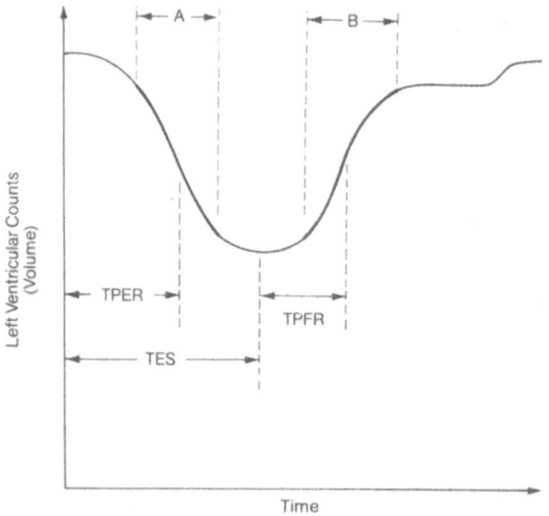

Figure 4. LV volume curve over time generated from the LV time activity curve showing the various timing intervals that can be measured to assess ventricular performance during systole and diastolic filling character- istics. The ejection rate and filling rate can be measured from A and B portions of the curve, respectively. TPER = time to peak ejection rate; TES = time to end-systole; TPFR = time to peak filling rate (from: Bonow et al.).

portion of the time-activity curve is constructed by combined forward-gating and reverse-gating from the R wave of the electrocardiogram. Peak rate of LV filling during the rapid filling phase of diastole is computed by fitting a third-order polynomial function to the rapid filling portion of the time-activity curve, using a least-squares technique. Peak filling rate is computed in counts per second, normalized for the number of counts at end-diastole, and expressed as end-diastolic volume per second (EDV/s). The time to peak filling rate is measured from end-systole to the time of peak left ventricular filling (figure 4). Relative LV diastolic filling volume during rapid diastolic filling and relative filling volume during atrial systole can also be computed.[3]

HEART FAILURE

Heart failure in patients with left ventricular hypertrophy can be related to abnormal LV systolic function with an increase in LVEDV, an increase in LVESV and reduction in LVEF or to abnormal diastolic compliance associated with an increase in LV end-diastolic pressure but normal or even small end-diastolic and end-systolic volumes. For example, a patient with chronic hypertension with LVH on the electrocardiogram and coronary artery disease may develop congestive heart failure on either basis. The radionuclide angiogram will be useful in determining whether abnormal systolic function or abnormal diastolic filling is the predominant pathophysiologic mechanism for the genesis of heart failure. Assessing ventricular performance non-invasively by radionuclide angiography can aid in decision making in such patients with heart failure. If a patient has abnormal LV compliance but has a normal LVEDV and small LVESV with an LVEF of > 60% a cardiac glycoside or other inotropic agents may not be very useful. In contrast, if the patient has an enlarged EDV and an increased ESV with an LVEF of 30%, an inotropic agent like digitalis may be helpful.

VALVULAR HEART DISEASE

The radionuclide angiogram is not routinely indicated in patients with valvular aortic stenosis since the degree of ventricular contraction does not reflect severity of the disease. In most instances, the LVEF returns to normal after valve replacement when the afterload stress is relieved. In certain critically ill patients with aortic stenosis, the radionuclide angiogram can substitute for the contrast ventriculogram thereby avoiding a dye load to the patient which might precipitate pulmonary edema. Excessive LVH is manifest as enhanced LV contraction on the radionuclide study except when the end-stage of the disease is reached, at which time a reduced LVEF can be observed with increases in the EDV and ESV. In those patients, the risk of surgery is higher and significant recovery of LV function not as great post-operatively. The radionuclide angiogram can be utilized to evaluate post-operative problems in patients with aortic stenosis, thus avoiding the need for repeat catheterization.

Cardiac blood pool imaging may be very useful in distinguishing hypertrophic cardiomyopathy from congestive and ischemic cardiomyopathy. As shown in figure 5, the gated blood pool scan in idiopathic hypertrophic

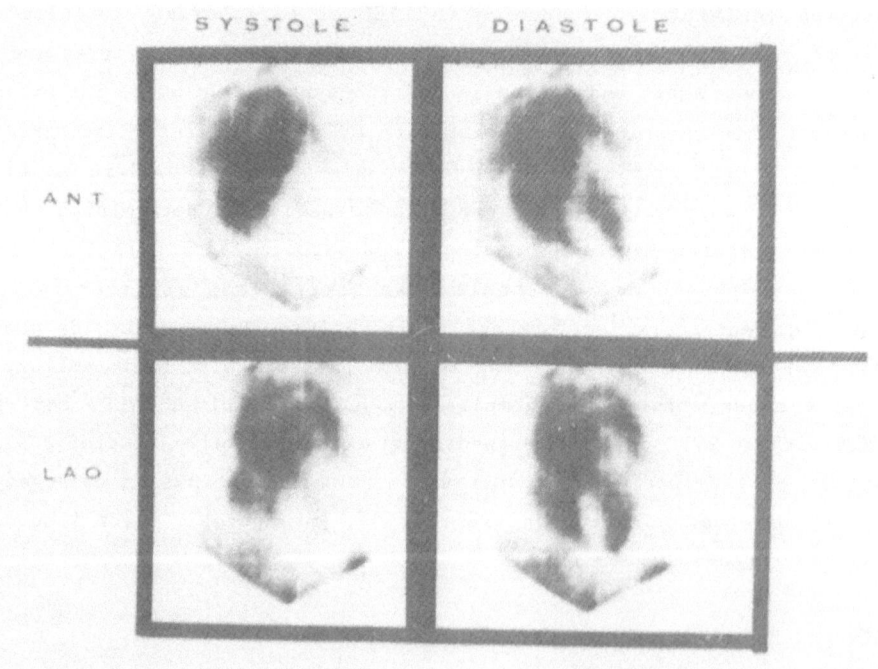

Figure 5. End-systolic and end-diastolic images of the left and right ventricular blood pools in the anterior (ANT) projection (upper panels) and the left anterior oblique (LAO) projection (lower panels) in a patient with hypertrophic cardiomyopathy. Note the thickened septum and the near LV cavity obliteration during systole.

subaortic stenosis demonstrates a small LVEDV, LV cavity obliteration during systole and a supranormal LVEF. Increased septal thickness can also be appreciated. Patients with congestive cardiomyopathy will demonstrate global hypokinesis on the gated scan with enlarged ventricular volumes and a reduced LVEF.

Radionuclide angiography at rest or with exercise might be useful in determining the severity of underlying LV dysfunction in patients with aortic insufficiency.[1,4-6] It has become increasingly evident in recent years that clinical symptoms, electrocardiographic changes and heart size on chest x-ray are not very predictive of the severity of left ventricular dysfunction in patients with aortic insufficiency. Efforts are being made to develop non-invasive criteria for timing of aortic valve replacement in such patients in order to achieve earlier selection of patients for operation before irreversible myocardial damage has occurred secondary to chronic volume overload. Radionuclide angiography at rest or with exercise may be of value in assessing aortic insufficiency patients for timing of valve replacement. As shown in figure 6 by Borer et al.,[4] in patients with symptomatic isolated aortic regurgitation, the ejection fraction response to exercise is depressed before operation and often remains depressed after operation. These investigators also found that exercise radionuclide angiography may unmask ventricular dysfunction not evident at rest.[5] They reported that all symptomatic patients with aortic regurgitation had an abnormal LVEF during supine exercise defined as a value below 0.55. However, 16 of 22 asymptomatic patients with aortic regurgitation had had abnormal LVEF response to exercise. The presence of an abnormal exercise LVEF was unrelated to symptoms or electrocardiographic evidence of left ventricular hypertrophy. These investigators suggested that patients with an exercise LVEF of below 0.55 might be considered candidates for early valve replacement despite absence of symptoms. Since the ejection fraction alone is both preload and afterload dependent, and ventricles with volume overload have abnormal loading conditions, indices of LV function that are more independent of preload than EF may also be important.

It has recently been reported that measurement of LV volume at rest and during exercise may give more information about LV functional reserve in

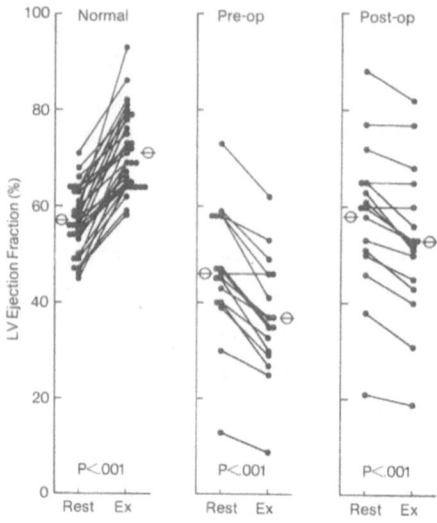

Figure 6. Left ventricular ejection fraction at rest and at peak exercise
(Ex) in normal subjects (left panel), in 16 symptomatic patients with
aortic regurgitation pre-operatively (center panel) and six months postoperatively in the same 16 patients. The open circles represent the mean
values (from Borer et al., <u>Am. J. Cardiol.</u>, 44, 1297, 1979).

patients with aortic regurgitation than do EF responses alone. Johnson
et al.[1] assessed changes in LVESV and LVEDV during upright bicycle
exercise in 27 asymptomatic and 22 symptomatic patients with aortic
regurgitation. They showed that in asymptomatic patients the LVEDV was
increased at rest but increased normally during exercise. The ESV was
also elevated at rest compared to controls but decreased by 30% during
exercise, a fall similar to that seen in control patients. In contrast,
symptomatic patients as a group showed no significant change in EDV
during exercise, but the mean ESV increased (100 $\pm$ 51 to 109 $\pm$ 73) in
association with a fall in LVEF (45 $\pm$ 15 to 42 $\pm$ 17%). Two subgroups of
symptomatic patients were identified. Seven of 22 symptomatic patients
demonstrated a normal decrease in ESV during exercise, whereas 8/22
patients showed and increase in both EDV and ESV during exercise, the
latter response indicating worsening failure. Similarly, certain asymptomatic patients showed an abnormal increase in LVESV from rest to exercise. Further prospective studies are warranted to determine the predictive value of these responses in determining improvement expected following valve replacement compared to assessment of ejection fraction alone.

Nevertheless, radionuclide angiography at rest and during exercise does provide a non-invasive means of evaluating LV functional reserve which cannot be measured by more conventional methods or by clinical symptoms.

RIGHT VENTRICULAR FUNCTION

Evaluation of right ventricular function has been difficult with contrast angiography because of the geometric complexities of the right ventricle. Radionuclide methods for measuring RVEF are less affected by geometric constraints than are the dye contrast studies performed at catheterization. The RVEF can be measured using either first-pass or equilibrium gated radionuclide techniques. The mean ($\pm$ SD) RVEF was 53 $\pm$ 6% in 20 normal subjects studied by Korr et al.[7] These investigators correlated the radionuclide measurement of RVEF with right heart hemodynamics in 60 patients and found a significant negative linear correlation between RVEF and mean pulmonary arterial pressure (figure 7; r = -0.82) and right ventricular end-diastolic pressure (r = -0.67). In 13 patients with an elevated right ventricular end-diastolic pressure, the average RVEF was 25 $\pm$ 8%, significantly lower than in patients with an elevated pulmonary pressure but a normal right ventricular end-diastolic pressure (38 $\pm$ 8%).

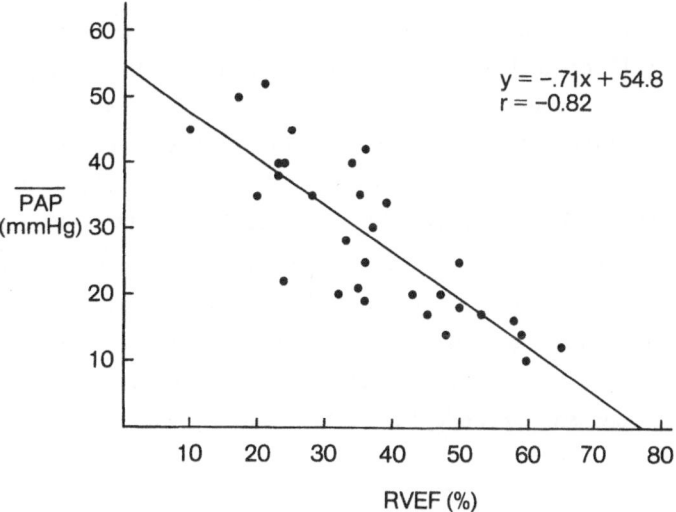

Figure 7. Relation between mean pulmonary artery pressure (PAP) and right ventricular ejection fraction (RVEF) in patients undergoing cardiac catheterization who had a wide range of findings (from Korr et al., Am. J. Cardiol., 49, 71, 1982).

Berger et al.[8] measured the RVEF by the first pass technique using a multicrystal scintillation camera with high count rate capabilities in patients with chronic obstructive pulmonary disease (COPD). In ten patients with cor pulmonale, RVEF averaged 35 $\pm$ 2% compared to normal individuals which ranged in RVEF from 45-65%. Interestingly, nine of 26 patients without clinical evidence of cor pulmonale had a depressed RVEF. In this study, arterial oxygen tension and forced expiratory volume were depressed significantly more in patients with an abnormal RVEF than in subjects with a normal RVEF. Thus, these studies demonstrate that radionuclide angiography can be employed to assess right ventricular function in disease states associated with right ventricular hypertrophy. Abnormal RVEF has also been reported in patients with mitral stenosis prior to valvular surgery and in patients with repair of a ventricular septal defect. Patients with COPD have also shown an abnormal RVEF response to exercise stress.

ABNORMALITIES OF LEFT VENTRICULAR FILLING

Impaired diastolic filling of the left ventricle can be detected by gated equilibrium radionuclide angiography. Bonow et al.[9] found that 70% of patients with hypertrophic cardiomyopathy had abnormal diastolic function evidenced by a peak LV filling rate of less than 2.5 EDV/s or a time to peak filling rate of greater than 180 ms. Verapamil increased the rate of peak LV filling and shortened the time to peak filling rate.[9] The same investigators subsequently demonstrated, using radionuclide angiography to calculate LV filling parameters, that patients with hypertrophic cardiomyopathy had a reduced LV filling volume during rapid diastolic filling and an increased contribution to LV filling by atrial systole.[3] The percent of LV stroke volume filled during rapid diastolic filling was 67 $\pm$ 17% compared to 83 $\pm$ 7% in normal subjects; the contribution of atrial systole was increased to 31 $\pm$ 18% compared to 16 $\pm$ 8% in normals. After verapamil the percent LV filling during rapid diastolic filling and percent LV filling during atrial systole reverted to normal.

Impaired diastolic filling of the hypertrophied left ventricle contributes to the symptoms of pulmonary vascular congestion and reduced cardiac output. Radionuclide angiography appears to be useful in detecting this abnormal diastolic filling and in assessing the effect of pharmacologic therapy directed at reversing this abnormality. Perhaps this approach can also be employed in patients with LVH to determine which patients might be at risk for severe hemodynamic decompensation if loss of atrial systole occurred as with the onset of atrial fibrillation.

THALLIUM-201 SCINTIGRAPHY

The myocardial mass of the left and right ventricle can be qualitatively assessed by rest thallium-201 (Tl-201) scintigraphy. The uptake of Tl-201 by myocardial tissue after intravenous injection is proportional to blood flow and the extraction fraction for the radioisotope. Myocardial visualization on Tl-201 images is also determined by relative myocardial mass. Usually, because of its smaller mass than the left ventricle, the right ventricle (RV) is not easily visualized by Tl-201 scintigraphy in the resting state. The RV is visualized during exercise when blood flow is augmented. Wackers et al.[10] (figure 8) showed in a canine model that Tl-201 uptake per gram of myocardial tissue was increased significantly with RV pressure overload induced by pulmonary artery constriction and by chronic RVH.

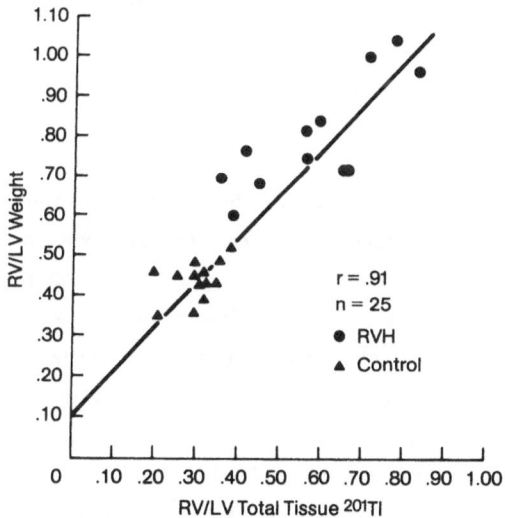

Figure 8. Correlation between the degree of RVH as calculated by RV/LV weight ratio and amount of RV thallium-201 myocardial tissue accumulation characterized by the RV/LV total tissue Tl-201 activity (from Wackers et al., Circulation, 64, 1256, 1981).

The total RV/LV Tl-201 tissue uptake rates correlated well with the degree of RVH (r = 0.91). Similarly, quantitative analysis of computerized Tl-201 images correlated well (r = 0.77) with the degree of RVH.

The degree of RV free wall Tl-201 visualization correlated well with hemodynamic indices of RV pressure overload in patients with a variety of disorders.[11] If RV Tl-201 activity is observed to be equal to or greater than LV activity on the 45° left anterior oblique image, the pulmonary vascular resistance usually exceeded 1,000 dynes.s.cm^{-5}. In this latter study, the sensitivity of Tl-201 scintigraphy for RVH was 93% compared to 81% for any of the electrocardiographic criteria of Sokolow and Lyon.

Tl-201 scintigraphy has been reported to be useful in detecting patients with hypertrophic cardiomyopathy.[12] Asymmetric septal hypertrophy was evident on Tl-201 scans in ten patients with idiopathic subaortic stenosis characterized by a ratio of septum to free wall thickness of 1.7 cm compared to 1.0 cm in normal volunteers (figure 9). Concentric LVH can often be recognized on resting or exercise Tl-201 scintigrams as an overall increase in Tl-201 counts in the myocardium after background subtraction as well as a small cavity size.

NMR IMAGING

In the future, imaging of the myocardium by nuclear magnetic resonance (NMR) should permit more accurate measurements of LV and RV volumes, myocardial wall thickness, systolic and diastolic function and myocardial mass than either echocardiographic or radionuclide imaging techniques. When subjected to a magnetic force, atomic particles line up in a north-south polar orientation. Radiosignals of predetermined frequency are beamed at these particles which causes perturbations in the protons altering their alignment in the magnetic field. When the radio signal is removed and protons come back into the position imposed by the magnetic field, they emit radiowaves. These radiowaves are characteristics of their substance. A computer picks up these signals, processes them and

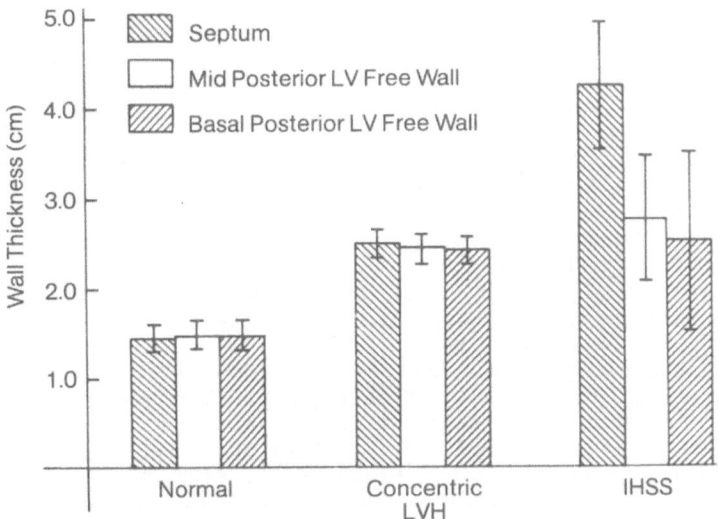

Figure 9. Relative wall thickness as measured from left anterior oblique thallium-201 scans in normal patients, in patients with concentric LVH and patients with idiopathic hypertrophic subaortic stenosis (IHSS) (from Bulkley et al., N. Engl. J. Med., 293, 1113, 1975).

depicts the results in an image. With gated NMR imaging, one can view the structure of the heart and great vessels in transverse, sagittal and coronal planes. Figure 10 shows an example of end-systolic and end-diastolic transverse images of the heart obtained by NMR imaging of protons in a normal human.

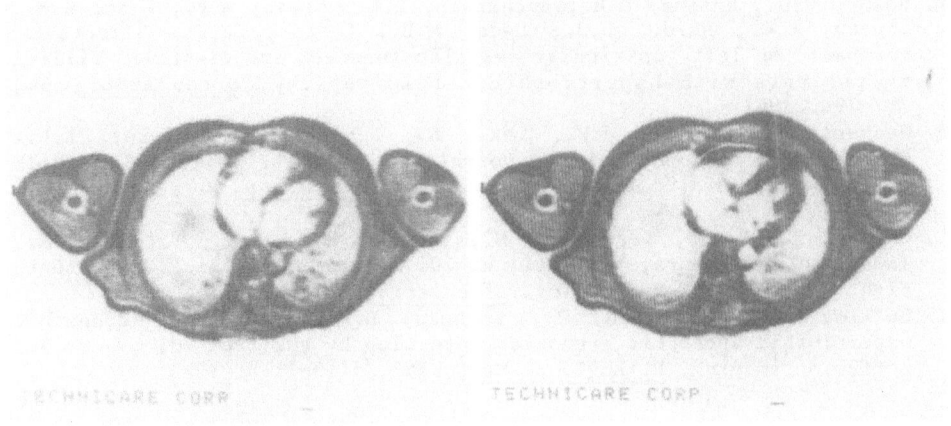

Figure 10. A. Transverse section NMR image of the heart during systole; B. transverse section NMR image of the heart during diastole (from Technicare Corporation).

REFERENCES

1. Johnson, L.L., Powers, E.R., Tzall, W.R., Feder, J., Sciacca, R.R., Eng, S.C.D., Cannon, P.S.: Left ventricular volume and ejection fraction response to exercise in aortic regurgitation, Am. J. Cardiol., 51, 1379-85, 1983

2. Bacharach, S.L., Green, M.V., Borer, J.S., Hyde, J.E., Farkas, S.P., Johnston, G.S.: Left ventricular peak ejection rate, filling rate, and ejection fraction: frame rate requirements at rest and exercise, J. Nucl. Med., 20, 189-193, 1979

3. Bonow, R.O., Frederick, T.M., Bacharach, S.L., Green, M.V., Goose, P.W., Maron, B.J., Rosing, D.R.: Atrial systole and left ventricular filling in hypertrophic cardiomyopathy: effect of verapamil, Am. J. Cardiol., 51, 1386-1391, 1983

4. Borer, J.S., Rosing, D.R., Kent, K.M., Bacharach, S.L., Green, M.V., McIntosh, C.J., Morrow, A.G., Epstein, S.E.: Left ventricular function at rest and during exercise after aortic valve replacement in patients with aortic regurgitation, Am. J. Cardiol., 44, 1297-1305, 1979

5. Borer, J.S., Bacharach, S.L., Green, M.V., Kent, M.V., Henry, W.L., Rosing, D.R., Seides, E.F., Johnston, G.S., Epstein, S.E.: Exercise-induced left ventricular dysfunction in symptomatic and asymptomatic patients with aortic regurgitation: assessment with radionuclide cineangiography, Am. J. Cardiol., 42, 351-357, 1978

6. Dehmer, G.J., Firth, B.G., Hillis, L.D., Corbett, J.R., Lewis, S.E., Parkey, R.W., Willerson, J.T.: Alterations in left ventricular volumes and ejection fraction at rest and during exercise in patients with aortic regurgitation, Am. J. Cardiol., 48, 17-27, 1981

7. Korr, K.S., Gandsman, E.J., Winkler, M.L., Shulman, R.S., Bough, E.W.: Hemodynamic correlates of right ventricular ejection fraction measured with gated radionuclide angiography, Am. J. Cardiol., 49, 71-77, 1982

8. Berger, H.J., Matthay, R.A., Loke, J., Marshall, R.C., Gottschalk, A., Zaret, B.L.: Assessment of cardiac performance with quantitative radionuclide angiocardiography: right ventricular ejection fraction with reference to findings in chronic obstructive pulmonary disease, Am. J. Cardiol., 41, 897-905, 1978

9. Bonow, R.O., Rosing, D.R., Bacharach, S.L., Green, M.V., Kent, K.M., Lipson, L.C., Maron, B.J., Leon, M.B., Epstein, S.E.: Effects of verapamil on left ventricular systolic function and diastolic filling in patients with hypertrophic cardiomyopathy, Circulation, 64, 787-796, 1981

10. Wackers, F.J., Klay, J.W., Laks, H., Schnitzer, J., Zaret, B.L., Geha, A.S.: Pathophysiologic correlates of right ventricular thallium-201 uptake in a canine model, Circulation, 64, 1256-1264, 1981

11. Ohsuzu, F., Handa, S., Kondo, M., Yamazki, H., Tsugu, T., Kubo, A., Takagi, Y., Nakamura, Y.: Thallium-201 myocardial imaging to evaluate right ventricular overloading, Circulation, 61, 620-625, 1980

12. Bulkley, B.H., Rouleau, J., Strauss, H.W., Pitt, B.: Idiopathic hypertrophic subaortic stenosis: detection by thallium-201 myocardial perfusion imaging, N. Engl. J. Med., 293, 1113-1116, 1975

THERAPEUTIC ASPECTS OF LEFT VENTRICULAR HYPERTROPHY

224

SUMMARY

Recent studies indicate that the prevalence of LVH in hypertensive patients assessed with the electrocardiogram and the chest X-ray is fairly low. The prevalence of echocardiographic LVH has been reported to be almost 50% in patients with mild to moderate hypertension.

An increasing number of studies have been published on the effect of antihypertensive therapy on the regression of cardiac muscle mass in patients with hypertension. Most studies have been performed in patients with mild or moderate hypertension who had not been selected on the basis of preexisting cardiac hypertrophy. The duration of antihypertensive therapy in these studies ranged between 1.5 and 60 months. Careful evaluation of the data reveals that neither the number of patients included in these studies nor the duration of therapy is related to the changes in cardiac muscle mass observed during antihypertensive therapy. In contrast, the degree of control of blood pressure is related to changes in cardiac muscle mass. In fact, the correlation between the changes in diastolic blood pressure and those in left ventricular mass as reported in the studies is significant. The correlation between changes in systolic blood pressure and changes in cardiac mass is even more impressive.

A decrease in muscle mass is most clearly, but not exclusively, found in patients with preexisting hypertrophy. Some studies reveal that moderate to marked decreases in blood pressure do not result in changes in cardiac muscle mass. Apparently, in these patients blood pressure probably is not the only determinant of cardiac hypertrophy.

The use of diuretics and vasodilatory agents in hypertension, although effectively lowering blood pressure, does not always lead to regression of cardiac muscle mass. Both classes of antihypertensive agents increase the activity of the renin-angiotensin system and the sympathetic nervous system. In turn, these factors are known to induce cardiac hypertrophy. In contrast, regression of hypertrophy has been observed during treatment with a combination of a diuretic and a centrally-acting sympatholytic agent. Sympatholytic agents, such as beta-adrenergic antagonists, also seem to reduce cardiac muscle mass, but the results are less conclusive. Recent data indicate that both calcium antagonists and converting enzyme inhibitors induce regression of hypertrophy.

MEDIATORS OF CHANGES IN LEFT VENTRICULAR MASS DURING ANTIHYPERTENSIVE THERAPY

DRAYER, J.I.M., WEBER, M.A., GARDIN, J.M.
Section of Clinical Pharmacology and Hypertension and Section of Cardiology, Veterans Administration Medical Center, Long Beach, California and the University of California, Irvine, California

INTRODUCTION

The evaluation of the anatomy of the heart has become routine in the workup of patients with hypertension. Non-invasive techniques such as electro-cardiography and radiologic examination of the chest are used in virtually all hypertensive patients. These examinations usually are performed prior to the start of the antihypertensive therapy as well as during its administration. The information gained in this way has been shown to provide data concerning the prognosis of the hypertensive patient. The presence of borderline or definitive cardiac left ventricular hypertrophy markedly increases morbidity and mortality in these patients[1]. Moreover, clinical data reveal that lowering of blood pressure will help to reduce the degree of cardiac hypertrophy measured by electrocardiography[2].

Recent studies indicate that the prevalence of left ventricular hypertrophy in hypertensive patients assessed using the electrocardiogram and the chest x-ray is fairly low. More sensitive techniques such as echocardiography now are often used to detect possible left ventricular hypertrophy. An increasing number of studies are being published on the use of echocardiography in the evaluation and followup of hypertensive patients. The results of these studies have recently been reviewed[3]. Blood pressure itself has been shown to be a major determinant of th development of cardiac hypertrophy. However, factors other than systolic and diastolic blood pressure levels have to be considered in the etiology of cardiac hypertrophy (table 1).[4-7] It seems reasonable to assume that blockage of these stimuli of hypertrophy might lead to regression of left ventricular hypertrophy.

METHODOLOGY

Standard M—mode echocardiographic techniques are used in the studies referenced in this paper. In some studies the M—mode tracing of the left ventricle was obtained using two—dimensional echocardiography as a guide. The techniques used differed slightly, but in all cases measurements of the interventricular septum, left ventricular posterior wall and left ventricular dimension measured during diastole have been used to calculate derived parameters of cardiac muscle mass; left ventricular cross-sectional area and left ventricular mass (see individual studies for details). In general, a septal thickness greater than 11 mm, a posterior wall thickness greater than 11 mm, and a left ventricular dimension greater than 56 mm are considered to be abnormal. However, each laboratory might use different values depending upon the normotensive control subjects studied in that center.

REGRESSION OF CARDIAC HYPERTROPHY: STUDIES IN ANIMALS

Data from animal studies have shown that a reduction in blood pressure does not necessarily lead to regression of cardiac hypertrophy as measured by changes in cardiac weight. Tarazi and coworkers have shown that blockade of sympathetic nervous system outflow is mandatory for regression of cardiac hypertrophy in the spontaneous hypertensive rat[5]. Both centrally acting sympatholytic agents and beta-adrenergic blocking agents are known to reduce sympathetic nervous system activity. However, the effects of treatment with centrally acting sympatholytic agents (e.g., alpha methyldopa) on cardiac muscle mass were more marked than those with beta-adrenergic blocking agents[5]. On the other hand, a reduction in blood pressure per se resulted in significant regression of cardiac hypertrophy in rats with renovascular hypertension and normal sympathetic nervous system activity. Moreover, diuretic treatment in DOCA hypertensive rats resulted in regression of hypertrophy despite a diuretic-induced increase in sympathetic nervous system activity and despite activation of the renin-angiotensin-aldosterone system[5]. The results of these and other studies in hypertensive animals reveal that, apart from blood pressure levels, the etiology of the hypertension and the pharmacology of

antihypertensive agents used are important factors both in the development and in the regression of cardiac hypertrophy. Animal studies also
suggest a role of age in the etiology of cardiac hypertrophy.

REGRESSION OF CARDIAC HYPERTROPHY IN PATIENTS WITH ESSENTIAL HYPERTENSION
Recent studies using M-mode echocardiography before and during antihypertensive therapy in man[8-18] appear to confirm the results from the
animal studies. The relationship between the percentage change in systolic or diastolic blood pressure and the change in echocardiographic
measurements of cardiac muscle mass is shown in Figure 1.

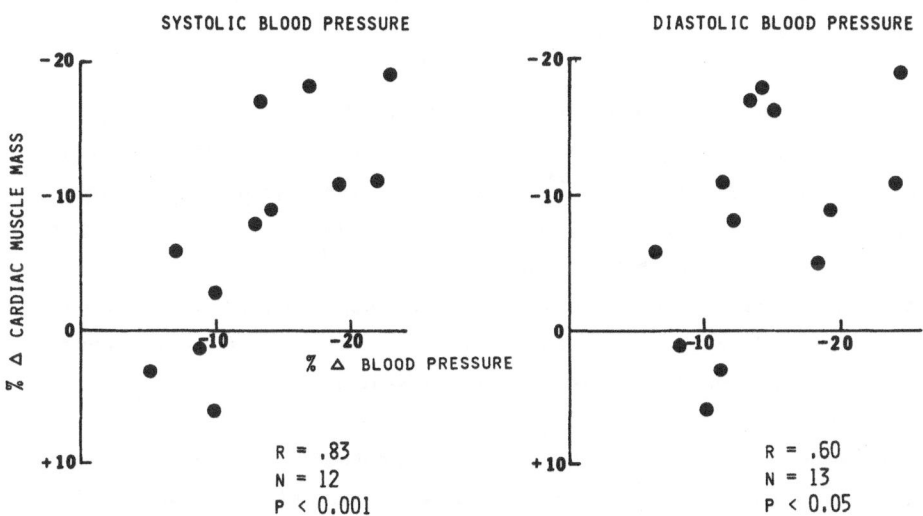

Figure 1. Relationship between drug-induced changes in systolic and
diastolic blood pressure and changes in echocardiograph cardiac muscle
mass in hypertensive patients. (Adapted from Drayer et al.[3]).

Each data point represents the relationship between the changes in
systolic or diastolic blood pressure and the changes in cardiac muscle
mass reported in each of these studies. Overall, a highly significant

correlation was found between the observed decreases in blood pressure and the decreases in cardiac muscle mass. This relationship was more pronounced for systolic blood pressure (r=.83) than for diastolic blood pressure (r=.60). However, in individual studies a significant correlation between the drug-induced changes in blood pressure and in muscle mass was not always observed. Therefore, these data show that a reduction in blood pressure is not the only factor determining regression of cardiac muscle mass, although a marked reduction in pressure often will lead to a reduction in muscle mass. Others have confirmed that chronic control of blood pressure resulted in regression of cardiac muscle mass, whereas in the absence of control of blood pressure decreases in cardiac mass do not occur[19]. In contrast, Fouad et al.[20] have shown that regression of hypertrophy may occur during antihypertensive therapy in the absence of a decrease in blood pressure. They claim that a drug-induced reduction in sympathetic nervous system activity may directly lead to regression of muscle mass.

It also has been observed that regression of hypertrophy occurs to the greatest extent in patients who have marked cardiac hypertrophy prior to the start of therapy[8,12,17,20]. Moreover, significant correlations have been observed between baseline measurements of cardiac muscle mass and drug-induced changes in cardiac muscle mass[10,14]. Preliminary results with the calcium channel blocker, nitrendipine, also revealed that drug-induced decreases in cardiac muscle mass were more pronounced in patients with greater baseline cardiac muscle mass.

Data from our own patients has revealed another factor related to drug-induced changes in cardiac muscle mass. The calcium channel blocker, nitrendipine, was given to 26 hypertensive patients whose ages ranged between 30 and 69 years. The calcium channel blocker lowered blood pressure significantly. Moreover, a decrease in echocardiographic left ventricular muscle mass was observed. It was noted that the changes in blood pressure did not correlate significantly with changes in cardiac muscle mass. However, a significant correlation was found between the ages of the patients and the drug-induced changes in cardiac muscle mass. Thus, the nitrendipine caused a more marked change in cardiac muscle mass in older than in younger patients. It is known that cardiac left ventricular hypertrophy is more often found in older hypertensive patients[1].

However, in our study, the age-related decrease in cardiac muscle mass was independent of the baseline measurements of cardiac mass. The greater response of cardiac muscle mass in older patients actually is surprising, since the composition of the myocardial tissue changes with age. Specifically, collagen deposition increases with age, and it seems unlikely that this process would be reversed during treatment with antihypertensive agents.

Thus, age, the degree of pretreatment cardiac hypertrophy, and the changes in blood pressure can be recognized as important determinants of the changes in cardiac muscle mass observed during antihypertensive therapy.

ANTIHYPERTENSIVE AGENTS AND REGRESSION OF CARDIAC HYPERTROPHY

Major factors related to the development of cardiac hypertrophy have been listed in Table 1. It seems likely that inhibition of these factors also helps determine the degree of regression of hypertrophy observed during antihypertensive therapy. Thus, the blood pressure level itself is directly related to the cardiac muscle mass, and a reduction in blood pressure may reduce the severity of the cardiac hypertrophy.

Table 1: Major determinants of cardiac hypertrophy

> Systolic blood pressure
> Diastolic blood pressure
> Cardiac output
> Sympathetic nervous system activity
> Renin-angiotensin-aldosterone activity
> Whole blood viscosity
> Cardiac cell metabolism
> Age.

However, other factors play a significant role. A reduction in sympathetic nervous system activity may lead to regression of cardiac hypertrophy even in the absence of effective blood pressure control[20]. Sympathetic nervous system activity probably is an important final determinant of the induction of adaptive cardiac hypertrophy[6]. Angiotensin II also is directly, or indirectly through stimulation of sympathetic nervous system activity or of adrenal catecholamine release, involved in the development of cardiac hypertrophy.

Careful analysis of the clinical studies show that regression of cardiac muscle mass may be influenced by drug-induced changes in any of the determinants of cardiac hypertrophy listed in Table 1.

The possible effects of commonly used antihypertensive agents on these factors are listed in Figure 2.

DRUG-INDUCED CHANGES IN MAJOR DETERMINANTS OF LVH

	BLOOD PRESSURE	CARDIAC OUTPUT	SNS ACTIVITY	RENIN ACTIVITY
DIURETICS	↓	—	↑	↑
BETA-ADRENERGIC ANTAGONISTS	↓	↓	↓	↓
CENTRALLY ACTING SYMPATHOLYTIC DRUGS	↓	↓	↓	↓
ANGIOTENSIN CONVERTING ENZYME INHIBITORS	↓	—	—	↓
VASODILATORS	↓	↑	↑	↑

Figure 2. Drug-induced changes in major determinants of cardiac left ventricular hypertrophy.

Diuretics: Diuretics are probably the most commonly used agents in the treatment of patients with hypertension. They effectively lower blood pressure but often stimulate sympathetic nervous system activity or renin release. Obviously, these latter effects could counteract the beneficial effects of the reduction of blood pressure on cardiac muscle mass. Indeed, smaller decreases in blood pressure in diuretic-treated patients do not necessarily result in a reduction in cardiac muscle mass[10]. However, marked reductions in blood pressure, especially in patients with preexisting cardiac hypertrophy, may cause a net reduction in cardiac muscle mass despite stimulation of the sympathetic nervous system or the renin-angiotensin system[17].

Combination therapy with a diuretic and the centrally-acting sympatholytic agent, alpha-methyldopa, often results in a significant reduction of
cardiac muscle mass[17,20,21]. These decreases in cardiac muscle mass are
observed even when blood pressures are only moderately reduced and can
occur in patients who do not have clear left ventricular hypertrophy
before therapy[9]. It is likely that blockade of the diuretic-induced
increase in sympathetic nervous system activity by alpha-methyldopa is a
factor in the observed decreases in muscle mass.

Beta-adrenergic blocking agents: Beta-blockers now are commonly used as
monotherapy in patients with mild hypertension. Beta-blockers lower blood
pressure effectively. Because they reduce cardiac output, renin activity
and sympathetic nervous sytem activity, these agents could be expected to
have a marked effect on cardiac muscle mass. However, initial studies
reveal that a significant reduction in muscle mass is not always observed
during beta-blocker therapy. Hill et al.[13] reported regression of hypertrophy during beta-blocker therapy only in patients with asymmetric or
concentric hypertrophy prior to the start of treatment. In contrast,
McKenna et al.[22] reported that reversal of cardiac hypertrophy during
beta-blocker treatment is not readily observed in patients with asymmetric hypertrophy. Only treatment with unusually high doses of propranolol
resulted in regression of hypertrophy in a few patients. Ibrahim et
al.[14] reported decreases in cardiac muscle mass during therapy with
atenolol, especially in patients with greater control values. Rowlands et
al.[18] reported a significant reduction in left ventricular hypertrophy
during treatment with timolol in seven patients without left ventricular
hypertrophy.

Combination therapy with a beta-blocker and a diuretic does not necessarily lead to regression of cardiac hypertrophy[3]. Thus, these studies
tend to relate regression of hypertrophy during beta-blocker therapy
to the presence of pre-existing hypertrophy rather than to specific
actions of the drug. It is of interest to note that Östman-Smith[6] suggests that certain characteristics of beta-blockers, such as intrinsic
sympathomimetic activity, may enhance rather than reverse the development
of cardiac hypertrophy. However, a broader experience using various
beta-adrenergic blocking agents is needed to define whether or not
beta-adrenergic blocking drugs cause regression of cardiac hypertrophy
independent of their blood pressure lowering effect or the presence of
pretreatment left ventricular hypertrophy.

<u>Centrally-acting Sympatholytic Agents</u>: Centrally-acting sympatholytic drugs have potent antihypertensive effects. They lower blood pressure through inhibition of sympathetic outflow. In addition, but to a lesser degree, they lower renin activity. The inhibition of sympathetic nervous system activity induced by these agents probably is more pronounced than that of beta-blockers. Conversely, beta-blockers cause a more marked reduction in renin activity than centrally-acting sympatholytic agents. These differences in characteristics between the two classes of anti-hypertensive agents might help to explain that regression of hypertrophy is more consistently reported in studies using the centrally-acting sympatholytic agent, alpha-methyldopa, than in studies using beta-adre-nergic blocking agents. Data from animal studies confirm this observa-tion[5].

Regression of cardiac muscle mass has been observed during monotherapy with alpha-methyldopa[8] as well as during treatment with the combination of a diuretic and alpha-methyldopa[17,20,21]. Another centrally-acting sympatholytic agent, clonidine, also has shown to cause regression of cardiac muscle mass in hypertensive patients (W. St. John LaCorte, personal communication).

<u>Angiotensin Converting Enzyme Inhibitor</u>: A new converting enzyme inhibi-tor, enalapril, has been shown to cause regression of cardiac muscle mass[22,23]. The regression of cardiac mass observed in these patients probably is related to both the drug-induced fall in blood pressure and the blockade of the renin-angiotensin-aldosterone system. In addition, the drug-induced decrease in angiotensin II levels might lead to a reduction in sympathetic nervous system activity. Thus, converting enzyme inhibitors attenuate the effects of at least three of the etiologic factors in the development of cardiac hypertrophy. The combination of these effects apparently does lead to regression of cardiac muscle mass in hypertensive patients.

<u>Vasodilators</u>: Treatment of hypertensive patients with a new vasodilator, trimazosin, did not result in a significant reduction in cardiac muscle mass[11]. A reduction in cardiac muscle mass also was not observed when the vasodilator was given to diuretic-treated patients[11] despite a significant fall in blood pressure. It is known that a vasodilator increases rather than decreases sympathetic nervous system activity and renin activity. Evidence from human[11] and animal studies[4,5] suggests

that stimulation of these humoral systems might be responsible for the lack of regression of cardiac hypertrophy observed during treatment with vasodilators. In fact, vasodilators and diuretics have qualitatively comparable effects on the major determinants of cardiac hypertrophy. Both drugs lower blood pressure, but at the same time enhance sympathetic nervous system activity and renin activity. Therefore, it is not surprising that regression of cardiac muscle mass is not always observed during treatment with these agents or their combination.

Calcium channel blockers lower blood pressure through mechanisms similar to those of vasodilators. However, preliminary results from our institution reveal that the calcium channel blocker nitrendipine does cause a significant reduction in cardiac muscle mass. The different effects of vasodilators and calcium channel blockers on cardiac muscle mass might be related to the fact that calcium channel blockers might cause a lesser degree of stimulation of the sympathetic nervous system. Preliminary pharmacologic studies have suggested that the calcium channel blockers might have inhibitory effects at alpha-adrenergic receptors, perhaps providing some peripheral blockade of sympathetic activity. In fact, increases in heart rate are believed to be less pronounced during therapy with a calcium channel blocker than during treatment with vasodilators such as hydralazine. Similarly, increases in renin activity seem to be less marked during therapy with a calcium channel blocker. A comparative study on the use of vasodilators and calcium channel blockers in hypertensive patients is needed to better define the possible different effects on cardiac muscle mass. Such a study should include careful measurements of catecholamine levels and renin activity before and during treatment with these agents.

GENERAL CONSIDERATIONS

The most important effects of commonly used antihypertensive agents on determinants of cardiac growth have been discussed in this paper. However, the effects of the various agents on factors such as blood viscosity and myocardial cell metabolism have not been described. It is known that blood viscosity increases during treatment with diuretics and decreases during treatment with the postsynaptic α-receptor blocker, prazosin. However, the relationship between these changes in blood viscosity and changes in cardiac muscle mass have not been studied. Blood viscosity has been related directly to the degree of cardiac hypertrophy

in hypertensive patients[7]. Thus, the diuretic-induced increase in blood
viscosity is yet another reason (in addition to those discussed earlier)
why regression of cardiac muscle mass is not generally observed during
such therapy.

Decreases in cardiac muscle mass have been reported with a variety of
antihypertensive agents. It is difficult to be certain which characteristics of the antihypertensive agents are important in causing regression
of muscle mass. Unfortunately, the available clinical data base is still
relatively small. Obviously, interrelations between the factors related
to growth of cardiac muscle cells ultimately will determine the degree of
cardiac hypertrophy.

Regression of cardiac muscle mass can readily be observed after normalization of blood pressure in patients with severe hypertension associated
with marked left ventricular hypertrophy. In such patients, regression of
cardiac mass may be induced irrespective of the therapy used. On the
other hand, changes in cardiac muscle mass might not occur during treatment of patients with mild hypertension associated with moderate cardiac
hypertrophy or in patients with mild hypertension without cardiac hypertrophy. Antihypertensive agents which attenuate hypertrophy-stimulating
factors are most likely to induce a beneficial readaptation of cardiac
muscle mass. Appropriate regression of hypertrophy or appropriate reduction in muscle mass in hypertensive patients with or without left ventricular hypertrophy then will result. Drugs which specifically decrease
sympathetic nervous system activity (centrally-acting sympatholytic
agents) or renin activity (converting enzyme inhibitors) induce regression of hypertrophy even in patients with milder forms of hypertension.
In contrast, drugs which enhance sympathetic nervous system activity and
renin activity (diuretics and vasodilators) are less likely to cause
regression of hypertrophy unless a marked decrease in blood pressure is
obtained.

The effect of beta-adrenergic blocking agents on cardiac muscle mass is
less well defined. It seems likely that the decrease in sympathetic
nervous activity and renin activity observed during beta-blocker therapy
will cause a reduction in cardiac muscle mass. However, the few studies
available are inconclusive. Beta-blockers are effective in hypertensive
patients with left ventricular hypertrophy, but only timolol has so far

been shown to reduce muscle mass in hypertensive patients without cardiac hypertrophy. Qualitative differences between centrally-acting sympatholytic agents, converting enzyme inhibitors and beta-adrenergic antagonists on the determinants of cardiac hypertrophy probably are responsible for the disparate effects of these agents on cardiac muscle mass. However, comparative studies using these agents have not been done.

The clinical data accumulated to date on the effect of antihypertensive agents on cardiac muscle mass suggest that knowledge of the effects of antihypertensive agents on determinants of cardiac muscle growth will help to define the most appropriate therapy in hypertensive patients. Long-term follow-up studies are needed to determine whether this approach leads to improvements in the control of cardiovascular complications in hypertensive patients.

REFERENCES

1. Kannel, W.B., Gordon, T., Castelli, W.P., Margolis, J.R.: Electrocardiographic left ventricular hypertrophy and risk of coronary heart disease, Ann. Int. Med., 72:813-822, 1970

2. Yamada, T., Kubota, T., Endo, T., Komatus, H., Oba, M., Nagata, H., Izumyama, T.: Effects of antihypertensive treatment on left ventricular hypertrophy in patients with essential hypertension, J. Am. Ger. Soc., 27:500-506, 1979

3. Drayer, J.I.M., Gardin, J.M., Weber, M.A.: Echocardiographic left ventricular hypertrophy in hypertension, Chest (in press), 1983

4. Frohlich, E.D., Tarazi, R.C.: Is arterial pressure the sole factor responsible for hypertensive cardiac hypertrophy? Am. J. Cardiol., 44:959-963, 1979

5. Tarazi, R.C., Saragoca, M., Khairallah, P.: The multifactorial role of catecholamines in hypertensive cardiac hypertrophy, Eur. Heart J., 3 (Suppl. A):103-110, 1982

6 Östman-Smith, I.: Cardiac sympathetic nerves as the final common pathway in the induction of adaptive cardiac hypertrophy, Clin. Sci., 61:265-272, 1981

7. Drayer, J.I.M., Devereux, R.B., De Young, J.L., Letcher, R.L., Chien, S., Pickering, T.G., Weber, M.A., Sealy, J.E., Laragh, J.H.,: Whole blood viscosity as a determinant of cardiac hypertrophy, Clin. Pharmacol Ther., 33:204, 1983

8. Corea, L., Bentivoglio, M., Verdecchia, P.: Reversal of left ventricular hypertrophy in essential hypertension by early and long-term treatment with methyldopa, Clin. Trials J., 18:380-394, 1981

9. Drayer, J.I.M., Weber, M.A., Gardin, J.M., Lipson, J.L.: The effect of chronic antihypertensive therapy on cardiac anatomy in patients with essential hypertension, Am. J. Med. (in press), 1983

10. Drayer, J.I.M., Gardin, J.M., Weber, M.A., Aronow, W.S.: Changes in ventricular septal thickness during diuretic therapy, Clin. Pharmacol. Ther., 32;283-288, 1982

11. Drayer, J.I.M., Gardin, J.M., Weber, M.A., Aronow, W.S.: Changes in cardiac muscle mass during vasodilation therapy of hypertension, Clin. Pharmacol. Ther. (in press), 1983

12. Dunn, F.G., Bastian B., Lawrie, T.D.V., Lorimer, A.R.: Effect of blood pressure control on left ventricular hypertrophy in patients with essential hypertension, Clin. Sci., 59:441-443, 1980

13. Hill, L.S., Monaghan, M., Richardson, P.J.: Regression of left ventricular hypertrophy during treatment with antihypertensive agents, Br. J. Clin. Pharmacol., 7:255S-259S, 1979

14. Ibrahim, M.M., Madkour, M.A., Mossallam Ragaa: Factors influencing cardiac hypertrophy in hypertensive patients, Clin. Sci., 61:105S-108S, 1981

15. Schlant, R.C., Felner, J.M., Heymsfield, S.B., Gilbert, C.A., Shulman, N.B., Tuttle, E.P., Blumenstein, B.A.: Echocardiographic studies of left ventricular anatomy and function in essential hypertension, Cardiovasc. Med., 2:477-491, 1977

16. Schlant, R.C., Felner, J.M., Blumenstein, B.A., Wollam, G.L., Hall, W.D., Schulman, N.B., Heymsfield S.B., Gilbert, C.A. Tuttle, E.P.: Echocardiographic documentation of regression of left ventricular hypertrophy in patients treated for essential hypertension, Eur. Heart J., 3 (Suppl. A):171-175, 1982

17. Reichek, N., Franklin, B.B., Chandler, T., Muhammad, A., Plappert, T., St.John-Sutton, M.: Reversal of left ventricular hypertrophy by antihypertensive therapy, Eur. Heart J. 3 (Suppl. A):165-169, 1982
18. Rowlands, D.B., Ireland, M.A., Glover, D.R., McLeay, A.B., Stallard, T.J., Littler, W.A.: The relationship between ambulatory blood pressure and echocardiographically assessed left ventricular hypertrophy, Clin. Sci., 61:101S-103S, 1981
19. Devereux, R.B.: Noninvasive evaluation of cardiac anatomy and function in patients with hypertension, Cardiovasc. Rev. Rep., 3:313-323, 1982
20. Fouad, F.M., Nakashima, Y., Tarazi, R.C., Salcedo, E.E.: Reversal of left ventricular hypertrophy in hypertensive patients treated with methyldopa, Am. J. Cardiol., 49:795-801, 1982
21. Drayer, J.I.M., Gardin, J.M., Weber, M.A., Aranow, W.S.: Changes in cardiac anatomy and function during therapy with alpha-methyldopa: an echocardiographic study, Curr. Ther. Res., 32:856-865, 1982
22. McKenna, W.J., Borggrefe, M., England, D., Deanfield, J., Oakley, C.M., Goodwin, J.F.: The natural history of left ventricular hypertrophy in hypertrophic cardiomyopathy: an electrocardiographic study, Circulation, 66:1233-1240, 1982
23. Fouad, F.M., Nakashima, Y., Tarazi, R.C., Bravo, E.L.: Left ventricular function with reversal of left ventricular hypertrophy in hypertensive patients, Clin. Pharmacol. Ther., 33:226, 1983
24. Dunn, F.G., Oigman, W., Ventura, H.O., Kobrin, I., Messerli, F.H., Frohlich, E.D.: Enalapril improves systemic and renal hemodynamics and regresses left ventricular mass in essential hypertension, J. Am. Coll. Cardiol., 1:611, 1983

SUMMARY

Twenty-five patients on a chronic hemodialysis program were studied by means of electrocardiography and echocardiography. In 18 patients a follow-up study lasting for eight months could be completed.

Four patients out of the original population showed ECG-LVH according to both the Bonner program and the Romhilt-Estes point score criterium. Two additional patients had LVH according to Bonner's point score only. On the echocardiogram nine out of 25 patients had either a septal wall thickness of more than 11 mm or a posterior wall thickness of more than 10 mm, or both. Eight patients had an increased left ventricular end-diastolic diameter over 60 mm. This demonstrated that electrocardiographic criteria for LVH are less sensitive than echocardiographic criteria. Electrocardiography is not a reliable method for the assessment of LVH in patients on chronic hemodialysis.

Left ventricular hypertrophy was clearly associated with diastolic hypertension before dialysis, and even more so with systolic hypertension. However, a direct relationship between degree of hypertension and LV-wall thickness was not found in several patients who still had one or two kidneys. Reduction of blood pressure during dialysis did not always lead to reversal of hypertrophy; wall thickness even increased in a few patients in whom blood pressure dropped after dialysis. This suggests that not only blood pressure but also volume load contribute to the development of left ventricular hypertrophy. Reversal of hypertrophy requires not only control of blood pressure but also correction of excess fluid load.

LEFT VENTRICULAR HYPERTROPHY IN PATIENTS ON CHRONIC HEMODIALYSIS:
A SIGN OF FLUID EXCESS

VOOGD, P.J., SCHICHT, I., BREDA VRIESMAN, P.C.J. VAN, MONSJOU, L.K.
Departments of Cardiology, Nephrology and Pathology,
Leiden University, Leiden, the Netherlands

INTRODUCTION

An increase in both preload and afterload may cause left ventricular hypertrophy albeit by differing mechanisms for enhanced afterload will cause an increase in wall thickness[2] whereas increases in preload will be accommodated by dilatations[3].

Patients on chronic hemodialysis are liable to develop left ventricular hypertrophy because an increase in preload as a consequence of anemia[4] and arteriovenous fistula[5] - necessary to obtain vascular access for hemodialysis - is invariably present. An expanded extracellular fluid volume - a not infrequent finding in these patients[6] - will give rise to an increase in preload as well as afterload[7]. Occasionally, hypertension of renal origin will be an additional cause of increased afterload. The purpose of this study was to investigate the prevalence of left ventricular hypertrophy in patients on chronic hemodialysis using M-mode echocardiography and electrocardiography as detection devices; next we related blood pressure to the degree of left ventricular hypertrophy in a longitudinal follow-up study.

MATERIAL AND METHODS

Twenty-five patients on a chronic hemodialysis program, who were without spontaneous symptoms indicative of cardiac disease and without pedal edema, were examined by non-invasive techniques. Of the 25 patients, two showed ECG changes compatible with a previously sustained inferior wall myocardial infarction and one patient had a pericardial effusion on echocardiography. Thus 22 patients were available for follow-up. One anephric patient with severe hypertension excepted, all patients were considered 'stable' by the nephrologists in charge, and no change in dialysis regimen was indicated. The follow-up period lasted for eight months. Of the 22 patients, five were lost to the follow-up, the reasons being: development of pericardial effusion (1); symptomatic coronary heart disease resulting in acute myocardial infarction (1); bypass surgery (1); renal transplant (1); technically unsatisfactory echocardiogram (1). Patients were hemodialyzed twice a week using regional heparinization. Access to the vasculature was by means of a fistula[23] or a Scribner shunt[2]; fistula or shunt was not changed during the follow-up period. Dialysis ultra-filtration was conducted in such a fashion that patients were either normotensive after dialysis or else close to their 'ideal' or 'minimal' weight. This weight was determined empirically by continuing dialysis ultra-filtration of patients with hypertension before dialysis until hypotension (systolic blood pressure < 90 mm Hg), or orthostatic hypotension (30 mm Hg difference in diastolic blood pressure between the upright and the supine position) developed. Alternatively, in the absence of predialysis hypertension, the heart rate at the end of dialysis had to increase by over 25% of the initial rate. Hemoglobin concentration was maintained between 2.5 and 3.7 mmol/l of blood using infrequent transfusion of packed erythrocytes if necessary. Blood pressure was measured with a cuff applied either to the arm without the fistula or to the ankle. Phase IV was taken as diastolic blood pressure. At entry and during follow-up, blood pressures were averaged every two or three months; the mean blood pressure was calculated by adding one third of the pulse pressure to the diastolic blood pressure. Standard 12-lead ECG's were read for the presence or absence of left ventricular hypertrophy by the criteria of Romhilt and Estes[8] using a point score system based on voltage (3 points), strain (3 points), P-wave changes (3 points), left axis deviation and prolongation of the QRS complex (3 points), and increased intrinsicoid deflection (1 point). ECG's were also read by means of a point score system used in computerized reading[9] for left ventricular hypertrophy, a system based primarily on voltage and ST-T changes.

Echocardiograms were taken in the left recumbent position using an Organon Technika 003 echocardiograph equipped with a multiscan and a 2.25 MHz single-element focussed transducer. After visualization of the cross-section through the long axis of the left ventricle, the transducer was positioned in the third, fourth or fifth interspace, depending on the findings of the two-dimensional examination. Complete M-mode scans[10] were performed in such fashion that the anterior wall of the aorta was as far as possible on the same horizontal level as the right septal endocardium. Left ventricular dimensions were measured slightly caudal to the mitral valves[10]. Left ventricular end-diastolic diameter and septal as well as posterior wall thickness were measured at the onset of the QRS complex. The largest end-diastolic diameter and the smallest wall thickness were taken as the true dimensions[10]. Left ventricular end-systolic diameter was measured at the peak of the inward motion of the posterior endocardial echo. Measurements were made at the anterior edge of each echo. Great care was taken not to incorporate the septal tricuspid leaflet into septal thickness; when desired, the right septal endocardial echo was visualized by means of contrast echocardiography[14], using a forceful injection of a 10-ml bolus of saline into the fistula or shunt. The left posterior endocardial echo was differentiated from the chordae tendineae by taking the thinnest line with the highest motion velocity as the endocardial echo. The gain setting was such that visceral and parietal perdicardial echoes were seen as separate lines. When desired, echocardiograms were read according to the 'Philadelphia' convention and left ventricular mass was calculated accordingly[12]. Echocardiograms were recorded on a Honeywell LSG fiberoptic recorder at paper speeds of 25 and 50 mm/second. Measurements were made with a caliper with calibrations 0.05 mm apart. M-mode dimensions were read to 1 mm accuracy. Because left ventricular end-diastolic inner dimension varies with heart rate[15], care was taken to exclude an effect of heart rate on the measurements by always making the echocardiograms prior to dialysis and using patients who were thoroughly familiar with the procedure.

In order to determine the magnitude of variability of the relevant echo dimensions used in this study, 25 patients from the chronic hemodialysis program at that time (including 13 patients from the follow-up study) were each investigated, within one half hour, by two different echocardiographers who were unaware of each other's transducer position and of the degree of the patient's recumbency. Next, each echocardiographer measured the echo dimensions of his own investigation independently. Variability of echo dimensions was expressed as twice the standard deviation of the difference between the measurements of the two observers.

RESULTS

Accuracy of echocardiographic measurements

In order to determine the reliability and reproducibility of the measurements made, the echocardiograms of the 25 patients were measured by two
observers independently of each other. Each observer made his own echocardiograms. The variability of the left ventricular end-diastolic
diameter was 3.4 mm, and of the septal and posterior wall thickness 2.6
mm (table 1). No significant systematic differences were found between
the two observers using the Student's t-test for paired data, so all
differences between the measurements made by the two observers were
random.

Table 1: Accuracy of echocardiographic measurements

	variability in mm*	difference in bias**	
left ventricular end-diastolic inner diameter	3.4	-0.48	(p < 0.18)
septal width	2.6	0.14	(p < 0.6)
posterial wall width	2.6	0.25	(p < 0.34)

Two independent observers measured left ventricular end-diastolic diameter and septal and posterior wall thickness at the onset of the QRS
complex.

* Variability was expressed as twice the standard deviation of differences in measurements made by both observers as follows:

$$SD (x-y) = \sqrt{\frac{\sum_{1}^{n}(x_1-y_1)^2}{n-1}}$$

where x: measurements by observer I
and y: measurements by observer II
n: number of measurements

** The difference in bias compared the measurements of two observers
   as follows: the mean of the measurements of observer I was subtracted
   from the mean of the measurements of observer II. Next the paired
   Student t-test was used in order to determine whether the measurements
   made by one observer differed significantly from the other (p < 0.05
   is significant).

Prevalence of left ventricular hypertrophy on entry

Four out of the 25 patients showed left ventricular hypertrophy on the
electrocardiogram using both the Bonner and the Romhilt and Estes point

scores. One of these patients also had ECG signs of an old inferior wall myocardial infarction. Two additional patients showed left ventricular hypertrophy according to the Bonner point score only. Of the four patients with a markedly increased left ventricular wall thickness (combined width 35 mm or over) and no left ventricular dilatation, two showed left ventricular hypertrophy on the ECG using the Bonner point score; with the Romhilt and Estes point score only one patient showed LVH (figure 1).

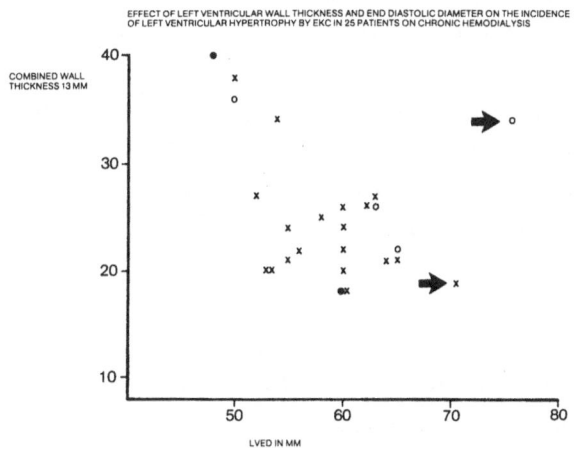

Figure 1. Left ventricular end-diastolic diameter (LVED) and posterior and septal wall thickness were measured echocardiographically. EKGs were read according to the Bonner computer program and according to Romhilt and Estes.[8]

O left ventricular hypertrophy present by both Bonner and Romhilt and Estes
• left ventricular hypertrophy present by Bonner only
x no left ventricular hypertrophy by EKG
→ indicates two patients with an old myocardial infarction

Eight of the 25 patients had increased left ventricular end-diastolic diameter (> 60 mm) by echocardiography and four of these eight showed left ventricular hypertrophy on the ECG; this was associated with echocardiographically normal left ventricular combined wall thickness (< 24 mm) in two of the four instances.

Clear-cut concentric increased left ventricular wall thickness (combined width > 30 mm) was associated with predialysis diastolic hypertension (> 90 mm Hg) in four out of five cases and with systolic hypertension (> 160 mm Hg) in all instances. None of the patients with a normal wall thickness proved to have diastolic or systolic hypertension prior to dialysis (table 2). Of the four patients with septal hypertrophy ($\geq$ 15 mm), three showed diastolic hypertension and one also systolic hypertension before dialysis (table 2).

After dialysis (table 3), the blood pressure decreased in four of the five patients with a concentric increase in left ventricular wall diameter and became normal in three, indicating that fluid excess contributed to, or mediated, the predialysis hypertension in these patients. Blood pressure decreased in all of the four patients with septal hypertrophy after dialysis; two of these patients were normotensive after dialysis. In these patients, too, fluid excess appeared to contribute to, or mediate, the hypertension.

LEFT VENTRICULAR WALL THICKNESS DURING FOLLOW-UP (figure 2)

Of the 25 patients, 18 were followed up for at least eight months without change in fistula or in dialysis regimen. Included in this series is one patient (patient T in figure 2) who had a subtotal parathyroidectomy because of persistent hypercalcemia within two months after entry into the study; since his fistula and his dialysis regimen were not changed he was not excluded from follow-up.

During the period of follow-up (figure 2), significant (> 5 mm) increases in combined left ventricular wall thickness occurred in four patients with one or two kidneys (patients BR, BE, VB, T in figure 2), which was associated with increases in mean blood pressure of 10 mm Hg (VB) and 5 mm Hg (BR), with no change in mean blood pressure (BE) and with an 8-mm Hg decrease in blood pressure (T). A decrease in mean blood pressure of 10 mm Hg (patient CR in figure 2), 8 mm Hg (DE) and 3 mm Hg (BN) was observed in those three patients with the greatest combined wall thickness at time of entry into the study. Among the anephric patients, a 10-mm decrease in combined left ventricular wall thickness was observed after treating patient VD with malignant hypertension with prolonged dialysis ultra-filtration.

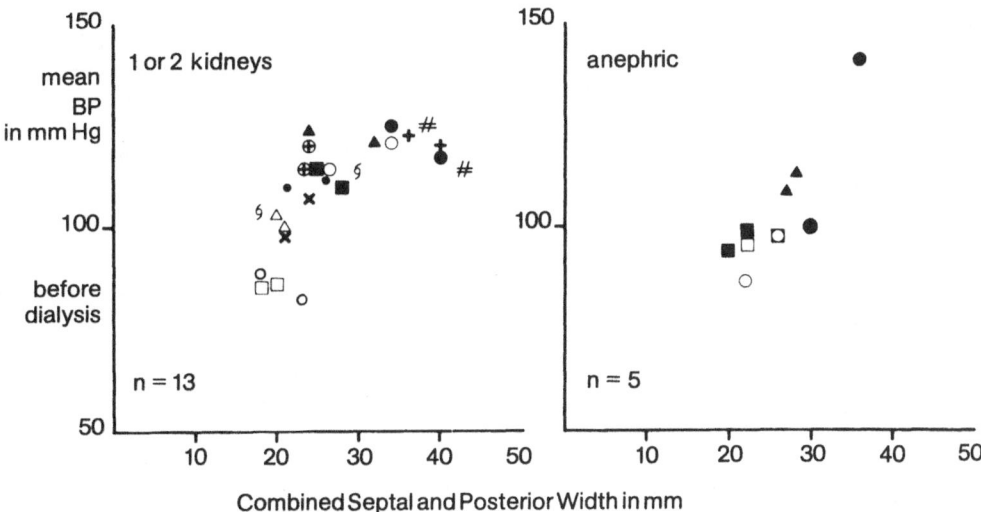

Relation Between Blood Pressure [1] and LV Wall Thickness in 18 Patients
on Chronic Hemodialysis[2]

Combined Septal and Posterior Width in mm

Figure 2. The relation between combined septal and posterior wall thickness and mean blood pressure in anephric patients (right-hand panel) and
in patients with one or two kidneys (left-hand panel). Mean blood pressure (diastolic pressure + 1/3 of the pulse pressure) was averaged over a
period of three months prior to echocardiography. Echocardiograms were
taken at entry into the study and after 7 to 13 months of follow-up.
Combined wall thickness was calculated from the echocardiogram.
Symbols indicate individual patients (left-hand panel: □ = B; θ = T;
X = D; ⨍ = VB; Δ = M; • = R; ⊕ = H; ■ = J; 0 = BR; ▲ = BE; ● = DE;
+ = BN; # = CR; right-hand panel: ■ = P; 0 = S; □ = F; ● = VD; ▲ = Z).

DISCUSSION

The main findings of this study are twofold: (i) the electrocardiographic
criteria for LVH are less sensitive than echocardiographic measurements
and are not reliable in patients on chronic hemodialysis; (ii) in patients on chronic hemodialysis the degree of concentric left ventricular
hypertrophy is not accurately predicted by the blood pressure measured
prior to dialysis.

Table 2. Effect of predialysis blood pressure on left ventricular wall thickness in 25 patients on chronic hemodialysis.

wall thickness in mm	N	MBP: mm Hg			DBP: mm Hg			SBP: mm Hg		
		<100	100-110	>110	<90	90-100	>100	<140	140-160	>160
IVS and LVPW ≥ 15	5	0	0	5	1	2	2	0	0	5
IVS > 15, LVPW < 15	4	0	1	3	1	2	1	0	3	1
IVS and LVPW 12-15	4	1	1	2	2	1	1	1	0	3
IVS < 12, LVPW < 11	12	10	2	0	12	0	0	8	4	0

Table 3. Effect of postdialysis blood pressure on left ventricular wall thickness in 25 patients on chronic hemodialysis.

wall thickness in mm	N	MBP: mm Hg			DBP: mm Hg			SBP: mm Hg		
		<100	100-110	>110	<90	90-100	>100	<140	140-160	>160
IVS and LVPW ≥ 15	5	1	3	1	3	2	0	1	2	2
IVS > 15, LVPW < 15	4	1	2	1	2	1	1	1	2	1
IVS and LVPW 12-15	4	2	1	1	4	0	0	2	1	1
IVS < 12, LVPW < 11	12	11	1	0	12	0	0	11	1	0

      N = number of patients
    MBP = mean blood pressure: DBP + 1/3 (SBP-DBP)
    DBP = diastolic blood pressure indicated by the switch from Korotkov III
          to IV
    SBP = systolic blood pressure
    IVS = septum and
   LVPW = posterior wall were measured at the end of diastole

Left ventricular hypertrophy can be expected to occur frequently in patients on chronic hemodialysis for two reasons. Adaptive increases in preload because of anemia and arteriovenous fistula may cause an increase in left ventricular mass due to dilatation. Increases in left ventricular wall thickness may also be expected to occur frequently because of renal hypertension or fluid overload. In the latter case, the left ventricular hypertrophy results from the conversion of a non-adaptive increase in preload into afterload[13]. The latter mechanism was most likely operative in those of our patients with marked increases in left ventricular wall thickness, since the hypertension observed before dialysis decreased or disappeared altogether after dialysis in all but one patient.

In agreement with others using angiographic techniques for measuring left ventricular mass[14], we observed, using echocardiographic techniques, that the criteria used for diagnosing left ventricular hypertrophy on the ECG provided an insensitive and unreliable measure for detecting symmetrical and asymmetrical increases in left ventricular wall thickness in our patients. This unreliability is probably accounted for by two observations. The left ventricular mass was measured on the echocardiogram according to the empirically obtained formula[12]:

$$LV_{mass} = 1.04 \ (LVID_{ed} + LVPW_{ed} + IVS_{ed})^3 - (LVID_{ed})^3 - 14 \ g$$

in which LV_{mass} = left ventricular mass
$LVID_{ed}$ = end-diastolic left ventricular diameter
$LVPW_{ed}$ = end-diastolic posterior wall thickness
IVS_{ed} = end-diastolic septal thickness

This formula reflects the fact that left ventricular hypertrophy is more efficiently brought about by an increase in wall thickness than by an increase in inner diameter. This observation should be considered together with the finding[14] that wall thickening that results in an increase in left ventricular mass usually does not lead to increased QRS voltages on the ECG unless a sufficient degree of chamber dilatation is present.

Sasayama[2] indicates that the ECG may particularly underestimate afterload-mediated left ventricular hypertrophy. Inclusion into the electrocardiographic point score of changes with limited specificity such as left axis deviation, ST-T changes or P-wave abnormalities, all of which are used in the Romhilt and Estes point score system[8], did not enhance the sensitivity of the ECG in detecting left ventricular hypertrophy.

Although the left ventricular wall thickness and inner diameters are easily and accurately measured echocardiographically, the echocardiograms could not be used for the accurate estimation of cardiac mass, because in our study the inter-observer variation in measuring wall thickness was 3 mm and also because the left ventricular inner diameter varies with the heart rate[15]. With these restrictions, the left ventricular mass of our patients - the infarcted ventricles and those with asymmetrical hypertrophy excepted - calculated echocardiographically according to Devereux[12] was in excess of 140 grams/m^2 which is well above the angiographically determined left ventricular mass for normal men and women of 120 and 80 g/m^2 respectively[16,17]. For the reasons outlined above, left ventricular wall thickness rather than calculated cardiac mass was used as a measure of afterload-mediated left ventricular hypertrophy during follow-up.

Although the data obtained at entry showed the presence of an increase in left ventricular wall thickness to be invariably associated with systolic or diastolic hypertension prior to dialysis, the follow-up data indicate that a direct relationship between the degree of hypertension after dialysis and the thickness of the left ventricular wall was not present in several patients with one or two kidneys. Firstly, a marked increase in left ventricular wall thickness developed in one patient who had only very mild hypertension before dialysis (VB in figure 2) and, secondly, increase in left ventricular hypertrophy was associated with a decrease of blood pressure in two patients. All these patients were normotensive after dialysis, suggesting that both hypertension[18] and left ventricular hypertrophy were secondary to excess of extracellular fluid. The increased left ventricular wall thickness in these patients does not appear to be due to edema since, after abolishing the predialysis hypertension by means of oral fluid restriction and prolonged ultra-filtration, we have found (unpublished observations) that it takes weeks to months before the left ventricular wall returns to normal thickness.

REFERENCES

1. Dodge, H.T., Frimer, M., Stewart, D.K.: Functional evaluation of the hypertrophical heart in man. Circ. Res. supplement II, 35, 122-127, 1974

2. Sasayma, S., Ross, J., Franklin, D., Bloor, C.M., Bishop, S., Dilley, B.D.: Adaptation of the left ventricle to chronic pressure overload. Circ. Res. 38, 172-178, 1976

3. Papadimitrion, J.M., Hopkins, B.E., Taylor, R.R.: Regression of left ventricular dilatation and hypertrophy after removal of volume overload, Circ. Res. 35, 127-135, 1974

4. Neff, M.S., Kim, K.E., Persoff, M., Onesti, G., Swartz, Ch.: Hemodymics of uremic anemia, Circulation 43, 876-883, 1971

5. Anderson, Ch.B., Codd, J.R., Graff, R.A., Groce, M.A., Harter, H.R., Newton, W.T.: Cardiac failure and upper extremity arteriovenous dialysis fistula, Arch. Intern Med. 136, 292-297, 1976

6. Omvik, P., Tarazi, R.C., Bravo, E.L.: Determination of extracellular fluid volume in uremic patients by oral administration of radiosulfate, Kidney International 15, 71-79, 1979

7. Coleman, C.T., Bower, J.D., Langford, H.G., Guyton, A.C.: Regulation of arterial pressure in the anephric state, Circulation, 42, 509-514, 1970

8. Romhilt, D.W., Estes, E.H.: A pointscore system for the E.C.G. diagnosis of left ventricular hypertrophy, Am. Heart J., 75, 752-758, 1968

9. Bailey, J.J., Itscoitz, S.B., Hirshfield, J.W., Graner, L.E., Horton, M.R.: A method for evaluating computer programs for electrocardiographic interpretation, Circulation, 50, 73-78, 1974

10. Feigenbaum, H., Chang, S.: Echocardiography, Lea and Febiger: 236, 311 and 464, Philadelphia, 1976

11. Allen, J.W., Sun June Kim, Edmiston, A.W., Venkataraman, K.: Problems in ultrasonic estimates of septal thickness, Am. J. of Card., 42, 289-296, 1979

12. Devereux, R.B., Reichek, N.: Echocardiographic determination of left ventricular mass in man, Circulation, 55: 613-618, 1977

13. Ross Jr., J.: Afterload mismatch and preload reserve: a conceptual framework for the analysis of ventricular function. Progress Cardiov. Disease, 28, 255-265, 1976

14. Antman, E.M., Green, L.H., Grossmann, W.: Physiologic determinants of the electrocardiographic diagnosis of left ventricular hypertrophy, Circulation, 60, 386-396, 1979

15. De Maria, A.N., Neuman, A., Schubart, P.J., Lee, G., Mason, D.T.: Systematic correlation of cardiac chamber size and ventricular performance determined with echocardiography and alterations in heart rate in normal persons, Am. J. of Card., 43, 1-10, 1979

16. Kennedy, J.W., Baxley, W.A., Figley, M.M., Dodge, H.T., Blackman, J.R.: Quantitative angiography I the normal ventricle in man, Circulation 34, 272-279, 1966

17. Kennedy, J.W., Reichenbach, D.D., Baxley, W.A., Dodge, H.T.: Left ventricular mass: a comparison of angiographic measurements with autopsy weight, Am. J. of Card., 19, 221-223, 1967

18. Brown, J.J., Curtis, L.R., Lever, A.F., Robertson, J.S., Wardener H.E. de, Wing, A.J.: Plasma renin concentration and the control of blood pressure in patients on maintenance haemodialysis, Nephron, 6, 329-349, 1969

250

SUMMARY

During open-heart surgery, the heart was formerly arrested at normal temperature by clamping the aorta. After such normothermic arrest, the risk of ischemic damage was high and occasionally patients died from ischemic contracture. Cooling of the heart after clamping offered better protection against ischemia, and even better results were obtained with cardioplegic procedures. Cardioplegia is obtained by rapid infusion of a solution containing a high concentration of potassium ions into the coronary arteries. This arrests the heart immediately, while the low temperature of the solution rapidly cools the heart. Controversies about the optimal composition of the cardioplegic solution still exist, but so far satisfactory results have been obtained with practically all types of solution, provided the temperature is low and the concentration of potassium ions is about 16 mmol/l.

Hypertrophic myocardium, probably because of its reduced vascular reserve, is more susceptible to ischemia than normal myocardium. The tolerance to ischemic arrest is therefore limited. The reduced tolerance to ischemia is especially a problem in aortic valve replacement. Even valve replacement under continuous normothermic perfusion of the coronary arteries with blood carries a considerable risk. The same is true for hypothermic ischemic arrest. Cold cardioplegia offers far better protection and reduces postoperative mortality to almost nil. As judged by metabolic and enzymatic parameters, continuous infusion of a cold cardioplegic solution containing blood probably offers the best protection.

A study was carried out in our center in which perioperative damage was assessed by means of a quantitative enzymatic technique. The quantity of the enzyme HBDH released during the first 36 h after surgery was 901 ± 319 U/l in the patients operated on under selective normothermic perfusion. Enzyme release fell to 106 ± 18 U/l in the group of patients operated on after cold cardioplegia. The study showed the usefulness of enzymatic quantification of myocardial damage, demonstrating the superiority of cold cardioplegia to normothermic selective perfusion.

PROTECTION OF THE HYPERTROPHIED HEART DURING OPEN-HEART SURGERY

LAARSE, A. VAN DER, HUYSMANS, H.A.*
Departments of Cardiology and Thoracic Surgery*, Leiden University, Leiden, the Netherlands

INTRODUCTION

In clinical open-heart surgery two conditions have to be met: first, good opportunity to perform the surgical procedure indicated and second, good myocardial protection during surgery. The surgeon desires a motionless, bloodless field with optimal access to the heart and sufficient time to perform the surgical procedure. In conflict with the surgeon's desires is the fact that normally myocardial tissue has a high rate of aerobic metabolism to maintain structure and function, made possible by a continuous supply of oxygen and metabolic substrates.

The simplest way for the surgeon to produce a motionless, bloodless operating field is aortic clamping after the patient has been connected to a cardiopulmonary bypass system. If a continous supply of oxygenated blood to a beating heart is interrupted in order to assist the surgeon, the period has to be short or the energy demands of the myocardium should be reduced to prevent the development of an energy deficit leading to myocardial injury. The combination of aortic clamping with hypothermia of the heart improves the length of the 'safe' period of cardiac arrest by reducing myocardial energy demands.

ISCHEMIC CARDIAC ARREST

Cooley's group[1] and Ebert et al.[2] qualified normothermic ischemic cardiac arrest to be a safe technique. Although these groups described good recovery of myocardial function after surgery, Cooley et al.[3] occasionally observed the occurrence of ischemic contracture ('stone heart') after normothermic ischemic cardiac arrest. Hearse et al.[4] demonstrated, in an isolated rat heart study, that ischemic contracture is initiated when the intracellular ATP level decreases below half its normal level.

INTERMITTENT CORONARY PERFUSION

During operations requiring more than 15-20 minutes of aortic cross-clamp time, the cross-clamp can be removed for some time to allow the myocardium to replenish myocardial energy reserves before initiating a new

period of ischemic arrest. Flameng et al.[5] described good results
in human heart surgery with a regimen of maximally 20 minutes of hypothermic ischemic cardiac arrest followed by at least 10 minutes of
intermittent perfusion of the coronary circulation. Levitsky et al.[6],
in canine hearts, showed only partial restoration of cellular ATP level
during five-minute periods of intermittent perfusion following 15-minute
ischemic periods, associated with amelioration of diastolic compliance of
the left ventricle. Braimbridge's group[7] (C̄anković-Darracott et al.[8])
as well as Follette et al.[9] compared different methods of cardiac preservation during open-heart surgery and came to the conclusion, on the
basis of biochemical, functional and ultrastructural parameters, that
ischemic cardiac arrest with intermittent aortic unclamping is associated
with injurious effects of ischemia and/or reperfusion on the myocardium.

CARDIOPLEGIA

Melrose et al.[10] proposed the concept of 'elective cardiac arrest'.
After occluding the aorta they rapidly injected a 2.5% solution of
potassium citrate in blood into the aortic root proximal to the cross-
clamp to arrest the heart. Elective cardiac arrest induced by chemical
additives to crystalloid solutions or blood is nowadays called 'cardioplegia'. The high potassium concentration in the coronary arteries
induces depolarization of cardiac cells, so preventing excitation and
contraction of cardiac cells. When the aortic cross-clamp is removed,
potassium ions are washed out of the coronary circulation and normal
beating resumes. McFarland et al.[11] demonstrated unusual areas of
necrosis in hearts of patients died from surgery with potassium citrate
arrest. With solutions being freshly prepared at the time of operation,
even more severe lesions in postmortem myocardium and an increased
mortality rate were found. Much later it was suggested by Gay and Ebert[12]
and Tyers et al.[13] that it was the extremely high concentration of
potassium citrate of over 250 mmol/l that was responsible for much of the
damage.

Long after the potassium citrate method was abandoned, other groups
trying to formulate a cardioplegic solution with good cardiac protection
qualities, switched to other mechanisms to arrest the hearts and to offer
protection against ischemia. A low-sodium, calcium-free, procaine-containing solution was proposed by Bretschneider[14] and a magnesium aspar-

tate-rich, sodium-free, calcium-free, procaine-containing solution by Kirsch et al.[15]. The group at St. Thomas' Hospital in London tested several cardioplegic solutions in different compositions experimentally, and proposed the principle that cardioplegic solutions should retain as closely as possible extracellular, rather than intracellular, concentrations of ions with only those additions which could be shown individually to be effective and, then, only in their optimal concentrations. A normal-sodium, normal-calcium, high-potassium (16 mmol/1), high-magnesium (16 mmol/1) and procaine-containing solution was introduced as St. Thomas' Hospital cardioplegic solution (Hearse et al.[16], Braimbridge et al.[17]).

A variant in American practice is the use of blood as the vehicle for infusing potassium into the coronary arteries, a concept introduced by Buckberg and coworkers (Follette et al.[9,18]; Buckberg,[19]). Blood was preferred to crystalloid solutions because of its better oxygenating and buffering capacities.

Nowadays the combination of moderate hypothermia and potassium cardioplegia, infused once or repeatedly (every 30-60 minutes), is most widely used although the debate on the optimal composition of the cardioplegic solution and the optimal conditions of its administration is still going on.

In addition to dextran, procaine, glucose, mannitol and insulin, a wide variety of organic compounds have been included in both experimental and clinical cardioplegic solutions. These include high-energy phosphates (Levitsky et al.[20]), steroids (Kirsh et al.[21]), albumin (Conti et al.[22]; Foglia et al.[23]), slow-channel calcium antagonists (Clark et al.[24]; Magee et al.[25]), chlorpromazine (Raju et al.[26]), histidine (Preusse et al.[27]), tryptophan (Preusse et al.[27]), gluconate (Tyers et al.[28]) and adenosine (Hearse et al.[16]).

Controversy about the optimal condition of administration of potassium cardioplegic solutions are concentrated around factors such as volume of solution infused, pressure at which the solution is infused, temperature of the infusate, and the interval between repeated infusions (single dose, multidose or continuous cardioplegia).

ADDITIONAL PROTECTION FACTORS

In addition to myocardial protection procedures, other factors are involved in determining the ultimate outcome of the heart after surgery, estimated by recovery of contractile function (i.e. external recovery) and recovery of cellular functional integrity (i.e. internal recovery). These factors include anesthesia, pre-, peri- or postoperatively adminis- tered pharmacological agents, handling, and surgical experience and skill. As far as anesthesia is concerned specific actions on the heart may be interpreted as protective (e.g. negative-inotropic action) or injurious (e.g. coronary vasoconstriction). Spieckermann et al.[29], Bretschneider et al.[30]) demonstrated that halothane anesthesia affor- ded considerably more protection to the ischemic heart than barbiturate anesthesia, by maintaining higher levels of ATP in the myocardial tissue for longer periods of ischemia.

Preoperative treatment of the patient with pharmacological agents such as β -blockers, slow-channel calcium antagonists, and steroids may lead to preconditioning of the myocardium, thus increasing the tolerance to ischemia. Postoperative treatment with pharmacological agents may help to improve both the overall rate and the overall extent of recovery. While catecholamines are still in use to counteract poor functional recovery after operation (low cardiac output), recently approaches have been developed which may enhance postischemic recovery through selective substrate provision or control of conditions during reperfusion.

REPERFUSION AFTER ISCHEMIA

Reperfusion of ischemic myocardium may, by itself, be injurious, the mechanism of which is closely related to myocardial cell swelling and cellular calcium overloading (Engelman et al.[31]). Administration of certain amino acids to the reperfusion blood was beneficial to the myocardium and improved postischemic contractile performance, as shown by Rau et al.[32]. Buckberg's group used hypocalcemic, hyperkalemic, alka- lotic blood to reperfuse the heart and to allow the myocardium to re- cover internally by channeling available energy away from electro- mechanical activity for repair and restitution (Follette et al.[18]. Postischemic treatment with normothermic blood having a cardioplegic potassium concentration is now used routinely by Buckberg and associates to condition the heart to resume normal function after restoration of normal coronary perfusion (Buckberg[19]).

PRESERVATION OF HYPERTROPHIC MYOCARDIUM

Coexisting cardiac disease may increase the risk of myocardial ischemia and necrosis. As far as left ventricular hypertrophy is concerned, the hypertrophic state of the myocardium as well as the anatomic substrate responsible for the hypertrophic process, if present, are factors which can seriously hamper adequate infusion or perfusion of the coronary arteries. Aortic insufficiency demands cannulation of individual coronary arteries, at the risk of dissection, gaseous emboli and ostial damage. Employing coronary perfusion by selective cannulation of the coronary arteries, Fishman et al.[33] reported on 18 cases autopsied after aortic valve replacement, and concluded that 10 of these deaths were related to problems associated with coronary perfusion. In postoperative deaths after valvular surgery, Henson et al.[34] found five types of myocardial lesions: contraction bands in the myocardial fibers, becoming more prominent near the subendocardium; subendocardial hemorrhage, occurring in areas where contraction bands were seen; coagulative necrosis, usually involving papillary muscles; fibrosis, found in hearts examined 16 or more days after surgery and, like the hemorrhage, restricted to the sub-endocardium involving either part, or the entire circumference, of the left ventricular myocardium; and calcification of damaged myocardial fibers, which mineralization was usually focal in distribution and appeared to be mitochondrial in location. In patients who died postoperatively after aortic valve replacement (n=33), after aortic and mitral valve replacement (n=11), or after aortic, mitral and tricuspid valve replacement (n=6), one or more of these lesions were seen in 82% of the hearts autopsied. In a clinical series of aortic valve replacement or aortic and mitral valve replacement, Braimbridge et al.[17] reported on the postoperative outcome of 69 patients who had continuous coronary perfusion at 32 $^{\circ}$C and 29 patients who had cold (below 25 $^{\circ}$C) cardio-plegic arrest. There were four deaths (7%) in the first group and no deaths in the second group. Myocardial preservation was assessed by cytochemical grading of myocardial biopsy specimens and also by the requirement for significant inotropic support postoperatively. In aortic valve replacements with an aortic occlusion time of 1.5 hours, both techniques afforded a similar degree of preservation, except that the inner half of the myocardium was markedly better preserved by cold cardioplegia. After two hours of double valve replacements, a single cardioplegic infusion was not so effective as continuous coronary per-fusion, but this could be corrected by a second infusion of the cardio-plegic solution after one hour.

Adams et al.[35], employing potassium-induced cardioplegia with hypo-thermia (myocardial temperature below 20 ^{o}C) in 54 patients undergoing aortic valve replacement, found neither deaths nor any electrocardio-graphic evidence of perioperative myocardial infarction. Enzymatic evidence of myocardial injury (postoperative peak CPK and GOT values in excess of 2,000 U/l and 200 U/l, respectively) occurred in 3.7% (2/54), and 3.7% (2/54) required postoperative inotropic support. The authors conclude that a combination of potassium-induced cardiac arrest and hypothermia is a practical and safe method of myocardial preservation during prolonged aortic cross-clamping.

Constant monitoring of intramural temperature is warranted to be able to assess the degree of rewarming of the heart, e.g. by non-coronary blood flow. Reinjection of cardioplegic solution at appropriate intervals will reinforce transmural cooling and will wash out this non-coronary collat-eral blood from the coronary tree.

Jacobs et al.[36], compared postoperative mortality in patients who under-went aortic valve replacement, using direct coronary perfusion († 7/93), cold cardioplegic arrest († 0/48), and ischemic arrest with topical hypothermia († 1/36).

Olin et al.[37] showed that selective coronary perfusion in 26 patients who underwent aortic valve replacement failed to protect the myocardium completely despite adequate coronary flow, as assessed by taking myocar-dial biopsy specimens, blood sampling from the coronary sinus and radial artery and, after operation, by serial determinations of myocardial enzymes. If three different cardioplegic methods (single-dose crystalloid potassium cardioplegia in 38 patients, single-dose blood cardioplegia in 15 patients, and continuous blood cardioplegia in 18 patients) were compared by metabolic and enzymatic parameters, the continuous blood cardioplegia method was most successful. Blood samples from the coronary sinus during the continuous cardioplegic infusion with high-potassium and high-magnesium cold blood showed that the heart extracted oxygen despite its relaxed state and the low temperature (15-18 ^{o}C). In addition, the myocardial biopsies also showed significantly less ATP and creatine phosphate decreases in the continuous cardioplegic infusion patients than in the other patients.

Čancović-Darracott et al.[8] compared five techniques of myocardial preservation during aortic valve replacement, and concluded that intermittent perfusion at 30 °C with a fibrillating heart was the worst means of preservation. Earlier, Buckberg's group (Hottenrott et al.[38]) presented a careful study of normal dogs and dogs in which left ventricular hypertrophy had been created by supravalvular aortic banding. They showed that, in spite of adequate coronary artery perfusion, normal and hypertrophic hearts behave differently during ventricular fibrillation. In contrast to normal dog hearts, oxygen consumption in the hypertrophic hearts failed to increase, vascular resistance rose progressively, and biochemical evidence of severe ischemia developed. This was due to relative underperfusion of the subendocardium in the thicker hearts. The preoperative function of a hypertrophic left ventricle is a factor also determining the postoperative outcome after aortic valve replacement. Thompson et al.[39] investigated the effect of preoperative left ventricular ejection fraction (EF) on early and late prognosis in 69 patients with aortic regurgitation who underwent aortic valve replacement. In 38 patients with EF > 0.45 there was one early death (2.6%) and two late deaths (5.3%) compared to two early deaths (6.5%) and seven late deaths (22.6%) in a group of 31 patients with EF $\leq$ 0.45, during a follow-up period of 13 to 98 months. Actuarial analysis showed a 94% survival at six years in patients with EF > 0.45, compared to 80% in patients with EF $\leq$ 0.45. The same group (Thompson et al.[40]) performed an identical study in 103 patients with aortic stenosis who underwent aortic valve replacement. In this patient group they found a poor correlation between clinical data and left ventricular function. They came to the conclusion that poor left ventricular function does not increase the risk of aortic valve replacement for aortic stenosis, and that improvement of left ventricular function can be expected in the majority of patients.

In 229 patients with aortic stenosis or mixed aortic valve disease, Forman et al.[41] reported that the three-year postoperative survival rate was not affected by the preoperative left ventricular EF, cardiac index, and left ventricular end-diastolic pressure. However, the patients with a combination of aortic regurgitation and a left ventricular EF < 0.50 had a significantly poorer three-year survival rate (64 $\pm$ 10%) compared to the whole group of patients (83 $\pm$ 4%). They conclude that monitoring left ventricular EF non-invasively in patients with aortic regurgitation is advisable and that aortic valve replacement should be advised before EF becomes severely depressed.

Bonow et al.[42] demonstrated that, in a group of symptomatic patients with chronic aortic regurgitation having preoperative left ventricular dysfunction, long-term prognosis after aortic valve replacement is excellent provided preoperative exercise capacity is preserved. In these patients, left ventricular dysfunction is likely to be reversible after operation. In patients with aortic regurgitation, aortic valve replacement after exercise capacity becomes limited will increase the likelihood of irreversible left ventricular dysfunction and reduce long-term postoperative prognosis.

IMPAIRED BALANCE BETWEEN ENERGY SUPPLY AND DEMAND IN HYPERTROPHIC MYOCARDIUM

As mentioned above, the hypertrophied state of ventricular myocardium adds difficulties to perioperative cardiac preservation. In hypertrophic rat hearts induced by chronic pressure overload, ischemic contracture develops after a significantly shorter duration of ischemia than in normal hearts. High-energy phosphate content is lower in hypertrophic hearts at baseline and at ischemic contracture initiation and completion than in normal hearts. These results emphasize the need for rapid cardiac arrest by the induction of ischemia in hypertrophic myocardium (Sink et al.[43]). Buckberg[44] indicated that the decreased tolerance to ischemia of hypertrophied myocardium is caused by a decreased energy supply/demand ratio. Ventricular hypertrophy is thought to cause resting vasodilatation and substantial reductions in the capacity of coronary arteries (especially in the subendocardial regions) to dilate and regulate blood flow proportionate to changing oxygen needs.

In ventricular hypertrophy, the coronary arteries must dilate to supply enough oxygenated blood to meet the raised oxygen demands of a heart which is either enlarged (Archie et al.[45]), producing high intra-myocardial tension, or performs increased pressure work or volume work. To get some insight into the energy supply/demand ratio of the left ventricle, Buckberg et al.[46] advocate the ratio of diastolic pressure time index (DPTI, the area between aortic diastolic and left atrial or pulmonary artery wedge pressure curves in diastole) to tension-time index (TTI, the area beneath the left ventricular systolic pressure curve). The ratio DPTI/TTI allows a beat-to-beat guide to the adequacy of subendocardial oxygenation. Subendocardial ischemia occurs when this ratio is less than 0.80 if blood oxygen content is normal. A low DPTI/TTI ratio

(< 0.80) before operation suggests increased susceptibility to subendocardial necrosis. Perioperative hypertension, for example induced by
anesthesia, should be avoided since high peripheral resistance markedly
raises left ventricular oxygen requirements (TTI) while left ventricular
emptying becomes impaired, leading to decreased DPTI and impaired
subendocardial blood flow. Pharmacological vasodilators may cause
marked improvement in the myocardial energy supply/demand balance despite
lowering coronary perfusion pressure. Marco et al.[47] demonstrated
that by selectively dilating the arterial system with hydralazine following aortic or mitral valve replacement, mean arterial pressure and
systemic vascular resistance fell, cardiac output increased, while
filling pressure remained stable.

Ventricular fibrillation during surgery impairs preservation of hypertrophied hearts, such as those with aortic or mitral disease or systemic
hypertension, which are not protected against ischemia even though
perfusion pressure is kept high and venting is adequate (Hottenrott et
al.[38]).

The increased vulnerability of hypertrophied myocardium to ischemia may
be due to the restriction of coronary arterial blood that perfuses the
subendocardial area of the myocardium, and may be attributable to reduced
coronary vascular reserve. Although oxygen consumption and coronary blood
flow per gram of myocardium are normal at rest in patients with left
ventricular hypertrophy (Trenouth et al.[48]), Pichard et al.[49] demonstrated that left ventricular hypertrophy is associated with a reduction
in coronary vascular reserve, by analyzing the hyperemic reaction to
selective injection of a contrast agent (a vasodilatory substance)
into the coronary arteries in 11 patients with aortic stenosis, left
ventricular hypertrophy (left ventricular mass > 200 g) and normal
coronary arteries. While the hyperemic response in these patients amounted to 49 $\pm$ 10%, in five patients with aortic stenosis and a left ventricular mass less than 200 g it amounted to 102 $\pm$ 10%. The hyperemic response showed a significant positive correlation with the diastolic left
ventricular aortic gradient and with aortic diastolic pressure, and a
significant negative correlation with left ventricular mass.

FACTORS FOR OPTIMAL MYOCARDIAL PROTECTION

On the basis of the knowledge available to date, optimal protection to the myocardium, and especially the hypertrophic myocardium, during open-heart surgery should be realized by:

1. Inducing rapid diastolic cardiac arrest in order to avoid wasting of substantial amounts of high-energy phosphates;

2. A combination of rapid diastolic cardiac arrest and hypothermia in order to minimize myocardial oxygen consumption;

3. Repeated infusion of cold cardioplegic solutions at appropriate intervals in order to reinforce transmural cooling and to wash out non-coronary collateral blood from the coronary tree;

4. Buffering the cardioplegic solution in order to counteract acidosis induced by ischemia;

5. Use of a cardioplegic solution which contains sufficient osmotic or oncotic pressure in order to counteract myocardial edema;

6. Addition of a calcium-entry blocker (verapamil, nifedipine, lidoflazine) in order to prevent calcium ions from flooding into myocardial cells during hypothermic aortic clamping as well as following aortic unclamping;

7. Scheduling aortic valve replacement surgery before left ventricular EF falls below 0.50, especially when left ventricular dysfunction is associated with limited exercise capacity;

8. An anesthetic regimen which avoids systemic hypertension and high heart rates.

QUANTIFICATION OF PERIOPERATIVE MYOCARDIAL DAMAGE TO TEST THE EFFECT OF NEW MYOCARDIAL PRESERVATION TECHNIQUES

In the Thoracic Surgery Department of our center we were able to demonstrate that changing myocardial protection procedures from selective coronary perfusion (10 patients) to cold potassium cardioplegia plus topical hypothermia (10 patients) improved the operative results of isolated aortic valve replacement (Davids et al.[50]). Although changing of the procedures increased the period of aortic cross-clamping from 48 $\pm$ 38 to 62 $\pm$ 14 minutes (difference not significant), the period of extracorporeal circulation decreased significantly from 156 $\pm$ 67 to 92 $\pm$ 15 minutes. Minimal body temperature was identical (28.3 $^{\circ}$C) in both groups. Perioperative myocardial infarction, diagnosed by the appearance of new or deeper Q-waves of at least 0.04 s duration, occurred in two out of 10 patients operated upon when selective coronary perfusion was used, and in none of the 10 patients operated upon when cold cardioplegia was used. Mortality in the first postoperative week decreased from one patient in the first group to none in the second group. Perioperative myocardial damage is quantified by calculating the total quantity of an enzyme, -hydroxybutyrate dehydrogenase (HBDH), released from the heart into the circulation. The quantity of HBDH released per liter of plasma over the first 36 hours after operation, denoted as $A_{HBDH}(36)$, is taken as a measure of myocardial tissue injury. In the selective coronary perfusion group $A_{HBDH}(36)$ was 901 ± 319 U/1, while in the cold cardioplegia group $A_{HBDH}(36)$ was 106 ± 18 U/1 ($P < 0.01$). So, this study demonstrates that by changing myocardial protection procedures from selective coronary perfusion to cold potassium cardioplegia plus topical hypothermia, cardiac injury after aortic valve replacement had decreased by an average of 88%.

CONCLUSIONS

In the seventies, myocardial preservation techniques were developed which offered the heart operated upon good protection for a considerable time. Optimal preservation is conferred by multi-dose crystalloid cardioplegia, multi-dose blood cardioplegia, and continuous blood cardioplegia, with potassium ions (16-20 mmol/1) as the cardiac arresting agent. The hypertrophic myocardium, through its limited coronary vascular reserve, is more susceptible to ischemia than the normal myocardium, and has, therefore, limited tolerance to cardioplegic procedures. Preparation of optimally formulated cardioplegic solutions and administration under specific conditions lead to excellent myocardial preservation, even in the hypertrophic heart.

A study carried out in the Leyden University Hospital shows the usefulness of enzymatic quantification of perioperative myocardial damage to assess the efficacy of the myocardial perservation techniques employed.

REFERENCES

1. Bloodwell, R.D., Gill, S.S., Pereyo, J.A., Hallman, G.L., DeBakey, M.E., Cooley, D.A.: Cardiac valve replacement without coronary perfusion (abstract). Circulation, 33 and 34, suppl. 3: 58-59, 1966
2. Ebert, P.A., Greenfield, L.J., Austen, E.G., Morrow, A.G.: Experimental comparison of methods for protecting the heart during aortic occlusion, Ann. Surg., 155: 25-32, 1962
3. Cooley, D.A., Reul, G.J., Wukasch, D.C.: Ischemic contracture of the heart: 'Stone heart', Am. J. Cardiol., 29: 575-577, 1972
4. Hearse, D.J., Garlick, P.B., Humphrey, S.M.: Ischemic contracture of the myocardium: Mechanisms and prevention, Am. J. Cardiol., 39: 986-993, 1977
5. Flameng, W., Borgers, M., Daenen, W., Stalpaert, G.: Ultrastructural and cytochemical correlates of myocardial protection by cardiac hypothermia in man, J. Thor. Cardiovasc. Surg., 79: 413-424, 1980
6. Levitsky, S., Wright, R.N., Rao, K.S., Holland, C., Roper, K., Engelman, R., Feinberg, H.: Does intermittent coronary perfusion offer greater, myocardial protection than continuous aortic cross-clamping? Surgery, 82: 51-59, 1977
7. Braimbridge, M.V., Darracott, S., Clement, A.J., Bitensky, L., Chayen, J.: Myocardial deterioration during aortic valve replacement assessed by cellular biological tests, J. Thor. Cardiovasc. Surg., 66: 241-246, 1973
8. Čanković-Darracott, S., Braimbridge, M.V., Williams, B.T., Bitensky, L., Chayen, J.: Myocardial preservation during aortic valve surgery, J. Thor. Cardiovasc. Surg., 73: 699-706, 1977
9. Follette, D.M., Mulder, D.G., Maloney Jr., J.V., Buckberg, G.D.: Advantages of blood cardioplegia over continuous coronary perfusion or intermittent ischemia, J. Thor. Cardiovasc. Surg., 76: 604-617, 1978b
10. Melrose, D.G., Dreyer, B., Bentall, H.H., Baker, J.B.E.: Elective cardiac arrest, Lancet, 2: 21-22, 1955
11. McFarland, J.A., Thomas, L.B., Gilbert, J.W., Morrow, A.G.: Myocardial necrosis following elective cardiac arrest induced with potassium citrate, J. Thor. Cardiovasc. Surg., 40: 200-208, 1960
12. Gay Jr., W.A., Ebert, P.A.: Functional, metabolic and morphologic effects of potassium-induced cardioplegia, Surgery, 74: 284-290, 1973
13. Tyers, G.F.O., Todd, G.J., Manley, N.J., Waldhausen, J.A.: The mechanism of myocardial damage following potassium citrate (Melrose) cardioplegia, Surgery, 78: 45-53, 1975
14. Bretschneider, H.J.: Überlebenszeit und Wiederbelebungszeit des Herzens bei Normo- und Hypothermie, Verh. Dtsch. Ges. Kreislauf-forsch., 30: 11-35, 1964
15. Kirsch, U., Rodewald, G., Kalmár, P.: Induced ischemic arrest, J. Thor. Cardiovasc. Surg., 63: 121-130, 1972
16. Hearse, D.J., Stewart, D.A., Braimbridge, M.V.: Cellular protection during myocardial ischema, Circulation, 54: 193-202, 1976
17. Braimbridge, M.V., Chayen, J., Bitensky, L., Hearse, D.J., Jynge, P., Čancović-Darracot, S.: Cold cardioplegia or continuous coronary perfusion? J. Thor. Cardiovasc. Surg., 74: 900-906, 1977
18. Follette, D.M., Fey, K., Steed, D.L., Foglia, R.P., Buckberg, G.D.: Reducing reperfusion injury with hypocalcemic, hyperkalemic, alkalotic blood during reoxygenation, Surg. Forum, 29: 284-286, 1978a

19. Buckberg, G.D.: A proposed 'solution' to the cardioplegic contro-
    versy, J. Thor. Cardiovasc. Surg., 77: 803-815, 1979
20. Levitsky, S., Feinberg, H.: Protection of the myocardium with high-
    energy solutions, Ann. Thor. Surg., 20: 86-90, 1975
21. Kirsh, M.M., Behrendt, D.M., Jochim, K.E.: Effects of methylpred-
    nisolone in cardioplegic solution during coronary bypass grafting,
    J. Thor. Cardiovasc. Surg., 77: 896-899, 1979.
22. Conti, V.R., Bertranou, E.G., Blackstone, E.H., Kirklin, J.W. Diger-
    ness, S.B.: Cold cardioplegia versus hypothermia for myocardial
    protection, J. Thor. Cardiovasc. Surg., 76: 577-589, 1978
23. Foglia, R.P., Steed, D.L., Follette, D.M., Deland, E., Buckberg,
    G.D.: Iatrogenic myocardial edema with potassium cardioplegia, J.
    Thor. Cardiovasc. Surg., 78: 217-222, 1979
24. Clark, R.E., Ferguson, T.B., West, P.N., Shuchleib, R.C., Henry,
    P.D.: Pharmacological preservation of the ischemic heart, Ann. Thor.
    Surg., 24: 307-314, 1977
25. Magee, P.G., Flaherty, J.T., Bixler, T.J., Glower, D., Gardner,
    T.J., Bulkley, B.H., Gott, V.L.: Comparison of myocardial protection
    with nifedipine and potassium, Circulation, 60 suppl. 1: 151-157,
    1979
26. Raju, S., Gibson, W.J., Heath, B., Lockhart, V., Conn, H.: Experi-
    mental evaluation of coronary infusates in dogs, Arch. Surg., 110:
    1374-1382, 1975
27. Preusse, C.J., Gebhard, M.M., Bretschneider, H.J.: Recovery of
    myocardial metabolism after a 210-minute cardiac arrest induced by
    Bretschneider cardioplegia (abstract), J. Mol. Cell. Cardiol., 11,
    suppl. 2: 46, 1979
28. Tyers, G.F.O., Manley, N.J., Williams, E.H., Shaffer, C.W., Williams,
    D.R., Kurusz, M.: Preliminary clinical experience with isotonic
    hypothermic potassium-induced arrest, J. Thor. Cardiovasc. Surg.,
    74: 674-681, 1977
29. Spieckermann, P.G.: Überlebens- und Wiederbelebungszeit des Herzens,
    Anästhesiol. Wiederbelebung, 66: 41-42, 1973
30. Bretschneider, H.J., Hubner, G., Knoll, D., Lohr, B., Nordbeck,
    H., Spiekermann, P.G.: Myocardial resistance and tolerance to is-
    chemia: Physiological and biochemical basis, J. Cardiovasc. Surg.,
    16: 241-260, 1975
31. Engelman, R.M., Chandra, R., Baumann, F.G., Goldman, R.A.: Myocar-
    dial reperfusion, a cause of ischemic injury during cardiopulmonary
    bypass, Surgery, 80: 266-276, 1976
32. Rau, E.E., Shine, K.I., Gervais, A. Douglas, A.M., Amos III, E.C.:
    Enhanced mechanical recovery of anoxic and ischemic myocardium by
    amino acid perfusion, Am. J. Physiol., 236: H873-H879, 1979
33. Fishman, N.H., Youker, J.E., Roe, B.B.: Mechanical injury to the
    coronary arteries during operative cannulation, Am. Heart J., 75:
    26-33, 1968
34. Henson, D.E., Najafi, H. Callaghan, R., Coogan, P., Julian, O.C.,
    Eisenstein, R.: Myocardial lesions following open heart surgery,
    Arch. Path., 88: 423-430, 1969
35. Adams, P.X., Cunningham Jr., J.N., Trehan, N.K., Brazier, J.R., Reed,
    G.E., Spencer, F.C.: Clinical experience using potassium-induced
    cardioplegia with hypothermia in aortic valve replacement, J. Thor.
    Cardiovasc. Surg., 75: 564-568, 1978
36. Jacobs, M.L., Fowler, B.N., Vezeridis, M.P., Jones, N., Daggett,
    W.M.: Aortic valve replacement: A 9-year experience, Ann. Thor.
    Surg., 30: 439-447, 1980

37. Olin, C.L., Bomfim, V., Vendz, R., Kaijser, L., Ström, S.J., Sylvén, C.H.: Myocardial protection during aortic valve replacement, J. Thor. Cardiovasc. Surg., 82: 837-847, 1981
38. Hottenrott, C.E., Towers, B., Kurkji, H.J., Maloney, J.V., Buckberg, G.: The hazard of ventricular fibrillation in hypertrophied ventricles during cardiopulmonary bypass, J. Thor. Cardiovasc. Surg., 66: 742-752, 1973
39. Thompson, R., Ahmed, M., Seabra-Gomes, R., Ilsley, C., Rickards, A., Towers, M., Yacoub, M.: Influence of preoperative left ventricular function on results of homograft replacement of the aortic valve for aortic regurgitation, J. Thor. Cardiovasc. Surg., 77: 411-421, 1979a
40. Thompson, R., Yacoub, M., Ahmed, M., Seabra-Gomes, R., Rickards, A. Towers, M.: Influence of preoperative left ventricular function on results of homograft replacement of the aortic valve for aortic stenosis, Am. J. Cardiol., 43: 929-938, 1979b
41. Forman, R., Firth, B.G., Barnard, M.S.: Prognostic significance of preoperative left ventricular ejection fraction and valve lesion in patients with aortic valve replacement, Am. J. Cardiol., 45: 1120-1125, 1980
42. Bonow, R.O., Rosing, D.R., Kent, K.M., Epstein, S.E.: Timing of operation for chronic aortic regurgitation, Am. J. Cardiol., 50: 325-336, 1982
43. Sink, J.D., Pellom, G.L., Currie, W.D., Hill, R.C., Olsen, C.O., Jones, R.N., Wechsler, A.S.: Response of hypertrophied myocardium to ischemia, J. Thor. Cardiovasc. Surg., 81: 865-872, 1981
44. Buckberg, G.D.: Left ventricular subendocardial necrosis, Ann. Thor. Surg., 24: 379-393, 1977
45. Archie, J.P., Fixler, D.E., Ullyot, D.J., Buckberg, G.D., Hoffman, J.I.E.: Regional myocardial blood flow in lambs with concentric right ventricular hypertrophy. Circ. Res., 34: 143-154, 1974
46. Buckberg, G.D., Fixler, D.E., Archie, J.P., Hoffman, J.I.E.: Experimental subendocardial ischemia in dogs with normal coronary arteries, Circ. Res., 30: 67-81, 1972
47. Marco, J.D., Standeven, J.W., Barner, H.B.,: Afterload reduction with hydralazine following valve replacement, J. Thor. Cardiovasc. Surg., 80: 50-53, 1980
48. Trenouth, R.S., Phelps, N.C., Neill, W.A.: Determinants of left ventricular hypertrophy and oxygen supply in chronic aortic valve disease, Circulation, 53: 644-650, 1976
49. Pichard, A.D., Gorlin, R., Smith, H., Ambrose, J. Meller, J.: Coronary flow studies in patients with left ventricular hypertrophy of the hypertensive type, Am. J. Cardiol., 47: 547-554, 1981
50. Davids, H.A., Hermens, W.Th., Hollaar, L., Laarse, A. van der, Huysmans, H.A.: Extent of myocardial damage after open-heart surgery assessed from serial plasma enzyme levels in either of two periods (1975 and 1980), Br. Heart J., 47: 167-172, 1982

SUMMARY

Twenty-three patients with isolated valvular aortic stenosis who under-went aortic valve replacement between January 1976 and January 1982 were studied before and after operation. Cardiothoracic ratio on chest X-ray, LVH criteria on the ECG, and echocardiographic measures were used to assess regression of left ventricular hypertrophy.

The disease was symptomatic in 18 patients, angina occurred in 10, syncopes in 9 and congestive heart failure in 10. Preoperative catheterization in 21 patients revealed peak systolic pressure differences across the valve from 40 to 130 mm Hg (mean value 90 mm Hg), and left ventricular end-diastolic pressure values from 6 to 32 mm Hg (mean value 17 mm Hg). There were no perioperative deaths, but three patients (13%) died of subsequent complications: one during reoperation for valve leakage and two from infectious endocarditis. Functional class (according to NYHA) of the remaining 20 patients improved from 2.30 ± 0.24 before to 1.35 ± 0.13 after operation. Left ventricular ejection time corrected for heart rate decreased from 115.6 ± 1.2% of normal preoperatively to 97.0 ± 1.2% after operation, indicating that pressure load on the ventricle was effectively reduced. CT ratio before and after operation did not differ significantly.

Electrocardiographic criteria of LVH could be assessed in 15 patients; LBBB or AV block prevented electrocardiographic assessment in most of the others. R and S wave voltages showed regression over a six-month period after operation. ST- and T-wave abnormalities were found in nine patients preoperatively and disappeared in six. Five patients had no abnormalities before and after operation and the remaining six were on chronic treatment with digitalis.

M-mode echocardiography was possible in 13 patients. Preoperatively LV wall thickening without LV dilation was common. Decrease of LV wall thickness, but not a complete normalization, occurred within 5.0 ± 0.6 months after operation (p < 0.02). Repeat measurements of LV wall thickness in eight patients 24.6 ± 1.7 months after operation showed no further change.

Data suggest that successful replacement of a stenotic aortic valve leads to reversal of left ventricular hypertrophy. Reduction of LV wall thickness is completed within six months of operation.

AORTIC VALVE REPLACEMENT IN AORTIC STENOSIS AND REGRESSION OF LEFT
VENTRICULAR HYPERTROPHY

DROST, H.
Department of Cardiology, Leiden University Hospital, Leiden, the Netherlands

INTRODUCTION

Chronic pressure overload in valvular aortic stenosis causes left ventricular hypertrophy[1], which can lead to myocardial ischemia, arrhythmias and cardiac failure. Patients with tight aortic stenosis may be
asymptomatic although they have severe obstruction of the aortic valve,
but with the onset of symptoms prognosis for a patient with aortic
stenosis is poor: without surgical intervention average survival rate is
less than five years when symptoms of angina, syncope or congestive heart
failure occur[2,3].

Surgical correction of valvular aortic stenosis often results in improvement of functional class, ventricular performance and survival rate[4-12].
Sasayama observed in dog experiments that abolishing of chronic pressure
overload could lead to (rapid) partial reduction of hypertrophy of the
left ventricle[1]. Other investigators showed regression of left ventricular hypertrophy after successful aortic valve replacement in aortic
stenosis in men[7-12]. There is however less information about rate of
regression in patients.

The aim of our study was to investigate the quantity and rate of regression of left ventricular hypertrophy in patients with aortic stenosis
after successful replacement of the diseased aortic valve. For this
purpose we used M-mode echocardiography as a 'direct' method to estimate
left ventricular wall thickness and 12-lead ECG recording as an indirect
measure for left ventricular hypertrophy. Devereux showed a good correlation between echocardiographically determined left ventricular mass and
post-mortem left ventricular mass by using measurements of septal wall
and posterior wall thickness and left ventricular internal dimension[13].
Because aortic stenosis mainly causes concentric hypertrophy, we were
especially interested in the time course of reversal of left ventricular
wall thickening after surgery.

An indirect measure for hypertrophy of the heart is the electrocardiogram. Enlargement of the left ventricle with increase of muscle mass adds strength to the left ventricular wave fronts, which results in greater amplitude of the R wave in the left lateral ECG leads and a deeper S wave in the right precordial leads. Sokolow and Romhilt already demonstrated that voltage criteria are of value in detecting left ventricular hypertrophy[14,15].

Left ventricular ejection time, calculated from carotid pulse tracing, increases with the degree of left ventricular outflow tract obstruction. We therefore estimated left ventricular ejection time to assess relief of obstruction.

PATIENTS AND METHODS

Patients

The patient population consisted of all patients who underwent aortic valve replacement for isolated valvular aortic stenosis between January 1976 and January 1982. Patients with coronary artery disease and patients with aortic regurgitation of less than 1+/4+, visualized by aortic root cineangiography, were included in this study. Excluded were patients with aortic regurgitation of more than 1+/4+ and patients with dysfunction of other heart valves.

Twenty-three patients met the selection criteria and were included in the present study. The clinical data of the patients are summarized in table 1. There were 18 men and five women, aged 18-78 (mean age 50.4 years). In 18 patients the disease was symptomatic. Ten patients had anginal complaints, nine suffered from dizzy spells or syncopes, and signs of congestive heart failure occurred in ten patients, two of whom even survived an attack of overt cardiac asthma.

All patients underwent preoperative catheterization, but in two the left ventricle could not be entered. In the remaining 21 patients systolic pressure drop across the aortic valve varied from 40 to 130 mm Hg (mean value 90 mm Hg). End-diastolic pressure in the left ventricle varied between 6 and 32 mm Hg (mean value 17 mm Hg). Significant narrowing of coronary arteries was found in only one case. This patient subsequently underwent a combined coronary bypass and valve replacement operation.

A Björk-Shiley prosthesis was implanted in 14 patients, eight received a Carpentier-Edwards and one a Hancock porcine valve.

Table 1 Clinical data of patients with aortic stenosis

No. of patients	23
Male/female	18/5
Age (years)	
Mean	50.4
Range	18-78
Preoperative symptoms	
Angina	10
Dizzy spells/syncope	9
Congestive heart failure	10
Cardiac asthma	2
Preoperative catheterization	
Aortic valve gradient (mm Hg)	
Mean	90
Range	40-130
LVEDP (mm Hg)	
Mean	17
Range	6-32
Prosthetic valve	
Björk-Shiley	14
Carpentier-Edwards	8
Hancock	1
Associated aorta-coronary bypass	1
Post-operative follow-up (months)	
Mean	36
Range	2-77

Methods

Functional class was assessed according to the NYHA classification[16]. Cardiothoracic (CT) ratio was measured from chest X-rays taken before and 6 to 12 months after operation.

The time interval between the start of the rapid upstroke to the dicrotic notch of the carotid pulse tracing was taken as the left ventricular ejection time. Ejection time was normalized for heart rate[17] (LVETc). Measurements of LVETc were performed prior to surgery and 6-12 months later.

QRS-voltages (SV_1+RV_5, RV_5, $R_{1/11}$ and RaVL) and degree of ST- and T-wave abnormalities (flat, diphasic or inverted T waves and ST-segment depressions of 0.5 mm or more) were measured on 12-lead ECG recordings[14,15]. Electrocardiograms were made before and at 1.3 ± 0.1, 2.4 ± 0.2, 5.3 ± 0.3, $13.4 + 0.7$ and $24.5 + 0.6$ months after operation (mean time interval $\pm$ SEM).

Left ventricular end-diastolic dimension (LVED), interventricular septal wall thickness (IVS) and left ventricular posterior wall thickness (LVPW) were estimated from M-mode echocardiography at the time of the Q-wave of the ECG. Left ventricular end-systolic dimension (LVES) was measured at the peak of the upward motion of the posterior left ventricular endocardium. Measurements were made from leading edge to leading edge with the ultrasonic beam directed at the chamber between the mitral valve echoes and the papillary muscle echoes[18]. For the sake of accuracy each dimension was calculated as the mean of three measurements taken on three different M-mode scans. A simple marking gauge permitted us to read dimensions to 0.1 mm exactly. In the group of patients in whom a good quality echocardiogram was obtained, estimations were done on echograms made before and 5.0 ± 0.6 months after operation. In a subgroup longer echocardiographic follow-up was available and measurements were taken on echocardiograms before and at 5.9 ± 0.3 and 24.6 ± 1.7 months after operation.

Data are reported as the mean ± SEM. Statistical analysis was performed with the t-test for paired data to assess significance of changes of CT ratio, LVETc, voltage levels on the ECG, and echocardiographic dimensions.

Total follow-up period in all 23 patients varied from 2 to 77 months (mean value 36 months).

RESULTS

Complications

There were no perioperative deaths. In none of the patients did new Q-waves on ECG develop after operation. However, in six patients postoperative cardiac enzymes were slightly but distinctly elevated (SGOT range 44-88 U/l and SLDH 431-808 U/l), indicating some myocardial damage. In the early postoperative phase 10 patients had transient supraventricular arrhythmias (six patients had atrial fibrillation, two patients atrial flutter and two patients atrial tachycardia). One patient had a ventricular tachycardia, requiring electrical cardioversion. Left bundle branch block on ECG was found in three patients and two patients had total atrioventricular block, all five already before operation. No new conduction disturbances developed. Valve dysfunction occurred in four patients: one patient had severe paravalvular leakage and died during reoperation, 10 months after original valve replacement, and three patients developed aortic regurgitation because of prosthetic valve endocarditis: two of them died two months postoperatively. In one of them infection could be controlled and till the time of study no reoperation had been necessary, although marked aortic regurgitation persisted. There were no thrombo-embolic events. (All patients with a Bjork-Shiley prosthesis are on life-long anticoagulant treatment, while in patients with a bioprosthesis anticoagulant therapy is withdrawn three months after operation.)

Functional class

The remaining 20 patients, who were alive at the time of the study, showed distinct symptomatic improvement (figure 1).

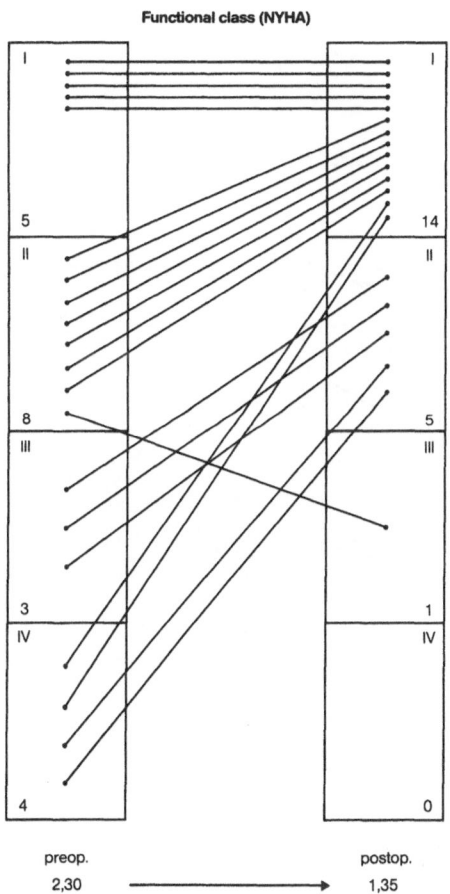

Figure 1. Functional class according to NYHA classification of 20 patients before and after aortic valve replacement. Mean value improved from 2.30 before to 1.35 after operation.

Their validity, according to NYHA classification, improved from 2.30 $\pm$ 0.24 to 1.35 $\pm$ 0.13. The only patient that got worse, from class II to III, was the patient who survived prosthetic valve endocarditis but developed paravalvular leakage with complaints of exertional dyspnea. Both patients with cardiac asthma showed improvement from class IV to II.

Chest X-ray

Pre- and postoperative chest X-rays were available of 18 out of 20 patients. There was no significant change in cardiothoracic ratio before and 6 to 12 months after operation CT ratio was 0.49 $\pm$ 0.02 before and 0.48 $\pm$ 0.02 after operation (figure 2).

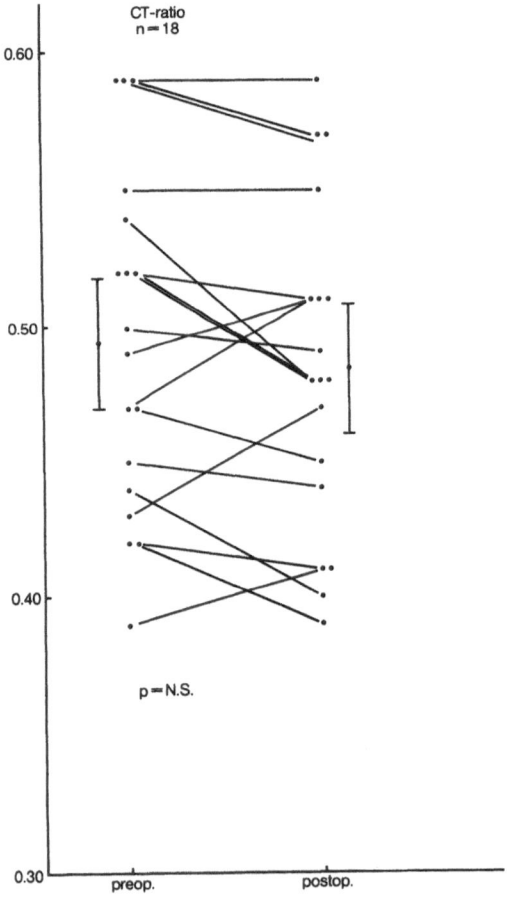

Figure 2. Cardiothoracic ratio measured from chest X-ray, taken before and between 6 and 12 months after aortic valve replacement in 18 patients.

Carotid pulse tracing

Carotid pulse tracings were available of 18 out of 20 patients. Preoperative LVETc was increased in all but one patient (mean value 115.6 ± 1.2% expressed as a percentage of normal). Six to twelve months after surgery ejection time dropped to normal in all patients, mean value 97.0 ± 1.2% (figure 3).

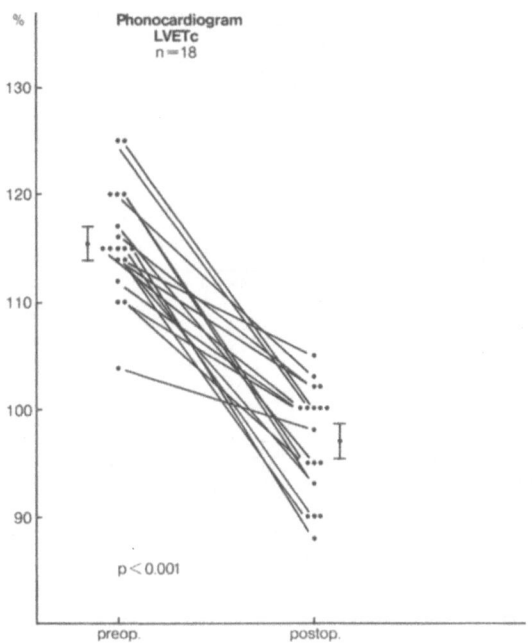

Figure 3. Left ventricular ejection time corrected for heart rate and expressed as a percentage of normal, derived from external carotid pulse tracings, in 18 patients, before and between 6 and 12 months after operation. Normal value 90-110%.

Electrocardiogram

Three out of 20 patients had left bundle branch block on ECG. One out of 20 patients had total atrioventricular block and of one patient only few ECG recordings were available. The remaining 15 patients showed marked regression of mean voltage amplitudes (figure 4 and table 2).Figure 5 shows that in almost all patients SV_1 + RV_5 decreased; only in two did the value of SV_1 + RV_5 increase after operation. Neither patient showed signs of perioperative myocardial damage. In both patients there was a reduction of left ventricular wall thickness as measured by M-mode echo-cardiogram, but in one there was a marked increase of left ventricular cavity dimension (from small to normal). Mean QRS-voltage levels decreased significantly up to 13.4 ± 0.7 months after operation (Wilcoxon matched paires ranked signs test). Data in figures 4 and 5 show that regression is almost completely within the first six months after operation.

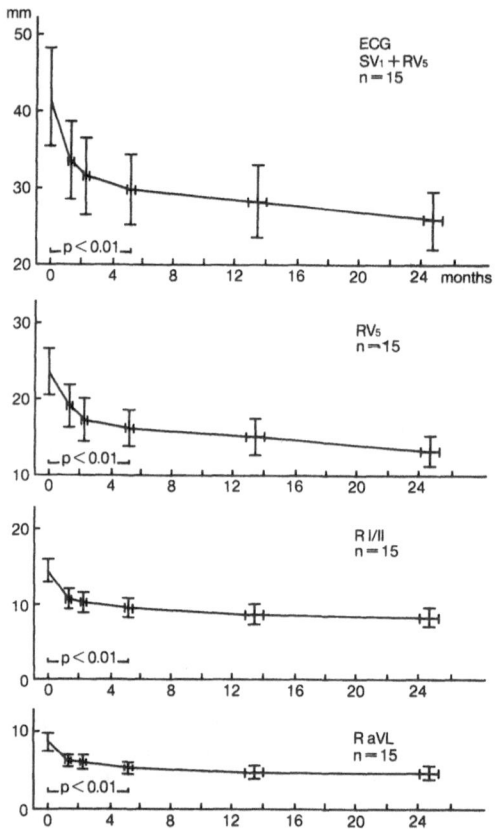

Figure 4. Course of mean voltage amplitudes on electrocardiograms in 15 patients before and at different times after aortic valve replacement. 0 indicates preoperative values.

ST- and T-wave abnormalities, suggesting myocardial ischemia, were present in nine out of 20 patients preoperatively. In six they subsequently disappeared. Six out of 20 patients were on chronic treatment with digitalis, so that ST- and T-wave abnormalities could not be assessed. The five remaining patients had normal ST-segments and T-waves before and after operation.

Table 2. Mean voltage amplitudes on 12-lead ECG recordings before and at different times after aortic valve replacement.

	preop.	1.3+0.1 months postop.	2.4+0.2 months postop.	5.3+0.3 months postop.	13.4+0.7 months postop.	24.5+0.6 months postop.
$SV_1 + RV_5$	41.4+6.3	33.3+4.9	31.3+4.8	29.7+4.5*	28.3+4.6	26.1+3.8
RV_5	23.3+3.0	19.0+2.7	17.2+2.7	16.3+2.3*	15.4+2.3	13.9+2.0
$R_{1/11}$	14.2+1.5	10.6+1.3	10.1+1.4	9.5+1.3*	8.9+1.3	8.8+1.2
RaVL	8.7+1.2	6.5+0.7	6.3+0.9	5.6+0.8*	5.4+0.8	5.7+0.9

Values in mm (mean ± SEM), n = 15 patients

* p < 0.01 compared to preoperative values

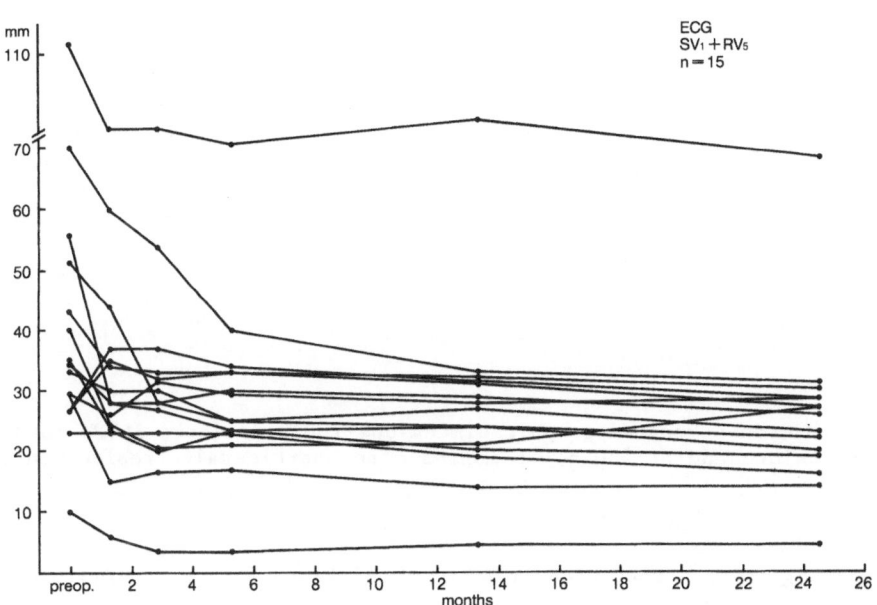

Figure 5. Course of $SV_1 + RV_5$ on ECG in 15 patients before and at different times after aortic valve replacement.

Echocardiography

M-mode echocardiography before and after operation was done in 17 patients. In three of them a good quality echocardiogram was not obtained.
Of the remaining 14 patients echocardiograms before and 5.0 $\pm$ 0.6 months
after operation were available (in one patient only LVPW could be measured). Of nine out of 14 patients also echograms of two years' follow-up
were available. Before operation there was marked thickening of both
septal and posterior wall in most patients, the septal wall being thickened most. In seven out of 13 patients IVS to LVPW ratio was more than 1.3,
in only one of them the ratio exceeded 1.5. In contrast, left ventricular
cavity dimensions were mostly normal.

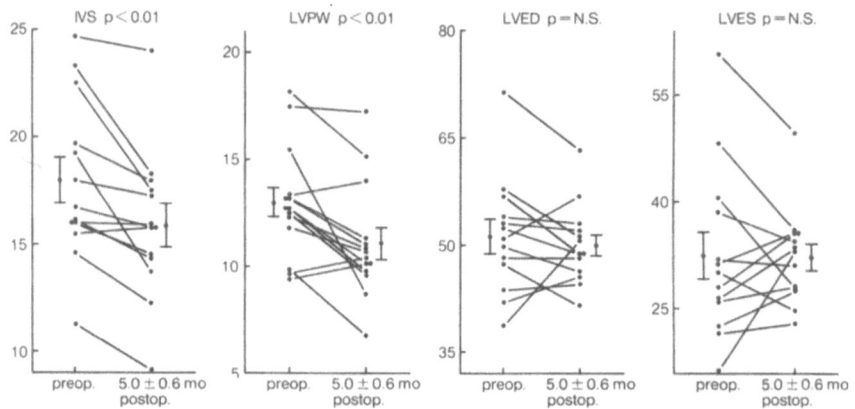

Figure 6. M-mode echocardiographic dimensions in 13 patients (LVPW in 14
patients) before and at 5.0 $\pm$ 0.6 months after aortic valve replacement.

There was significant reduction of LV wall thickness (IVS and LVPW) 5.0 $\pm$
0.6 months after valve replacement, but no complete normalization (figure
6 and table 3a). In the nine patients with a two-year follow-up we noted
no significant further reduction after 5.9 $\pm$ 0.3 months (figure 7 and
table 3b). Left ventricular end-diastolic and end-systolic dimensions
did not differ significantly before and after operation.

Table 3a. Mean echocardiographic measurements before and after aortic valve replacement in 13 patients (LVPW in 14 patients) in whom a good quality echocardiogram was obtained.

	preop.	5.0 + 0.6 mo. postoperatively	p value
IVS	18.0 + 1.1	15.9 + 1.0	< 0.01
LVPW	13.0 + 0.7	11.1 + 0.7	< 0.01
LVED	51.2 + 2.3	50.2 + 1.6	N.S.
LVES	32.5 + 3.3	32.5 + 1.9	N.S.

values in mm (mean + SEM)
IVS = interventricular septal wall thickness
LVPW = left ventricular posterior wall thickness
LVED = left ventricular end-diastolic dimension
LVES = left ventricular end-systolic dimension

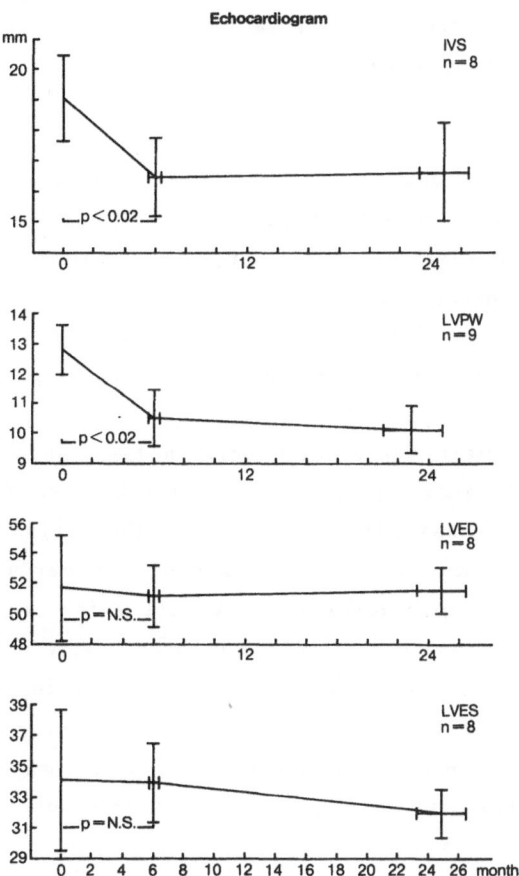

Figure 7. Mean M-mode echocardiographic dimensions in eight patients (LVPW in nine patients) before and at different times after aortic valve replacement.
0 indicates preoperative values.

Table 3b. Mean echocardiographic measurements before and at different times after aortic valve replacement in eight patients (LVPW in nine patients) of whom echocardiograms of two-year follow-up were available.

	preop.	5.9 + 0.3 mo. postoperatively	24.6 + 1.7 mo. postoperatively
IVS	19.1 + 1.4	16.5 + 1.3*	16.6 + 1.6°
LVPW	12.8 + 0.8	10.5 + 0.9*	10.1 + 0.8°
LVED	51.7 + 3.5	51.1 + 2.0**	51.5 + 1.5°
LVES	34.1 + 4.6	33.9 + 2.6**	31.9 + 1.6°

legend: see also table 3a.

for LVPW 23.3 + 1.9 months postoperatively

* p < 0.02, compared to preoperative values

** p = N.S., compared to preoperative values

o p = N.S., compared to 5.9 + 0.3 months postoperatively

DISCUSSION

It appears from our study that aortic valve replacement for valvular aortic stenosis can result in marked improvement in patient validity, even in two patients who suffered from an attack of cardiac asthma. There were no perioperative deaths but late valve-related mortality was 13%. Before operation conduction disturbances existed but no new ones developed. Arrhythmias occurred only in the early postoperative phase.

As shown by the LVETc, left ventricular outflow tract obstruction was greatly decreased after valve replacement in all patients. Although low cardiac output also decreases LVETc, in none of the patients who were alive at the time of study were there signs of low cardiac output. Because aortic stenosis mainly results in LV wall thickening, over-all heart size on chest X-ray was not markedly increased before operation, as expected. Therefore, CT ratio is no great help in estimating the results of aortic valve replacement in patients with aortic stenosis. Preoperative echocardiographic measurements of our patients showed that left ventricular wall thickening is common in valvular aortic stenosis.

The disproportional septal wall thickening in seven of 13 patients was a remarkable finding. It has been suggested that in these patients asymmetric septal thickening is due to coexistence of secondary hypertrophy and hypertrophic cardiomyopathy[19,20]. By assessing myocardial histologic features in patients with aortic stenosis and asymmetric septal hypertrophy Hess and coworkers showed that there were no typical signs of hypertrophic cardiomyopathy, such as fiber disarray or severely hypertrophied muscle fibers with vacuoles and degenerated mitochondria[21,22].

Asymmetrical septal hypertrophy in patients with aortic stenosis is probably an adaptive mechanism for the long-standing pressure overload, and it may be a result of asymmetrical distribution of wall stress by which the septal wall is stressed most.

In contrast to left ventricular thickness, left ventricular internal cavity dimensions were mostly normal. Thus our study confirms other observations that the left ventricle responds to severe pressure overload only by thickening its walls[1]. Elimination of the pressure overload leads to regression of LV wall thickness in our study patients as shown in M-mode echocardiograms. There appeared to be a reduction, but not a complete normalization, of left ventricular wall thickness. Regression seemed to be almost completed within six months.

Voltage criteria on the electrocardiogram, although highly specific for left ventricular hypertrophy, are known to be of low sensitivity in detecting LVH, as pointed out by Romhilt in an autopsy-controlled study[15]. However, reduction of voltage amplitude in an individual patient seems to be a good measure of regression of LVH. From the time course of the voltage amplitudes we can deduce that regression of LVH is fastest in the first two to three months after operation and is almost completed after six months, which is in agreement with our echocardiographic findings.

It is obvious that improvement in ventricular performance and regression of LVH largely depends on the extent of pre- and perioperative (irreversible) myocardial damage. Importantly, the two patients with cardiac asthma also showed improvement in functional class and regression of LVH, which is in agreement with the observations by Smith et al., who achieved good results with aortic valve replacement also in patients with severe aortic stenosis associated with impaired left ventricular function[6].

REFERENCES

1. Sasayma, S., Ross Jr., J., Franklin, D., Bloor, C.M., Bishop, S., Dilley, R.B.: Adaptations of the left ventricle to chronic pressure overload, Circ. Res., 38: 172-178, 1976
2. Frank, S., Johnson, A., Ross Jr., J.: Natural history of valvular aortic stenosis, Br. Heart J., 35: 41-46, 1973
3. Rapaport, E.: Natural history of aortic and mitral valve disease. Am. J. Cardiol., 35: 221-227, 1975
4. Bamhorst, D.A., Oxman, H.A., Connolly, D.C., Pluth, J.R., Danielson, G.R., Wallace, R.B., McGoon, D.C.: Long-term follow-up of isolated replacement of the aortic or mitral valve with the Starr-Edwards prosthesis, Am. J. Cardiol 35: 228-233, 1975
5. Bristow, J.D., Kremkau, E.L.: Hemodynamic changes after valve replacement with Starr-Edwards prosthesis, Am. J. Cardiol., 35: 716-724, 1975
6. Smith, N., McAnulty, J.H., Rachimtoola, S.H.: Severe aortic stenosis with impaired left ventricular function and clinical heart failure: results of valve replacement, Circulation, 58: 255-264, 1978
7. Krayenbuehl, H.P., Turina, M., Hess, O.M., Rothlin, M., Senning, A.: Pre- and postoperative left ventricular contractile function in patients with aortic valve disease, Br. Heart J., 41: 204-213, 1979
8. Henry, W.L., Bonow, R.O., Borer, J.S., Kent, K.M., Ware, J.H., Redwood, J.R. Itscoitz, S.B., McIntosh, C.L., Morrow, A.G., Epstein, S.E.: Evaluation of aortic valve replacement in patients with valvular aortic stenosis, Circulation, 61: 814-825, 1980
9. Pantely, G., Morton, M., Rahimtoola, S.M.: Effects of successful, uncomplicated valve replacement on ventricular hypertrophy, volume and performance in aortic stenosis and in aortic incompetence, J. Thorac Cardiovasc Surg., 75: 383-391, 1978
10. Kennedy, J.W., Doces, J., Stewart, D.K.: Left ventricular function before and following aortic valve replacement, Circulation, 56: 944-950, 1977
11. Schwarz, F., Flameng, W., Thormann, J., Sesto, M., Langebartels, F., Hehrlein, F., Schlepper, M.: Recovery from myocardial failure after aortic valve replacement, J. Thorac Cardiovasc. Surg., 75: 854--864, 1978
12. Drobinski, G., Kellessides, C., Thomas, D., Evans, J.I., Bejean Lebuisson, A., Laurenceau, J.L., Grosgogeat, Y.: Etude echocardiographique du ventricle gauche après remplacement monovalvulaire aortique, Arch.Mal Coeur, 73: 683-690, 1980
13. Devereux, R.B., Reichek, N.: Echocardiographic determination of left ventricular mass in man: anatomic validation of the method, Circulation, 55: 613-618, 1977
14. Sokolow, M., Lyon, Th.P.: The ventricular complex in left ventricular hypertrophy as obtained by unipolar precordial and limb leads, Am. Heart J., 37: 161-186, 1949
15. Romhilt, D.W., Bove, K.E., Norris, R.J., Conyers, E., Conradi, S., Rowlands, D.T., Scott, R.C.: A critical appraisal of the electrocardiographic criteria for the diagnosis of left ventricular hypertrophy, Circulation, 40: 185-195, 1969
16. The criteria committee of the New York Heart Association: Nomenclature and criteria for diagnosis of diseases of the heart and the great vessels, 7th ed., Little, Brown and Company, Boston, 1973
17. Meiners, S.: Meβ-Methoden zur Analyse der Herz- und Kreislaufdynamik, 1. Freiburger Colloquium München, Gräfelfing, 1958
18. Feigenbaum, H.: Echocardiography, 3rd ed., Philadelphia, Lea and Febiger, chapter 3: Echocardiographic evaluation of cardiac chambers, 1981

19. Nanda, N.C., Gramiak, R., Shah, P.M., Stewart, S., De Weese, J.A.: Echocardiography in the diagnosis of idiopathic hypertrophic sub-aortic stenosis coexisting with aortic valve disease, Circulation, 50: 752-757, 1974
20. Parker, D.P., Kaplan, M.A., Connolly, J.E.: Co-existent aortic valvu lar and functional subaortic stenosis: clinical, physiologic and angiographic aspects, Am. J. Cardiol., 24: 307-317, 1969
21. Hess, O.M., Schneider, J., Turina, M., Carroll, J.D., Rothlin, M., Krayenbuehl, H.P.: Asymmetric septal hypertrophy in patients with aortic stenosis: an adaptive mechanism or a coexistence of hyper-trophic cardiomyopathy? J. Am. Coll. Cardiol., 1: 783-789, 1983
22. Ferraus, V.J., Morrow, A.G., Roberts, W.G.: Myocardial ultrastructure in idiopathic hypertrophic subaortic stenosis, Circulation, 45: 769-772, 1972

Index